AF680625

Frontiers in Anti-Infective Agents

(Volume 1)

(Current Perspectives on Anti- Infective Agents)

Edited by

K. Tamreihao, Saikat Mukherjee & Debananda S. Ningthoujam

Advanced Level State Biotech Hub, Microbial Biotechnology Research Laboratory, Department of Biochemistry, Manipur University, Canchipur - 795003, India

Frontiers in Anti-Infective Agents

Volume # 1

Current Perspectives on Anti-Infective Agents

Editors: K. Tamreihao, Saikat Mukherjee & Debananda S. Ningthoujam

ISBN (Online): 978-981-14-3273-6

ISBN (Print): 978-981-14-3272-9

© 2019, Bentham eBooks imprint.

Published by Bentham Science Publishers Pte. Ltd. Singapore. All Rights Reserved.

BENTHAM SCIENCE PUBLISHERS LTD.

End User License Agreement (for non-institutional, personal use)

This is an agreement between you and Bentham Science Publishers Ltd. Please read this License Agreement carefully before using the ebook/echapter/ejournal (**"Work"**). Your use of the Work constitutes your agreement to the terms and conditions set forth in this License Agreement. If you do not agree to these terms and conditions then you should not use the Work.

Bentham Science Publishers agrees to grant you a non-exclusive, non-transferable limited license to use the Work subject to and in accordance with the following terms and conditions. This License Agreement is for non-library, personal use only. For a library / institutional / multi user license in respect of the Work, please contact: permission@benthamscience.net.

Usage Rules:

1. All rights reserved: The Work is the subject of copyright and Bentham Science Publishers either owns the Work (and the copyright in it) or is licensed to distribute the Work. You shall not copy, reproduce, modify, remove, delete, augment, add to, publish, transmit, sell, resell, create derivative works from, or in any way exploit the Work or make the Work available for others to do any of the same, in any form or by any means, in whole or in part, in each case without the prior written permission of Bentham Science Publishers, unless stated otherwise in this License Agreement.
2. You may download a copy of the Work on one occasion to one personal computer (including tablet, laptop, desktop, or other such devices). You may make one back-up copy of the Work to avoid losing it.
3. The unauthorised use or distribution of copyrighted or other proprietary content is illegal and could subject you to liability for substantial money damages. You will be liable for any damage resulting from your misuse of the Work or any violation of this License Agreement, including any infringement by you of copyrights or proprietary rights.

Disclaimer:

Bentham Science Publishers does not guarantee that the information in the Work is error-free, or warrant that it will meet your requirements or that access to the Work will be uninterrupted or error-free. The Work is provided "as is" without warranty of any kind, either express or implied or statutory, including, without limitation, implied warranties of merchantability and fitness for a particular purpose. The entire risk as to the results and performance of the Work is assumed by you. No responsibility is assumed by Bentham Science Publishers, its staff, editors and/or authors for any injury and/or damage to persons or property as a matter of products liability, negligence or otherwise, or from any use or operation of any methods, products instruction, advertisements or ideas contained in the Work.

Limitation of Liability:

In no event will Bentham Science Publishers, its staff, editors and/or authors, be liable for any damages, including, without limitation, special, incidental and/or consequential damages and/or damages for lost data and/or profits arising out of (whether directly or indirectly) the use or inability to use the Work. The entire liability of Bentham Science Publishers shall be limited to the amount actually paid by you for the Work.

General:

1. Any dispute or claim arising out of or in connection with this License Agreement or the Work (including non-contractual disputes or claims) will be governed by and construed in accordance with the laws of Singapore. Each party agrees that the courts of the state of Singapore shall have exclusive jurisdiction to settle any dispute or claim arising out of or in connection with this License Agreement or the Work (including non-contractual disputes or claims).
2. Your rights under this License Agreement will automatically terminate without notice and without the

need for a court order if at any point you breach any terms of this License Agreement. In no event will any delay or failure by Bentham Science Publishers in enforcing your compliance with this License Agreement constitute a waiver of any of its rights.

3. You acknowledge that you have read this License Agreement, and agree to be bound by its terms and conditions. To the extent that any other terms and conditions presented on any website of Bentham Science Publishers conflict with, or are inconsistent with, the terms and conditions set out in this License Agreement, you acknowledge that the terms and conditions set out in this License Agreement shall prevail.

Bentham Science Publishers Pte. Ltd.
80 Robinson Road #02-00
Singapore 068898
Singapore
Email: subscriptions@benthamscience.net

BENTHAM SCIENCE

CONTENTS

PREFACE I

The last century has achieved remarkable breakthroughs in controlling various infectious diseases by synthesizing and modifying antibiotics. However, the present century has been witnessing emergence of drug resistant virulent organisms, specially the ESCAPE pathogens comprising *Enterococcus faecium, Staphylococcus aureus, Klebsiella pneumonia, Acinetobacter baumanii, Pseudomonus aeruginosa, and Enterobacter sp.* Besides, major infectious diseases like tuberculosis, kala-azar, malaria, elephantiasis, polio, leprosy, *etc* (from tropical countries), which could have been controlled in the last century by large-scale eradication program or chemotherapy are re-emerging, causing outbreaks due to the virulence of existing organisms or accumulation of susceptible hosts. Besides, new viruses have been emerged, such as SARS, Ebola, Hendra, Hanata, *etc.* causing deaths wordwide. The WHO has been updating the list of all priority organisms which have been emerged as a global healthcare threat.

Antibiotic resistance is an alarming agenda in healthcare sectors. Increased mortality rates, nosocomial infections, and reduced drug availability against such resistance organisms have generated an urgency for new antimicrobial agents. New approaches are being undertaken to control these WHO priority organisms, such as genome mining approach, one strain-many compound approach, repurposing of old drugs, phage therapy, usage of immunobiotics and probiotics.

Many natural sources are also under investigation for extracting new anti-microbial agents. Actinomycetes synthesize various secondary metabolites which have been successfully used for decades as anti-infective agents such as antibiotics, antifungal agents, *etc.* Majority of these actinomycetes are Streptomyces sp. producing anti-tuberculosis drugs like Chyrsomycin A, Hytramycin, *etc.* New actinomycetes are now being searched from unexplored or underexplored ecosystems for the development of new antimicrobials against disease organisms. New therapeutic molecules need to be searched from unexplored or underexplored ecosystem. For diseases like AIDS where successful chemotherapy is still not possible, new challenges exist in controlling opportunistic infections, such as skin and mouth infections, nervous subsystem disorders, respiratory disorders, as well as cancers. Fusion inhibitors, pharmacokinetic enhancers, fixed dose anti-retrovirals, and combination therapy are new promising anti-infective agents. Such combination therapy exists for treating malaria as well, such as the use of quinone, chloroquines, sulphonamides, *etc.* Medicinal plants have proven to play an important role in generating anti-malarial medications. Antimalarials such as quinone, artemesinin, *etc.* have been extracted from medicinal plants and these anti-infective agents have shown promising results clinically against malaria. New medicinal plants are being investigated for the possible extraction of new antimalarial medications from bark, leaves, roots and aerial parts of the plants. Similarly, the silk protein sericin has been found to have anti-microbial activities and new methodologies using nanotechnology are being developed for loading and targeting Sericin as a human medicine.

Another important group of anti-infective agents, such as Bioactive Peptides are also being synthesized in by enzymatic hydrolysis or microbial fermentation methods. Antimicrobial peptides have important roles in innate immunity and can directly or indirectly kill a pathogen and the mechanism of action is different from conventional antibiotics.

In this book, the authors have provided a comprehensive documentation on various major infectious diseases, from tropical countries, such as Tuberculosis, Kala-azar, Elephantiasis, Malaria, Leprosy and various fungal disorders. The chapters have focused on the pathogenesis and etiology of the diseases, updated WHO reports wherever applicable, conventional drugs and their pharmacokinetics as well as new approaches to develop anti-infective agents. Moreover, one chapter has also addressed emergent viral diseases causing serious threat to healthcare globally and healthcare agenda being taken up by the WHO, Center for Drug and Disease Control and other healthcare institutions for controlling them.

In one of the chapters, the authors have given a detailed report on the Superbugs and new measures being taken up to eradicate them. Our book also focuses on new antimicrobials, such as bioactive peptides and silk protein sericin and the approaches undertaken by scientists and healthcare professionals for successful targeting of these molecules as a human medicine. This book will be essential for general readers as well as healthcare professionals who are actively involved in research on infectious diseases and anti-therapeutic drugs.

The editors wish to thank all the authors for their dedicated efforts to bring this book into realization. The authors would also like to acknowledge the Department of Biotechnology (DBT), Govt. of India and the Department of Science and Technology (DST), Government of India, for the constant support and encouragement by funding various research projects.

The editors would also like to thank the parent Institution, Manipur University, for infrastructural support.

Thank you.

K. Tamreihao
Advanced Level State Biotech Hub, Microbial Biotechnology
Research Laboratory, Department of Biochemistry,
Manipur University, Canchipur - 795003,
India

PREFACE II

Healthcare sectors are facing an alarming condition due to the emergence of new viruses and re-emergence of drug resistant organisms, causing outbreaks globally in recent years. The WHO has been continuously updating the list of such newly emergent virulent pathogens. Pathogenesis and mode of transmission of these pathogens need careful documentation and controlled therapeutic measures should be planned according to specified guidelines. While the last century witnessed the eradication of polio using the attenuated polio vaccine; mutated and infectious polio strains have recently emerged resulting in epidemics. Similar situations were also witnessed for major infectious diseases especially in the tropical countries. Excessive use of antibiotics and other anti-infective agents has resulted in disease-resistant Superbugs, such as Methicillin Resistant Staphylococcus aureus (MRSA) causing nosocomial infections, leading to increased mortality. In the last decade, many new zoonotic viral diseases have re-emerged, such as Ebola, SARS, MERS, *etc.* Unusual vectors have been reported for disease transmission, such as infected bats spreading Ebola. Similarly, novel modes of transmissions of such viruses, such as through handling bushmeats viruses have also been reported.

Therefore, we need to redesign our antimicrobial arsenal. Conventional antibiotic therapies need to be supplemented with additional methodologies involving immunobiotics, probiotics, gene editing technologies, *etc.* Unexplored and underexplored ecosystems should be searched for new microbial species which can synthesize novel anti-microbials as secondary metabolites. Traditional and advanced instrumentation needs a co-operational search to extract novel anti-infective agents from medicinal plants, actinomycetes, and other diverse sources with antimicrobial activity, such as platypus milk.

Lastly, appropriate guidelines should be specified by the WHO and other concerned authorities for the controlled use of new anti-infective drugs as the English author Celia Rees has quoted rightfully "Those that can heal can harm; those that can cure can kill."

Professor Debananda S. Ningthoujam
Advanced Level State Biotech Hub,
Microbial Biotechnology Research Laboratory,
Department of Biochemistry,
Manipur University,
Canchipur - 795003,
India

List of Contributors

Debananda S. Ningthoujam	Advanced Level State Biotech Hub, Microbial Biotechnology Research Laboratory (MBRL), Department of Biochemistry, Manipur University, Canchipur - 795003, India
Dollyca Ningombam	Department of Life Science, Manipur University, Canchipur-79500, India
Elangbam Shanta Singh	Advanced Level State Biotech Hub, Microbial Biotechnology Research Laboratory (MBRL), Department of Biochemistry, Manipur University, Imphal, Canchipur – 795003, India
Ibemhal D Asem	Advanced Level State Biotech Hub, Microbial Biotechnology Research Laboratory (MBRL), Department of Biochemistry, Manipur University, Imphal, Canchipur – 795003, India
Khullakpam Shaheen	Advanced Level State Biotech Hub, Microbial Biotechnology Research Laboratory (MBRL), Department of Biochemistry, Manipur University, Imphal, Canchipur – 795003, India
K. Tamreihao	Advanced Level State Biotech Hub, Microbial Biotechnology Research Laboratory (MBRL), Department of Biochemistry, Manipur University, Canchipur - 795003, India ICAR Research Complex for NEH Region, Manipur Centre, Imphal-795004, India
Laishram Jaya Devi	Microbial Biotechnology Research Laboratory (MBRL), Department of Biochemistry, Manipur University, Advanced Level State Biotech Hub, Canchipur-795003, India
Laishram Somenkumar Singh	Department of Obstetrics and Gynaecology, Regional Institute of Medical Science (RIMS), Imphal, Manipur-795004, India
Laishram Rupachandra Singh	Protein Biochemistry Laboratory, Microbial Biotechnology Research Laboratory (MBRL), Department of Biochemistry, Manipur University, Manipur, India
Pintubala Kshetri	ICAR Complex for NEH region, Manipur Centre, Lamphelpat 795004, India
Rakhi Khunjamayum	Advanced Level State Biotech Hub, Microbial Biotechnology Research Laboratory (MBRL), Department of Biochemistry, Manipur University, Imphal, Canchipur – 795003, India
Roshan Singh Asem	Advanced Level State Biotech Hub, Microbial Biotechnology Research Laboratory (MBRL), Department of Biochemistry, Manipur University, Imphal, Canchipur – 795003, India
Sanjenbam Kunjeshwori Devi	Protein Biochemistry Laboratory, Microbial Biotechnology Research Laboratory (MBRL), Department of Biochemistry, Manipur University, Manipur, India
Shamjetshabam Babeeta Chanu	Protein Biochemistry Laboratory, Microbial Biotechnology Research Laboratory (MBRL), Department of Biochemistry, Manipur University, Manipur, India
Saikat Mukherjee	Advanced Level State Biotech Hub, Microbial Biotechnology Research Laboratory (MBRL), Department of Biochemistry, Manipur University, Imphal, Canchipur – 795003, India

Subhra Saikat Roy	ICAR Research Complex for NEH Region, Manipur Centre, Imphal-795004, India
Sumita Banerjee	Department of Oral Pathology & Microbiology, Dental College, Regional Institute of Medical Sciences, Imphal, Manipur - 795004, India
Thangjam Surchandra Singh	ICAR Complex for NEH region, Manipur Centre, Lamphelpat 795004, India

CHAPTER 1

Prospects of Actinobacteria from Underexplored Ecosystems as Anti-infective Agents against *Mycobacterium tuberculosis*

K. Tamreihao[1,2,*], **Saikat Mukherjee**[1], **Debananda S. Ningthoujam**[1] and **Subhra Saikat Roy**[2]

[1] *Advanced Level State Biotech Hub, Microbial Biotechnology Research Laboratory (MBRL), Department of Biochemistry, Manipur University, Canchipur - 795003, India*

[2] *ICAR Research Complex for NEH Region, Manipur Centre, Imphal-795004, India*

Abstract: About one-third of the world's population is infected with a deadly communicable disease called Tuberculosis (TB), caused by *Mycobacterium tuberculosis*. A majority of this infected population is confined in South-East Asia, especially India. With the emergence of multi-drug resistant (MDR) strains through the sequential accumulation of chromosomal mutations, the disease has become the 9th leading cause of death worldwide. The need of the hour is to discover new anti-infective drugs that have low toxicity, potent activity, are cost-effective, and have a novel target against the MDR *M. Tuberculosis* strain, to combat the dreaded disease. Actinobacteria can be a good candidate for the discovery of new anti-TB drugs as they are prolific producers of antibiotics that can be used for the treatment of different infectious diseases. The exploration of anti-infective agents from soil actinobacteria is exhausting, and the frequency of extracting novel compounds is declining because of the redundancy in the isolation of bioactive actinobacteria. Nevertheless, there is great prospect for the discovery of effective anti-TB drugs from actinobacteria that are isolated from unique, extreme and unexplored/under-explored ecosystems, such as marine, cave, endophytes from medicinal plants, *etc*. Anti-TB compounds extracted from actinobacteria, especially *Streptomyces* sp., associated with medicinal plants, marine *etc*. display good activity against MDR *M. tuberculosis* and low toxicity towards macrophage and normal cells. Further exploration of new anti-TB agents from novel and rare actinobacteria from unique, extreme and unexplored/under-explored ecosystems that have a novel target against MDR strain, is the need of the hour to suppress the dissemination and development of TB.

[*] **Corresponding Author K. Tamreihao:** Advanced Level State Biotech Hub, Microbial Biotechnology Research Laboratory (MBRL), Department of Biochemistry, Manipur University, Canchipur - 795003, India; Tel: +91 897 400 9605; E-mail: tammasi2009@gmail.com

K. Tamreihao, Saikat Mukherjee and Debananda S. Ningthoujam (Eds.)
All rights reserved-© 2019 Bentham Science Publishers

Keywords: Antibiotics, Actinobacteria, Anti-TB Agents, Endophyte, Marine, Macrophage, Medicinal Plants, Multidrug Resistant, *Mycobacterium tuberculosis*, Novel, South-East Asia, *Streptomyces* sp., Tuberculosis, Unexplored/under-explored Ecosystem.

INTRODUCTION

Tuberculosis (TB) is a potentially deadly disease caused by *Mycobacterium tuberculosis* (*M. tuberculosis*). About one-third of total world's entire population is latently infected with *M. tuberculosis* [1]. The disease is the 9th leading cause of death worldwide as a result of a single infectious agent, ranking above AIDS. The dreaded disease infected over 10.4 million people (90% adults; 65% male; 10% HIV positive) in the year 2016, out of which 56% belonged to the South-East Asian countries, especially India, Indonesia, China, the Philippines and Pakistan. South-East Asia was closely followed by Africa (25%) and the Western Pacific (17%). However, mild infection cases occurred in the Eastern Mediterranean (7%), Europe (3%) and America (3%) [2]. An estimated 1.3 million HIV-negative and an additional 3,74,000 HIV-positive people died of TB in 2016, and India accounted for the largest percentage of deaths. TB infection in South-East Asia is enhanced by several factors such as rapid urbanization, high population density, and a rise in diabetes. The use of tobacco, occupational lung disease, indoor and outdoor air pollution due to burning of wood and cow dung also enhances the infection [3 - 7]. Three lists of 30 high burden countries infected with TB, MDR-TB, and HIV-positive TB that will be used by the WHO 2016-2020 are illustrated in Fig. (**1**).

It was Robert Koch, who, in 1882, announced the discovery of *M. tuberculosis*, the cause of TB [8]. Most of the *Mycobacterium* species are ubiquitous environmental saprophytes belonging to actinomycetes taxon, that include most of the antibiotic-producing *Streptomyces* species [9, 10].

Universal mortality due to TB steadily dropped during the 20th century in the developed world. This was aided by improvement in the public health practice, development, and the use of *Mycobacterium bovis* (*M. bovis*) BCG vaccine as well as the development of the antibiotics streptomycin and *p*-aminosalicylic acid during the 1950s. Many more TB drugs were developed in the so-called golden age of antibiotics (1940s-1960s). The introduction of other TB drugs such as isoniazid, ethambutol, rifampicin and pyrazinamide played a significant role in the decline of TB incidence during the 1960s. However, due to poverty, a burgeoning increase in population, and the emergence of AIDS along with the development of drug-resistant *M. tuberculosis* strain, TB cases increased during the 1980s [11, 12]. In 2016, there were over 6,00,000 TB cases, which exhibited resistance to the most effective first-line drug, rifampicin. Out of these, over 4,90,000 TB cases exhibited multidrug-resistance. Most of these cases (47%) were found in India, China and the Russian Federation [2].

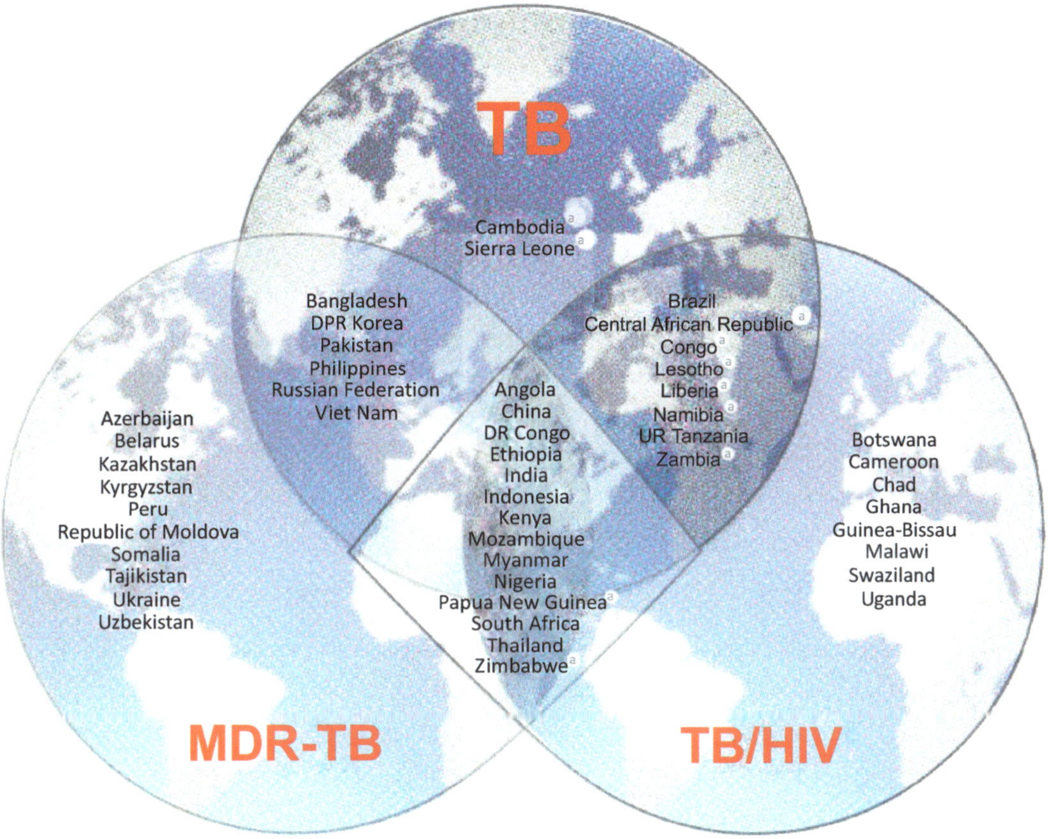

Fig. (1). The three "high burden country" lists of 30 countries that will be used by WHO 2016-2020 {Adapted from WHO [2]}.

This chapter deals with some of the bioactive compounds extracted from actinomycete strains from various ecosystems that display a potent activity against *M. tuberculosis*. It also deals with the discovery of new actinobacterial anti-TB compounds from unexplored/under-explored ecosystems having a novel target against MDR *M. tuberculosis*, since the discovery of new and effective anti-TB compounds from soil actinobacteria is declining rapidly due to the redundancy in isolating novel bioactive actinobacteria.

Infection and Evolution of Drug-Resistance by *M. tuberculosis*

TB is a communicable airborne disease and infected people are the main carriers of the infection. The disease is spread when the bacteria are released into the air from an infected person while coughing, sneezing, or spitting, and the saliva droplets are inhaled by a nearby person. The bacteria then enter the uninfected person through the respiratory route [13]. The probability of the infection depends on several factors such as closeness of the contact, amount of bacteria inhaled, and immune status of the host. The infection of *M. tuberculosis* and the development of the pulmonary form of TB can be summarised into four successive steps: ingestion of the bacilli by macrophages; multiplication of the bacilli in macrophages and regional lymph nodes; the latent stage of infection, metabolically active, multiplication, dissemination; and, finally, the development of TB [13, 14].

Evolution of drug resistance by *M. tuberculosis* depends on several factors: short treatment of drugs, carelessness/noncompliance to the prescribed drugs and prolonged application of the same few drugs. These factors created a selective pressure condition for rapid evolution of bacilli from mono-drug resistant to multidrug resistant (MDR), extensively drug resistant (XDR), and eventually totally drug resistant (TDR) to all available TB drugs, through the sequential accumulation of chromosomal mutation [12, 15 - 22]. Lists of anti-TB drugs and the development of drug-resistance through sequential chromosomal mutations are shown in Table **1**.

Table 1. TB drugs, target genes and drug-resistance through chromosomal mutation by *M. tuberculosis*.

Drug	Drug Mode of Action	Target Gene	Gene Encoded Protein	Resistant Mechanism	References
Isoniazid	Inhibiting mycolic acid biosynthesis and other metabolic processes	*kat*G	Catalase-peroxidase	Abrogated prodrug activation	[19]
		*inh*A	Enoyl ACP reductase	Drug target alteration	[20 - 21]
Ethionamide	Inhibiting mycolate biosynthesis	*inh*A	Enoyl ACP reductase	Drug target alteration	[20 - 21]
		*eth*A	Flavin monoxygenase	Abrogated prodrug activation	[22]
Pyrazinamide	Inhibiting trans-translation	*pnc*A	Pyrazinamidase	Abrogated drug activation	[23, 24]
Ethambutol	Inhibiting arabinogalactan synthesis	*emb*B	Arabinosyltransferases	Drug target alteration	[25]

(Table 1) cont.....

Streptomycin	Inhibiting protein synthesis	*rrs*	16S rRNA	Drug target alteration	[26, 27]
		*rps*L	S12 ribosomal protein	Drug target alteration	[26, 28]
Amikacin/Kanamycin	Inhibiting protein synthesis	*rrs*	16S ribosomal RNA	Drug target alteration	[27, 29]
		eis	Aminoglycoside acetyltransferase	Overexpression of drug inactivating enzyme	[30]
Fluoroquinolones	Inhibiting DNA gyrase	*gyr*A	DNA gyrase subunit A	Drug target alteration	[31 - 33]
D-Cycloserine	Inhibiting peptidoglycan synthesis	*alr*A	D-Alanine racemase	Drug target alteration	[34]
		*cyc*A	D-alanine ligase		
p-Aminosalicylic acid	Inhibiting folate biosynthesis	*thyA*	Thymidylate synthase A	Drug target bypassing	[35, 36]
		*fol*C	Dihydrofolate synthase	Abrogation of prodrug activation	
Capreomycin	Inhibiting protein synthesis	*rrs*	16S ribosomal RNA	Drug target alteration	[27]
		*tly*A	rRNA methyltrans-ferase	Abrogation of drug target methylation	[37]

Perspective of Actinobacteria as Anti-TB Agents

Actinobacteria are Gram-positive, spore-forming bacteria, containing high cytosine-guanine (57-75%) in their genome that grow as branching filament consisting of vegetative mycelia and aerial hyphae. They are found everywhere and can survive in various ecosystems, even in harsh environmental conditions through the formation of spore [38, 39]. Actinobacteria are prolific producers of different classes of antibiotics that can be used to treat various infectious diseases. They produce more than 45% of all known antibiotics and 90% of antibiotics for treating various diseases available in the market [40, 41]. Majority of the antibiotic producers belong to genera *Streptomyces*.

A number of research literature have been reported for anti-TB compounds extracted from plants/medicinal plants belonging to class; alkaloids, flavonoids, chalcones, quinines, coumarin, lignin, phenols, terpenoids, chromones, *etc* [42 - 55]. Similarly, there are many literature reports on anti-TB compounds from different genera of fungi [56 - 62]. Research on the extraction of bioactive compounds possessing potent activity against *M. tuberculosis* is underway to discover new compounds that can be used as effective anti-TB drugs. As a prolific producer of antibiotics that can survive in different ecosystems, actinobacteria have great potential for discovering novel anti-TB drugs. There is also great prospect for isolating new actinobacteria from various unexplored/under-explored ecosystems for discovering effective anti-TB compounds that can have a potential novel target mechanism against MDR *M. tuberculosis*.

With the discovery of anti-TB drug, streptomycin, from *S. griseus*, other drugs such as kanamycin and rifampicin were extracted from actinobacteria isolated from soil. Secondary metabolites present in a cell-free filtrate of *Streptomyces lydicus*, isolated from soil showed inhibition against *M. tuberculosis* H37Ra with MIC of 130 µg/mL [63]. Out of 35,000 actinobacteria screened for activity against *M. tuberculosis* H37R, antimycobacterial compounds, hytramycins V and I, extracted from *Streptomyces hygroscopicus* exhibited good antimycobacterial activity with MIC of 2.4 and 1.5 µg/mL, respectively. The MIC of the compounds was in the same range as the commonly used TB drugs, capreomycin and streptomycin. The bioactivity of the compounds was bacteriostatic rather than bacterial agents [64]. Similarly, of 492 *Streptomyces* isolates from the soil, 155 isolates exhibited antimycobacterial activity. Antibiotic treponemycin produced by *Streptomyces mutabilis* exhibited potent activity against *M. tuberculosis* [65]. Antimycobacterial antibiotics produced by *Streptomyces* sp. isolated from soil displayed antimycobacterial activity against *M. tuberculosis* and *M. smegmatis* [66, 67]. Antimycobacterial compound extracted from actinobacteria are shown in Table **2**.

Table 2. Antimycobacterial compound from actinobacteria.

Actinobacteria	Source	Compound	Target	MIC/IC$_{50}$ (µg/mL)	Reference
Streptomyces sp.	Soil	Chyrsomycin A	*M. tuberculosis* H37Rv	MIC 3.12	[41]
Streptomyces hygroscopicus		Hytramycin 1	*M. tuberculosis* H37Rv	MIC 2.4	[64]
		Hytramycin 2	*M. tuberculosis* H37Rv	MIC 1.5	
Streptomyces mutabilis	Soil		*M. tuberculosis*	MIC 4.17	[65]
Streptomyces sp.	-	Svetamycins A	*M. tuberculosis* H37Rv	IC$_{80}$ 65	[66]
		Svetamycins C		IC$_{80}$ 54	

(Table 2) cont.....

Streptomyces lydicus	Soil	Lydiamycins	*M. tuberculosis* H37Rv	MIC 12.5	[67]
			M. smegmatis	MIC 100.1	
Streptomyces sp.	Medicinal plant	Munumbicins B	*M. tuberculosis* H37Rv	IC_{50} 46	[77]
			SHRE resistant *M. tuberculosis*	IC_{50} 10	
Streptomyces sp.	Medicinal plant	-	*M. tuberculosis* H37Rv	IC_{50} 62.48	[81]
Streptomyces sp.				IC_{50} 74.7	
Streptomyces sp.	Plant	(2E,4E)-5-(3-hydroxyphenyl- penta-- -4- dienamide	*M. tuberculosis*	MIC 128	[82]
		Ergosterol		MIC 64	
		Ergosterol peroxide		MIC 32	
		Halolitoralin		MIC 64	
Streptomyces sp.	Marine	Lobophorin G	*M. bovis* BCG	MIC 1.56	[83]
		Lobophorin A		MIC 1.56	
		Lobophorin B		MIC 0.78	
		Lobophorin G	*M. tuberculosis* H37Rv	MIC 32	
		Lobophorin A		MIC 32	
		Lobophorin B		MIC 16	
Streptomyces sp.	Marine water	Streptcytosine A	*M. smegmatis*	MIC 32	[85]
		Bamicetin		MIC 16	
		Amicetin		MIC 8	
Streptomyces sp.	Marine sediment	Aranciamycins I	*M. bovis* BCG	IC50 0.8	[86]
		Aranciamycins J		IC50 0.7	
		Aranciamycins A		IC50 1.1	
		Aranciamycins		IC50 1.7	
Micromonospora sp.	Marine sediment	Phocoenamicin	*M. tuberculosis* H37Rv	MIC 16-32	[89]
Micromonospora sp.	Marine sediment	Sporalactam B	*M. tuberculosis*	-	[90]

(Table 2) cont.....

Streptomyces luridus	Soil	Spiramycin	*M. tuberculosis* H37Rv	MIC 64	[91]
Streptomyces sp.	Cave	Phenoxazinone (class)	*M. tuberculosis* H37Rv	MIC 6.25	[92]
			SHRE sensitive and resistant *M. tuberculosis*	MIC 25	
Streptomyces sp.	Tissue of mollusc	Lobophorins 2 -5	*M. tuberculosis* H37Rv	MIC 1.3 – 7.8	[95]
Micromonospora sp.	Lake sediment	Diazaquinomycin H	*M. tuberculosis* H37Rv	MIC 0.04	[96]
		Diazaquinomycin J		MIC 0.07	
Streptomyces xinghaiensis	Coalmine	Reductiomycin	*M. tuberculosis* H37Rv	MIC 128	[98]
Nonomuraea rhodomycinica	Swamp forest	7-deoxy-13-dihydrocarminomycinone	*M. tuberculosis* H37Ra	MIC 50	[99]

Need for Exploration of Actinobacteria from Unexplored/Under-Explored Ecosystem

Soil actinobacteria have been the most frequently screened bacteria for bioactive compounds against infectious disease. However, exploration of anti-infective agents from soil has depleted and the frequency of extracting new, effective compounds is declining rapidly because of the redundancy in the isolation of novel bacteria [40]. With the emergence of drug resistant pathogens in recent years, the search for novel, economically affordable, low toxicity, and more effective antimicrobial agents is an urgent need to combat emerging MDR *M. tuberculosis* [68]. Bacteria especially actinobacteria from unique, extreme and unexplored/under-explored ecosystems like medicinal plants, marine, caves, mountain, forest, deep ocean, desert, and forest can be a great candidate for discovering effective anti-infective agents against *M. tuberculosis*.

Antimycobacterial Agents from Actinobacteria Associated with Medicinal Plants

Humans have been exploiting plants for thousands of years as the chief source of natural products for use as antibiotics or chemotherapeutic agents [69]. The frequency of discovering novel bioactive compounds is still promising as only 10-15% of the existing higher plants have been screened for biologically active compounds [70, 71]. Approximately 80% of the world's population, particularly from developing countries, still rely on plants for primary health care [72]. There are about 300,000 higher plant species on earth and each individual plant (in billions) may host one or more beneficial endophytes [69]. Endophytic bacteria associated with higher plants, especially medicinal plants, have recently generated significant interest in the search for antibiotics due to their immense potential to contribute to the discovery of new bioactive compounds. Endophytic bacteria have been reported to possess wide spectrum activity against many pathogenic fungi and bacteria [73 - 78].

Due to the close biological association between endophytes and their host plant, there is more potential for discovering greater number of bioactive molecules as compared to epiphytes or soil related bacteria. Also, due to a long association with the host plants, endophytes may participate in metabolic pathways or some genetic information may be transferred from the host to produce the same important bioactive compounds as their host plants [78]. For example, production of the same medically important bioactive compound produced by endophytes as the host plant is an anticancer compound taxol by a fungus, *Taxomyces andreanae*, associated with plant *Taxus brevifolia* [79]. The antibiotics produced by endophytes are also likely to possess reduced cell toxicity as the bioactive compounds may not affect the eukaryotic host cell due to the symbiotic relationship between endophytes and host plants. This is of significance to the medical community as potential anti-TB drugs may not adversely affect human cells [80].

A large number of plants are required for the extraction of bioactive compounds for treating infectious disease. Moreover, most of the important anti-infective compounds are isolated from endangered or highly endemic plants. Plant tissue culture may offer a solution but the cost of production is exorbitant [71]. Moreover, plants are slow-growing and are generally distributed in a particular geographical area. However, extraction of bioactive metabolites from endophytes that produce the same important bioactive compounds as host plants can save the plants/trees from being cut-down and protect the indigenous rare medicinal plants from extinction while also conserving biodiversity as well as reducing environmental damage. Using endophytic bacteria for large scale production of bioactive compounds can be easier, cost-effective and can be done in a short duration of time. There is great prospect for the extraction of potent anti-TB compounds from endophytes that are associated with previously known indigenous plants having antimycobacterial activity. The need of the hour is to further explore plants from unexplored/under-explored ecosystems for antimycobacterial activity and extraction of anti-TB compounds from endophytes associated with them.

Snake vine has been used as a medicinal plant by Australian Aborigines for many decades. Different parts of the plant are harvested- a fresh stem piece is placed on hot coal for a short time, mashed into a pulp, and then applied as a sticky paste to treat cuts, wounds and infection. Antibiotic munumbicins B extracted from endophytic *Streptomyces* sp., associated with snakevine, inhibits MDR and drug sensitive *M. tuberculosis* with IC_{50} of 10 and 46 μg/mL, respectively. The IC_{50} value of the antibiotic was more potent than rifampicin (>150 μg/mL) [77]. Of 18 endophytic bacteria isolated from enthobotanically medicinal plant *Solanum xanthocarpum*, crude extract from 3 isolates exhibited antimycobacterial activity against *M. smegmatis*. Two isolates belonging to *Streptomyces* sp. exhibited antimycobacterial activity against *M. tuberculosis* H37Rv and attenuated *M. bovis* BCG [81]. Antibiotics (2E,4E)-5-(3-hydroxyphenyl-penta-2,4-dienamide, ergosterol, ergosterol peroxide and halolitoralin B extracted from endophytic *Streptomyces* sp. displayed good activity against *M. tuberculosis* [82].

Antimycobacterial Agents from Actinobacteria from Other Under-Explored Ecosystems

Under-explored ecosystems such as marine, cave, ocean, peat swamp *etc*., can be a good source for the isolation of rare and new species of actinobacteria that can produce effective bioactive compounds and, that can have novel target mechanisms against MDR *M. tuberculosis*. Bacteria living in marine ecosystems may have gained diverse metabolic and genetic capabilities in order to survive the extreme environment. Due to this, marine bacteria may have a high potential for discovering novel antibiotics to fight against contagious disease infection. Although a search on the production of anti-infective agents by marine actinobacteria is still in an early stage, the discovery rate of novel bioactive compounds has recently surpassed that of their terrestrial counterparts [83]. The antibiotics may also be more efficient in treating the disease as the terrestrial pathogens may not have developed a resistant against the novel antibiotics produced by the marine bacteria [84]. Antibiotics produced by *Streptomyces* spp. derived from marine ecosystems have been reported to display potent antimycobacterial activity [83, 85, 86]. A rare actinobacteria *Microployspora* sp., isolated from marine sediment has been reported to show potent antimycobacterial activity showing inhibition zone of 20 and 18 mm against *M. tuberculosis* and *M. smegmatis,* respectively [87]. Similarly, out of 49 actinobacteria obtained from marine sediment, crude metabolites from 41 isolates reduced the growth of one of the three *M. tuberculosis* H37Rv, SHRE sensitive and resistant *M. tuberculosis*. Crude metabolites from 5 actinobacteria strain exhibited good activity showing reduction by more than 90% against the three *Mycobacterium* strains. The bioactive strains belong to *Streptomyces* sp., *Micromonospora* sp., *Actinosynnema* sp., and some rare actinobacteria. A majority of the bioactive strains belong to *Streptomyces* sp [88]. Phocoenamicin 1, 2 and 3 extracted from *Micromonospora* sp., derived from marine sediments, displayed an inhibitory effect against *M. tuberculosis* H37R and *M. bovis*. Compound 3 displayed the highest inhibitory effect against *M. tuberculosis* H37R. All the compounds exhibited negligible activity against *M. bovis* [89].

About one-third of the world population is latently infected with *M. tuberculosis*. Discovery of drugs that are active against latent *M. tuberculosis* growing in macrophages cells and possessing low toxicity to macrophage and normal cells is urgently required to combat the dissemination and development of TB. Sporalactam B producing *Micromonospora* sp. isolated from marine sediment exhibits potent activity against *M. tuberculosis*. The compound is active against *M. tuberculosis* growing intracellularly in macrophage cells, but is not toxic to the macrophage cells at an effective anti-*M. tuberculosis* dose [90]. Anti-TB drugs/antibiotics that are non-toxic to normal cells are also important to control the adverse effect of drugs on human health. Antibiotic spiramycin purified from *Streptomyces luridus* exhibits antitubercular activity. The antitubercular activity of the antibiotic was comparable to rifampicin. The anti-tubular compound is non-mutagenic at the concentration of 1000 μg/mL and non-cytotoxic to normal cells. As the compound is comparable with the rifampicin, it can be used as novel alternative anti-TB drug [91]. *Streptomyces* sp. producing antimycobacterial antibiotic; chrysomycin A, exhibits potent activity against *M. tuberculosis* with MIC of 3.125 μg/mL. The MIC of the antibiotic was better than the two first-line anti-TB drugs, rthambutol (4 μg/mL) and pyrazinamide (16 μg/mL), but comparable to rifampicin (1 μg/mL). The bioactivity of the compound is bactericidal in nature. *M. tuberculosis* growth was completely inhibited at a concentration of 3.125 μg/mL after 24 hours. It can also inhibit intracellularly growing bacilli in macrophages and its activity at macrophage cells was comparable to the standard drug rifampicin. The macrophage cells remained unharmed by treating the compound at MIC (3.125 μg/mL). The compound can also display activity against *M. smegmatis* at 1 μg/mL. The treatment of human cell line remained unaffected at 31.25 μg/mL. Human erythrocytes remained unharmed even at a concentration ten times the MIC against *M. tuberculosis* [41].

Streptomyces sp. was derived from the cave displayed activity against *M. tuberculosis* H37Rv, SHRE sensitive and resistant *M. tuberculosis*. The compound was soluble in acid and alkali, and a peak appeared at 440 nm revealing that the bioactive compound contains phenoxazinone chromophore [92].

Radhakrishnan *et al.* [93] tested 15 actinomycete strains isolated from various ecosystems such as desert, coffee plantation, alkaline soil, plant leaves and marine sediments for bioactivity against *M. tuberculosis* H37Rv, SHRE sensitive and resistant *M. tuberculosis*. Culture filtrate of 7 isolates and crude metabolites extracted from mycelia of 10 isolates showed good activity against all the three *Mycobacterium* strain. Five strains were found to be the most potent for antimycobacterial activity. Majority of the bioactive strains belong to *Streptomyces*. Out of 128 psychrophilic actinobacteria obtained from ice cold mountain, strain *Streptomyces* sp., *Micromonospora* sp. and *Micropolyspora* sp. were active against *M. tuberculosis*. Among the bioactive strains, *Micropolyspora* sp. was the most potent displaying inhibition zone of 28 mm [94]. *Streptomyces* sp. isolated from the tissue of molluscs species *Lienardia totopotens*, produced an antimycobacterial compound, lobophorins 1-5. All the compounds except 1, showed strong inhibitory activity against *M. tuberculosis* H37Ra with MIC values ranging from 1.3 to 7.8 μM [95]. Similarly, *Micromonospora* sp. isolated from fresh lake sediment produced antibiotic diazaquinomycin H and J that inhibited the drug resistant *M. tuberculosis* H37Rv with MIC of 0.04 and 0.07 μg/mL. The antimycobacterial activities of the antibiotics were better in comparison to the standard TB drugs such as rifampicin, isoniazid and streptomycin [96]. Out of 54 actinobacteria isolated from different less explored ecosystems such as desert, forest, mountain and coffee plantation; crude extract from 34 isolates inhibited one or more drug sensitive and drug-resistant *M. tuberculosis* H37Rv [97]. Antibiotic reductiomycin extracted from *Streptomyces xinghaiensis* isolated from coalmine at the depth of 100m exhibited activity against multidrug-resistant *M. tuberculosis* H37Rv [98].

Rare actinobacteria from unexplored biotopes are a promising source for discovering novel anti-TB drugs. For example, *Nonomuraea rhodomycinica* a rare actinomycete isolated from peat swamp forest produced 7-deoxy-13-dihydrocarminomycinone inhibiting the growth of *Mycobacterium tuberculosis* H37Ra. The compound exhibited low cytotoxicity against normal cells in the range of 17.33 to >50 μg/mL [99]. This compound has also been extracted from *Actinomodura reseoviolacea* [100].

CONCLUSION

Most deaths due to *M. tuberculosis* infection can be prevented with early diagnosis and appropriate treatment. A currently recommended treatment for drug-susceptible TB cases is a 6-month regimen of four first-line drugs *viz.*, isoniazid, rifampicin, ethambutol and pyrazinamide [2]. However, sequential chromosomal accumulation of mutation has resulted in the development of MDR *M. tuberculosis* strains, that are resistant to available anti-TB drugs. Now, the major issues for the elimination of the dreaded TB disease are the non-discovery of novel compounds/drugs that have a novel mechanism of action against MDR strain. The alarming increase of MDR-TB cases, therefore, requires an urgent development of new anti-TB agents that exhibits extensive activity and novel target mechanisms against MDR *M. tuberculosis* and, low toxicity to normal and macrophage cells in order to reduce the duration of treatment and, suppress the dissemination and development of TB.

As actinobacteria are the prolific producers of various antibiotics and can survive in different ecosystems, there is a great perspective for discovering novel, effective antibiotics that can act as efficient agents to combat the most dreaded infectious TB disease. Exploration of anti-infective agents from soil actinobacteria has become exhausted and the frequency of extracting novel compounds is declining rapidly because of the redundancy in the isolation of bacteria; the need of the hour is to explore bioactive actinobacteria from unexplored/under-explored ecosystems. Exploration of rare and novel actinobacteria from unique, extreme and unexplored/under-explored ecosystem should be encouraged in order to discover effective anti-TB agents.

CONSENT FOR PUBLICATION

Not applicable.

CONFLICT OF INTEREST

The authors confirm that this chapter contents have no conflict of interest.

ACKNOWLEDGEMENTS

Authors acknowledge the Department of Biotechnology (DBT), Government of India (GOI), for the grant given to Advanced Level State Biotech Hub (AdvSBT Hub) (BT/04/NE/2009).

REFERENCES

[1] Global tuberculosis control: surveillance, planning and financing WHO/HTM/ TB/2009411, WHO. Geneva, Switzerland 2009.

[2] Global tuberculosis report 2017 2017.http://creativecommons.org/licenses/by-nc-sa/3.0/igo

[3] Gajalakshmi V, Peto R, Kanaka TS, Jha P. Smoking and mortality from tuberculosis and other diseases in India: retrospective study of 43000 adult male deaths and 35000 controls. Lancet 2003; 362(9383): 507-15.
[http://dx.doi.org/10.1016/S0140-6736(03)14109-8] [PMID: 12932381]

[4] Sanghani RN, Udwadia ZF. The association of diabetes and tuberculosis: impact on treatment and post-treatment outcomes. Thorax 2013; 68(3): 202-3.
[http://dx.doi.org/10.1136/thoraxjnl-2012-202976] [PMID: 23400366]

[5] Hwang SS, Kang S, Lee JY, *et al.* Impact of outdoor air pollution on the incidence of tuberculosis in the Seoul metropolitan area, South Korea. Korean J Intern Med (Korean Assoc Intern Med) 2014; 29(2): 183-90.
[http://dx.doi.org/10.3904/kjim.2014.29.2.183] [PMID: 24648801]

[6] Lakshmi PV, Virdi NK, Thakur JS, Smith KR, Bates MN, Kumar R. Biomass fuel and risk of tuberculosis: a case-control study from Northern India. J Epidemiol Community Health 2012; 66(5): 457-61.
[http://dx.doi.org/10.1136/jech.2010.115840] [PMID: 21118950]

[7] Basnyat B, Caws M, Udwadia Z. Tuberculosis in South Asia: a tide in the affairs of men. Multidiscip Respir Med 2018; 13: 10.
[http://dx.doi.org/10.1186/s40248-018-0122-y] [PMID: 29599974]

[8] Keshavjee S, Farmer PE. Tuberculosis, drug resistance, and the history of modern medicine. N Engl J Med 2012; 367(10): 931-6.
[http://dx.doi.org/10.1056/NEJMra1205429] [PMID: 22931261]

[9] Cosma CL, Sherman DR, Ramakrishnan L. The secret lives of the pathogenic mycobacteria. Annu Rev Microbiol 2003; 57: 641-76.
[http://dx.doi.org/10.1146/annurev.micro.57.030502.091033] [PMID: 14527294]

[10] Morris RP, Nguyen L, Gatfield J, *et al.* Ancestral antibiotic resistance in Mycobacterium tuberculosis. Proc Natl Acad Sci USA 2005; 102(34): 12200-5.
[http://dx.doi.org/10.1073/pnas.0505446102] [PMID: 16103351]

[11] Smith I. Mycobacterium tuberculosis pathogenesis and molecular determinants of virulence. Clin Microbiol Rev 2003; 16(3): 463-96.
[http://dx.doi.org/10.1128/CMR.16.3.463-496.2003] [PMID: 12857778]

[12] Nguyen L. Antibiotic resistance mechanisms in *M. tuberculosis*: an update. Arch Toxicol 2016; 90(7): 1585-604.
[http://dx.doi.org/10.1007/s00204-016-1727-6] [PMID: 27161440]

[13] Bañuls A-L, Sanou A, Anh NTV, Godreuil S. *Mycobacterium tuberculosis*: ecology and evolution of a human bacterium. J Med Microbiol 2015; 64(11): 1261-9.
[http://dx.doi.org/10.1099/jmm.0.000171] [PMID: 26385049]

[14] Getahun H, Matteelli A, Chaisson RE, Raviglione M. Latent *Mycobacterium tuberculosis* infection. N Engl J Med 2015; 372(22): 2127-35.
[http://dx.doi.org/10.1056/NEJMra1405427] [PMID: 26017823]

[15] Dorman SE, Chaisson RE. From magic bullets back to the magic mountain: the rise of extensively drug-resistant tuberculosis. Nat Med 2007; 13(3): 295-8.
[http://dx.doi.org/10.1038/nm0307-295] [PMID: 17342143]

[16] Ormerod LP. Multidrug-resistant tuberculosis (MDR-TB): epidemiology, prevention and treatment. Br Med Bull 2005; 73-74(74): 17-24.
[http://dx.doi.org/10.1093/bmb/ldh047] [PMID: 15956357]

[17] Udwadia ZF. MDR, XDR, TDR tuberculosis: ominous progression. Thorax 2012; 67(4): 286-8.
[http://dx.doi.org/10.1136/thoraxjnl-2012-201663] [PMID: 22427352]

[18] Gygli SM, Borrell S, Trauner A, Gagneux S. Antimicrobial resistance in *Mycobacterium tuberculosis*: mechanistic and evolutionary perspectives. FEMS Microbiol Rev 2017; 41(3): 354-73.
[http://dx.doi.org/10.1093/femsre/fux011] [PMID: 28369307]

[19] Heym B, Alzari PM, Honoré N, Cole ST. Missense mutations in the catalase-peroxidase gene, *kat*G, are associated with isoniazid resistance in *Mycobacterium tuberculosis.* Mol Microbiol 1995; 15(2): 235-45.
[http://dx.doi.org/10.1111/j.1365-2958.1995.tb02238.x] [PMID: 7746145]

[20] Banerjee A, Dubnau E, Quemard A, *et al. inh*A, a gene encoding a target for isoniazid and ethionamide in *Mycobacterium tuberculosis*. Science 1994; 263(5144): 227-30. [http://dx.doi.org/10.1126/science.8284673] [PMID: 8284673]

[21] Morlock GP, Metchock B, Sikes D, Crawford JT, Cooksey RC. *eth*A, *inh*A, and *kat*G loci of ethionamide-resistant clinical *Mycobacterium tuberculosis* isolates. Antimicrob Agents Chemother 2003; 47(12): 3799-805. [http://dx.doi.org/10.1128/AAC.47.12.3799-3805.2003] [PMID: 14638486]

[22] Telenti A, Imboden P, Marchesi F, *et al.* Detection of rifampicin-resistance mutations in *Mycobacterium tuberculosis*. Lancet 1993; 341(8846): 647-50. [http://dx.doi.org/10.1016/0140-6736(93)90417-F] [PMID: 8095569]

[23] Konno K, Feldmann FM, McDermott W. Pyrazinamide susceptibility and amidase activity of tubercle bacilli. Am Rev Respir Dis 1967; 95(3): 461-9. [PMID: 4225184]

[24] Scorpio A, Zhang Y. Mutations in *pnc*A, a gene encoding pyrazinamidase/nicotinamidase, cause resistance to the antituberculous drug pyrazinamide in tubercle bacillus. Nat Med 1996; 2(6): 662-7. [http://dx.doi.org/10.1038/nm0696-662] [PMID: 8640557]

[25] Sreevatsan S, Stockbauer KE, Pan X, *et al.* Ethambutol resistance in *Mycobacterium tuberculosis*: critical role of embB mutations. Antimicrob Agents Chemother 1997; 41(8): 1677-81. [http://dx.doi.org/10.1128/AAC.41.8.1677] [PMID: 9257740]

[26] Meier A, Kirschner P, Bange FC, Vogel U, Böttger EC. Genetic alterations in streptomycin-resistant *Mycobacterium tuberculosis*: mapping of mutations conferring resistance. Antimicrob Agents Chemother 1994; 38(2): 228-33. [http://dx.doi.org/10.1128/AAC.38.2.228] [PMID: 8192448]

[27] Maus CE, Plikaytis BB, Shinnick TM. Molecular analysis of cross-resistance to capreomycin, kanamycin, amikacin, and viomycin in *Mycobacterium tuberculosis*. Antimicrob Agents Chemother 2005; 49(8): 3192-7. [http://dx.doi.org/10.1128/AAC.49.8.3192-3197.2005] [PMID: 16048924]

[28] Nair J, Rouse DA, Bai GH, Morris SL. The *rps*L gene and streptomycin resistance in single and multiple drug-resistant strains of *Mycobacterium tuberculosis*. Mol Microbiol 1993; 10(3): 521-7. [http://dx.doi.org/10.1111/j.1365-2958.1993.tb00924.x] [PMID: 7968530]

[29] Alangaden GJ, Kreiswirth BN, Aouad A, *et al.* Mechanism of resistance to amikacin and kanamycin in *Mycobacterium tuberculosis*. Antimicrob Agents Chemother 1998; 42(5): 1295-7. [http://dx.doi.org/10.1128/AAC.42.5.1295] [PMID: 9593173]

[30] Kambli P, Ajbani K, Nikam C, *et al.* Correlating *rrs* and *eis* promoter mutations in clinical isolates of *Mycobacterium tuberculosis* with phenotypic susceptibility levels to the second-line injectables. Int J Mycobacteriol 2016; 5(1): 1-6. [http://dx.doi.org/10.1016/j.ijmyco.2015.09.001] [PMID: 26927983]

[31] Takiff HE, Salazar L, Guerrero C, *et al.* Cloning and nucleotide sequence of *Mycobacterium tuberculosis gyr*A and *gyr*B genes and detection of quinolone resistance mutations. Antimicrob Agents Chemother 1994; 38(4): 773-80. [http://dx.doi.org/10.1128/AAC.38.4.773] [PMID: 8031045]

[32] Xu C, Kreiswirth BN, Sreevatsan S, Musser JM, Drlica K. Fluoroquinolone resistance associated with specific gyrase mutations in clinical isolates of multidrug-resistant *Mycobacterium tuberculosis*. J Infect Dis 1996; 174(5): 1127-30. [http://dx.doi.org/10.1093/infdis/174.5.1127] [PMID: 8896523]

[33] Malik S, Willby M, Sikes D, Tsodikov OV, Posey JE. New insights into fluoroquinolone resistance in *Mycobacterium tuberculosis*: functional genetic analysis of *gyr*A and *gyr*B mutations. PLoS One 2012; 7(6)e39754

[http://dx.doi.org/10.1371/journal.pone.0039754] [PMID: 22761889]

[34] Desjardins CA, Cohen KA, Munsamy V, *et al.* Genomic and functional analyses of *Mycobacterium tuberculosis* strains implicate ald in D-cycloserine resistance. Nat Genet 2016; 48(5): 544-51. [http://dx.doi.org/10.1038/ng.3548] [PMID: 27064254]

[35] Zhao F, Wang XD, Erber LN, *et al.* Binding pocket alterations in dihydrofolate synthase confer resistance to para-aminosalicylic acid in clinical isolates of *Mycobacterium tuberculosis.* Antimicrob Agents Chemother 2014; 58(3): 1479-87. [http://dx.doi.org/10.1128/AAC.01775-13] [PMID: 24366731]

[36] Minato Y, Thiede JM, Kordus SL, McKlveen EJ, Turman BJ, Baughn AD. *Mycobacterium tuberculosis* folate metabolism and the mechanistic basis for para-aminosalicylic acid susceptibility and resistance. Antimicrob Agents Chemother 2015; 59(9): 5097-106. [http://dx.doi.org/10.1128/AAC.00647-15] [PMID: 26033719]

[37] Maus CE, Plikaytis BB, Shinnick TM. Mutation of *tly*A confers capreomycin resistance in *Mycobacterium tuberculosis.* Antimicrob Agents Chemother 2005; 49(2): 571-7. [http://dx.doi.org/10.1128/AAC.49.2.571-577.2005] [PMID: 15673735]

[38] de Jesus Sousa JA, Olivares FL. Plant growth promotion by streptomycetes: ecophysilogy, mechanisms and applications. Chem Biol Technol Agric 2016; 3: 24. [http://dx.doi.org/10.1186/s40538-016-0073-5]

[39] Franco-Correa M, Quintana A, Duque C, Saurez C, Rodríguez MX, Barea J-M. Evaluation of actinomycete strains for key traits related with plant growth promotion and mycorrhiza helping activities. Appl Soil Ecol 2010; 45(3): 209-17. [http://dx.doi.org/10.1016/j.apsoil.2010.04.007]

[40] Bérdy J. Bioactive microbial metabolites. J Antibiot (Tokyo) 2005; 58(1): 1-26. [http://dx.doi.org/10.1038/ja.2005.1] [PMID: 15813176]

[41] Muralikrishnan B, Dan VM, Vinodh JS, *et al.* Anti-microbial activity of chrysomycin A produced by *Streptomyces* sp. against *Mycobacterium tuberculosis.* RSC Advances 2017; 7: 36335-9. [http://dx.doi.org/10.1039/C7RA05576E]

[42] Ignacimuthu S, Shanmugam N. Antimycobacterial activity of two natural alkaloids, vasicine acetate and 2-acetyl benzylamine, isolated from Indian shrub *Adhatoda vasica* Ness. leaves. J Biosci 2010; 35(4): 565-70. [http://dx.doi.org/10.1007/s12038-010-0065-8] [PMID: 21289439]

[43] Pallant CA, Cromarty AD, Steenkamp V. Effect of an alkaloidal fraction of *Tabernaemontana elegans* (Stapf.) on selected micro-organisms. J Ethnopharmacol 2012; 140(2): 398-404. [http://dx.doi.org/10.1016/j.jep.2012.01.036] [PMID: 22313627]

[44] Lin YM, Zhou Y, Flavin MT, Zhou LM, Nie W, Chen FC. Chalcones and flavonoids as anti-tuberculosis agents. Bioorg Med Chem 2002; 10(8): 2795-802. [http://dx.doi.org/10.1016/S0968-0896(02)00094-9] [PMID: 12057669]

[45] Fushiya S, Kishi Y, Hattori K, *et al.* Flavonoids from *Cleome droserifolia* suppress NO production in activated macrophages *in vitro.* Planta Med 1999; 65(5): 404-7. [http://dx.doi.org/10.1055/s-1999-14084] [PMID: 10418324]

[46] Lall N, Das Sarma M, Hazra B, Meyer JJ. Antimycobacterial activity of diospyrin derivatives and a structural analogue of diospyrin against *Mycobacterium tuberculosisinin vitro.* J Antimicrob Chemother 2003; 51(2): 435-8. [http://dx.doi.org/10.1093/jac/dkg068] [PMID: 12562718]

[47] Mahapatra A, Mativandlela SPN, Binneman B, *et al.* Activity of 7-methyljuglone derivatives against *Mycobacterium tuberculosis* and as subversive substrates for mycothiol disulfide reductase. Bioorg Med Chem 2007; 15(24): 7638-46. [http://dx.doi.org/10.1016/j.bmc.2007.08.064] [PMID: 17888665]

[48] Chen JJ, Lin WJ, Shieh PC, Chen IS, Peng CF, Sung PJ. A new long-chain alkene and antituberculosis constituents from the leaves of *Pourthiaea lucida.* Chem Biodivers 2010; 7(3): 717-21. [http://dx.doi.org/10.1002/cbdv.200900198] [PMID: 20232337]

[49] Chiang CC, Cheng MJ, Peng CF, Huang HY, Chen IS. A novel dimeric coumarin analog and antimycobacterial constituents from *Fatoua pilosa.* Chem Biodivers 2010; 7(7): 1728-36. [http://dx.doi.org/10.1002/cbdv.200900326] [PMID: 20658660]

[50] Baquero E, Quiñones W, Ribon W, Caldas ML, Sarmiento L, Echeverri F. Effect of an oxadiazoline and a lignin on mycolic acid biosynthesis and ultrastructural changes of *Mycobacterium tuberculosis.* Tuberc Res Treat 2011; 2011986409 [http://dx.doi.org/10.1155/2011/986409] [PMID: 22567272]

[51] Singh S, Kumar JK, Saikia D, *et al.* A bioactive labdane diterpenoid from Curcuma amada and its semisynthetic analogues as antitubercular agents. Eur J Med Chem 2010; 45(9): 4379-82. [http://dx.doi.org/10.1016/j.ejmech.2010.06.006] [PMID: 20584563]

[52] Gua JQ, Wang Y, Franzblau SG, Montenegro G, Timmermann BN. Constituents of *Quinchamalium majus* with potential antitubercular activity. Z Natforsch C J Biosci 2004; 59(11-12): 797-802. [http://dx.doi.org/10.1515/znc-2004-11-1206] [PMID: 15666537]

[53] Wu MC, Peng CF, Chen IS, Tsai IL. Antitubercular chromones and flavonoids from Pisonia aculeata. J Nat Prod 2011; 74(5): 976-82. [http://dx.doi.org/10.1021/np1008575] [PMID: 21542597]

[54] Deng JZ, Starck SR, Hecht SM. Pentacyclic triterpenoids from *Freziera* sp. that inhibit DNA polymerase beta. Bioorg Med Chem 2000; 8(1): 247-50. [http://dx.doi.org/10.1016/S0968-0896(99)00276-X] [PMID: 10968284]

[55] Changtam C, Hongmanee P, Suksamrarn A. Isoxazole analogs of curcuminoids with highly potent multidrug-resistant antimycobacterial activity. Eur J Med Chem 2010; 45(10): 4446-57. [http://dx.doi.org/10.1016/j.ejmech.2010.07.003] [PMID: 20691508]

[56] Wijeratne EM, He H, Franzblau SG, Hoffman AM, Gunatilaka AA. Phomapyrrolidones A-C, antitubercular alkaloids from the endophytic fungus *Phoma* sp. NRRL 46751. J Nat Prod 2013; 76(10): 1860-5. [http://dx.doi.org/10.1021/np400391p] [PMID: 24079882]

[57] Kornsakulkarn J, Dolsophon K, Boonyuen N, *et al.* Dihydronaphthalenones from endophytic fungus *Fusarium* sp. BCC14842. Tetrahedron 2011; 67(39): 7540-7. [http://dx.doi.org/10.1016/j.tet.2011.07.078]

[58] Pan JH, Chen Y, Huang YH, *et al.* Antimycobacterial activity of fusaric acid from a mangrove endophyte and its metal complexes. Arch Pharm Res 2011; 34(7): 1177-81. [http://dx.doi.org/10.1007/s12272-011-0716-9] [PMID: 21811925]

[59] Cheng M-J, Wu M-D, Yanai H, *et al.* Secondary metabolites from the endophytic fungus *Biscogniauxia formosana* and their antimycobacterial activity. Phytochem Lett 2012; 5(3): 467-72. [http://dx.doi.org/10.1016/j.phytol.2012.04.007]

[60] Sommart U, Rukachaisirikul V, Sukpondma Y, Phongpaichit S, Sakayaroj J, Kirtikara K. Hydronaphthalenones and a dihydroramulosin from the endophytic fungus PSU-N24. Chem Pharm Bull (Tokyo) 2008; 56(12): 1687-90. [http://dx.doi.org/10.1248/cpb.56.1687] [PMID: 19043240]

[61] Wang QX, Bao L, Yang XL, *et al.* Ophiobolins P-T, five new cytotoxic and antibacterial sesterterpenes from the endolichenic fungus Ulocladium sp. Fitoterapia 2013; 90: 220-7. [http://dx.doi.org/10.1016/j.fitote.2013.08.002] [PMID: 23954177]

[62] Verma VC, Lobkovsky E, Gange AC, Singh SK, Prakash S. Piperine production by endophytic fungus *Periconia* sp. isolated from *Piper longum* L. J Antibiot (Tokyo) 2011; 64(6): 427-31. [http://dx.doi.org/10.1038/ja.2011.27] [PMID: 21505472]

[63] Lertcanawanichakul M, Chawawisit K, Damnadee N, Thiengtham N, Rittirak N. Anti-tubercular activity and mutagenicity of bioactive compounds in culture broth (CBPs) of *Streptomyces lydicus* A2. Int J Pharm Tech Res 2017; 10(2): 89-95.
[http://dx.doi.org/10.20902/IJPTR.2017.10113]

[64] Cai G, Napolitano JG, McAlpine JB, *et al.* Hytramycins V and I, anti-Mycobacterium tuberculosis hexapeptides from a *Streptomyces hygroscopicus* strain. J Nat Prod 2013; 76(11): 2009-18.
[http://dx.doi.org/10.1021/np400145u] [PMID: 24224794]

[65] Yassien MA, Abdallah HM, El-Halawany AM, Jiman-Fatani AAM. Anti-tuberculous activity of treponemycin produced by a *streptomyces* strain MS-6-6 isolated from Saudi Arabia. Molecules 2015; 20(2): 2576-90.
[http://dx.doi.org/10.3390/molecules20022576] [PMID: 25648598]

[66] Dardić D, Lauro G, Bifulco G, *et al.* Svetamycins A-G, unusual piperazic acid-containing peptides from *Streptomyces* sp. J Org Chem 2017; 82(12): 6032-43.
[http://dx.doi.org/10.1021/acs.joc.7b00228] [PMID: 28489377]

[67] Huang X, Roemer E, Sattler I, Moellmann U, Christner A, Grabley S. Lydiamycins A-D: cyclodepsipetides with antimycobacterial properties. Angew Chem Int Ed Engl 2006; 45(19): 3067-72.
[http://dx.doi.org/10.1002/anie.200503381] [PMID: 16619323]

[68] Corbett EL, Watt CJ, Walker N, *et al.* The growing burden of tuberculosis: global trends and interactions with the HIV epidemic. Arch Intern Med 2003; 163(9): 1009-21.
[http://dx.doi.org/10.1001/archinte.163.9.1009] [PMID: 12742798]

[69] Strobel G, Daisy B, Castillo U, Harper J. Natural products from endophytic microorganisms. J Nat Prod 2004; 67(2): 257-68.
[http://dx.doi.org/10.1021/np030397v] [PMID: 14987067]

[70] Bisht D, Owais M, Venkatesan K. Potential of plant-derived products in the treatment of mycobacterial infections.Modern phytomedicine: turning medicinal plants into drugs. Weinheim: Wiley-VCH 2006.
[http://dx.doi.org/10.1002/9783527609987.ch14]

[71] Alvin A, Miller KI, Neilan BA. Exploring the potential of endophytes from medicinal plants as sources of antimycobacterial compounds. Microbiol Res 2014; 169(7-8): 483-95.
[http://dx.doi.org/10.1016/j.micres.2013.12.009] [PMID: 24582778]

[72] Gurib-Fakim A. Medicinal plants: traditions of yesterday and drugs of tomorrow. Mol Aspects Med 2006; 27(1): 1-93.
[http://dx.doi.org/10.1016/j.mam.2005.07.008] [PMID: 16105678]

[73] Qin S, Wang HB, Chen HH, *et al. Glycomyces endophyticus* sp. nov., an endophytic actinomycete isolated from the root of *Carex baccans* Nees. Int J Syst Evol Microbiol 2008; 58(Pt 11): 2525-8.
[http://dx.doi.org/10.1099/ijs.0.2008/000398-0] [PMID: 18984687]

[74] Gos FMWR, Savi DC, Shaaban KA, *et al.* Antibacterial activity of endophytic actinomycetes isolated from the medicinal plant *Vochysia divergens* (Pantanal, Brazil). Front Microbiol 2017; 8: 1642.
[http://dx.doi.org/10.3389/fmicb.2017.01642] [PMID: 28932210]

[75] Kafur A, Khan AB. Isolation of endophytic actinomycetes from *Catharanthes roseus* (L.) G. Don leaves and their antimicrobial activity. Iranian J Biotechnol 2011; 9(4): 302-6.

[76] Rao HCY, Rakshith D, Satish S. Antimicrobial properties of endophytic actinomycetes isolated from *Combretum latifolium* Blume, a medicinal shrub from Western Ghats of India. Front Bio 2015; 10(6): 528-36.
[http://dx.doi.org/10.1007/s11515-015-1377-8]

[77] Castillo UF, Strobel GA, Ford EJ, *et al.* Munumbicins, wide-spectrum antibiotics produced by Streptomyces NRRL 30562, endophytic on Kennedia nigriscans. Microbiology 2002; 148(Pt 9): 2675-85.

[http://dx.doi.org/10.1099/00221287-148-9-2675] [PMID: 12213914]

[78] Golinska P, Wypij M, Agarkar G, Rathod D, Dahm H, Rai M. Endophytic actinobacteria of medicinal plants: diversity and bioactivity. Antonie van Leeuwenhoek 2015; 108(2): 267-89. [http://dx.doi.org/10.1007/s10482-015-0502-7] [PMID: 26093915]

[79] Stierle A, Strobel G, Stierle D. Taxol and taxane production by Taxomyces andreanae, an endophytic fungus of Pacific yew. Science 1993; 260(5105): 214-6. [http://dx.doi.org/10.1126/science.8097061] [PMID: 8097061]

[80] Strobel G, Daisy B. Bioprospecting for microbial endophytes and their natural products. Microbiol Mol Biol Rev 2003; 67(4): 491-502. [http://dx.doi.org/10.1128/MMBR.67.4.491-502.2003] [PMID: 14665674]

[81] Khunjamayum R, Tamreihao K, Ningthoujam DS, *et al.* In-vitro antimycobacterial activities of endophytic bacteria associated with medicinal plant of Manipur. J Bacteriol Mycol Open Access 2017 2017; 4(4): 00097.

[82] Zhou H, Zhao L, Li W, Yang Y, Xu L, Ding Z. Anti-Mycobacterium tuberculosis active metabolites from an endophytic *Streptomyces* sp. YIM65484. Rec Nat Prod 2015; 9(2): 196-200.

[83] Chen C, Wang J, Guo H, *et al.* Three antimycobacterial metabolites identified from a marine-derived *Streptomyces* sp. MS100061. Appl Microbiol Biotechnol 2013; 97(9): 3885-92. [http://dx.doi.org/10.1007/s00253-012-4681-0] [PMID: 23324803]

[84] Saha M, Jaisankar P, Das S, *et al.* Production and purification of a bioactive substance inhibiting multiple drug resistant bacteria and human leukemia cells from a salt-tolerant marine Actinobacterium sp. isolated from the Bay of Bengal. Biotechnol Lett 2006; 28(14): 1083-8. [http://dx.doi.org/10.1007/s10529-006-9054-2] [PMID: 16788738]

[85] Bu Y-Y, Yamazaki H, Ukai K, Namikoshi M. Anti-mycobacterial nucleoside antibiotics from a marine-derived *Streptomyces* sp. TPU1236A. Mar Drugs 2014; 12(12): 6102-12. [http://dx.doi.org/10.3390/md12126102] [PMID: 25522318]

[86] Khalil ZG, Raju R, Piggott AM, Salim AA, Blumenthal A, Capon RJ. Aranciamycins I and J, antimycobacterial anthracyclines from an Australian marine-derived *Streptomyces* sp. J Nat Prod 2015; 78(4): 949-52. [http://dx.doi.org/10.1021/acs.jnatprod.5b00095] [PMID: 25789410]

[87] Gajalakshmi P, Raja A, James RA. Study on antimycobacterial activity of marine actinomycetes from coromondal coastal region of southern India. Int J Pharm Pharm Sci 2014; 6(7): 144-7.

[88] Radhakrishnan M, Balagurunathan R, Selvakumar N, Doble M, Kumar V. Bioprospecting of marine derived actinomycetes with special reference to antimycobacterial activity. Ind J Mar Sci 2011; 40(3): 407-10.

[89] Pérez-Bonilla M, Oves-Costales D, de la Cruz M, *et al.* Phocoenamicins B and C, new antibacterial spirotetronates isolated from a marine Micromonospora sp. Mar Drugs 2018; 16(3): 95. [http://dx.doi.org/10.3390/md16030095] [PMID: 29547589]

[90] Williams DE, Dalisay DS, Chen J, *et al.* Aminorifamycins and sporalactams produced in culture by a *Micromonospora* sp. isolated from a Northeastern-Pacific marine sediment are potent antibiotics. Org Lett 2017; 19(4): 766-9. [http://dx.doi.org/10.1021/acs.orglett.6b03619] [PMID: 28164711]

[91] Anuradha S, Kumar KS, Bhama S, Kishan V. Fermentation, isolation, purification and characterization of an antitubercular antibiotic from *Streptomyces luridus* MTCC 4402. Indian J Exp Biol 2016; 54(9): 577-85. [PMID: 28699723]

[92] Radhakrishnan M, Raman VA, Bharathi S, Balagurunathan R, Kumar V. Anti MRSA and antitubercular activity of phenoxazinone containing molecule from Borra caves *Streptomyces* sp. BCAI. IJPSR 2014; 5(12): 5342-8.

[93] Radhakrishnan M, Suganya S, Balagurunathan R, Kumar V. Preliminary screening for antibacterial and antimycobacterial activity of actinomycetes from less explored ecosystems. World J Microbiol Biotechnol 2010; 26: 561-6.
[http://dx.doi.org/10.1007/s11274-009-0198-9]

[94] Raja A, Prabakaran P. Preliminary screening of antimycobacterial effect of psychrophillic actinomycetes isolated from Manali ice point: Himachal predesh. J Microbiol Antimicrob 2011; 3(2): 41-6.

[95] Lin Z, Koch M, Pond CD, *et al.* Lobophorins with antimycobacterial activity from a turrid mollusc-associated *Streptomyces* sp. J Antibiot (Tokyo) 2014; 67(1): 121-6.
[http://dx.doi.org/10.1038/ja.2013.115] [PMID: 24220110]

[96] Mullowney MW, Hwang CH, Newsome AG, *et al.* Diaza-anthracene antibiotics from a freshwater-derived actinomycete with selective antibacterial activity toward *Mycobacterium tuberculosis.* ACS Infect Dis 2015; 1(4): 168-74.
[http://dx.doi.org/10.1021/acsinfecdis.5b00005] [PMID: 26594660]

[97] Manikkam R, Venugopal G, Subramaniam B, Ramasamy B, Kumar V. Bioactive potential of actinomycetes from less explored ecosystems against Mycobacterium tuberculosis and other nonmycobacterial pathogens. Int Scholar Res Not 2014; p. 812974.

[98] Kumar KS, Anuradha S, Sarma GR, Venkateshwarlu Y, Kishan V. Screening, isolation, taxonomy and fermentation of an antibiotic producer *Streptomyces xinghaiensis* from soil capable of acting against linezolid resistant strains. Indian J Exp Biol 2012; 50(10): 718-28.
[PMID: 23214266]

[99] Supong K, Sripreechasak P, Phongsopitanun W, *et al.* Antimicrobial substances from the rare actinomycete *Nonomuraea rhodomycinica* NR4-ASC07^T. Nat Prod Res 2018.
[http://dx.doi.org/10.1080/14786419.2018.1440223] [PMID: 29451019]

[100] Nakagawa M, Hayakawa Y, Kawai H, *et al.* A new anthracycline antibiotic N-formyl-13-dihydrocarminomycin. J Antibiot (Tokyo) 1983; 36(4): 457-8.
[http://dx.doi.org/10.7164/antibiotics.36.457] [PMID: 6574126]

CHAPTER 2

Protozoan and Helminth Infections: Epidemiology and Anti Infective Therapy

Saikat Mukherjee[1,*], **K. Tamreihao**[1], **Rakhi Khunjamayum**[1], **Khullakpam Shaheen**[1], **Elangbam Shanta Singh**[1], **Debananda S. Ningthoujam**[1] and **Sumita Banerjee**[2]

[1] *Advanced Level State Biotech Hub, Microbial Biotechnology Research Laboratory (MBRL), Department of Biochemistry, Manipur University, Imphal, Canchipur – 795003, India*

[2] *Department of Oral Pathology & Microbiology, Dental College, Regional Institute of Medical Sciences, Imphal, Manipur - 795004, India*

Abstract: Our book chapter discusses the two most important protozoan and helminth infections: Leishmaniasis and Elephantiasis. Both of these communicable diseases are a major concern for tropical and subtropical countries. Leishmaniasis has been responsible for frequent epidemics, while elephantiasis is the second most important vector borne disease after malaria. Here, we discuss in detail the vectors transmitting these diseases, the mode of transmission, disease pathogenesis, and conventional/ target based therapeutic approaches.

Keywords: Anti-filarial drugs, Anti-leishmanial drugs, Combination chemotherapy, Elephantiasis, Leishmaniasis.

Section A: Protozoan Infections: Epidemiology and Antiprotozoan Drugs (Special Emphasis on Leishmaniasis)

INTRODUCTION

Protozoans cause various communicable diseases in human, such as trypanosomiasis, leprosy, malaria, filarial, schistosomiasis, and leishmaniasis. Our book chapter will focus on the major protozoan diseases in tropical countries: Leishmaniasis and Elephantiasis.

* **Corresponding author Saikat Mukherjee:** Advanced Level State Biotech Hub, Microbial Biotechnology Research Laboratory (MBRL), Department of Biochemistry, Manipur University, Imphal, Canchipur – 795003, India; Tel: +91 878 7490 855; Fax: +91 385 243 5145; E-mail: mukherjee.saikat7@gmail.com

K. Tamreihao, Saikat Mukherjee and Debananda S. Ningthoujam (Eds.)
All rights reserved-© 2019 Bentham Science Publishers

Leishmaniasis

Leishmanias comprises a group of protozoan parasites of vertebrates, which are transmitted from host to host by the bite of blood sucking sand fly vectors. *Leishmania sp.* exists in two forms; as an extracellular flagellated form, also known as promastigotes, in the digestive tract of the insect vector and as an intracellular, non-motile form or amastigote form in the lysosomal compartment of macrophage within the susceptible vertebrate host.

A wide variety of *Leishmania sp.* infects reptiles and mammals causing a spectrum of diseases in humans, collectively known as leishmaniasis [1].

General Description

Leishmania sp. is an obligate intracellular pathogen invading the phagocytic host cell. Over 30 different species of Phlebotomine sand flies transmit this parasite either zoonotically or anthroponotically or through their bites. The disease Leishmaniasis affects poor people living around the Mediterranean Basin, East Africa, the Americas, and Southeast Asia. Leishmaniasis is reported to be the second most dangerous neglected tropical diseases ranking only after malaria in parasitic causes of death. People carry some species of *Leishmania* for a long period without becoming ill, and the symptoms depend on the forms of the disease.

There are two types of leishmaniasis; cutaneous and visceral. Visceral leishmaniasis was known in India as lethal "Kala Azar" long before its parasitic nature was known. Russian army physician Borovsky (1889) discovered the parasitic nature of the disease and it was Leishman (1903) who discovered that the protozoa is related to Trypanosomes. Donovan, in the same year made similar observations in samples from India. The causative agent was then named as *Leishmania donovani.*

The WHO recognized leishmaniasis as one of the six major communicable diseases along with trypanosomiasis, leprosy, malaria, filarial, and schistosomiasis [2].

Kala–azar or visceral leishmaniasis has periodically appeared as an endemic throughout India, particularly in Eastern India. The first recorded epidemic dates back to 1824 in Jessore district of Bengal (Now Bangladesh), which gradually spread to Nadia district in 1832, Hooghly district in 1857, and subsequently to Burdwan district (Now in West Bengal, India) in 1862, and to the Garo Hills of Assam in 1963. It was a full blown epidemic in Assam between 1890 and 1900 and has appeared as epidemics in Bihar for a number of times [3].

In the post DDT era, incidence of Kala–azar had declined, along with other vector transmitted diseases like malaria, primarily due to the elimination of the vector by pesticides. Resurgence of leishmaniasis along with malaria took place after withdrawal of the insecticide word wide. In 1991, there were large epidemics in India affecting almost two hundred thousand people, which killed seventy-five thousand people. Based on the pathogenesis, leishmaniasis can be classified into three major classes [4]:

A. Kala-azar: It is a lethal systemic disease of reticulo-endothelial system, particularly affecting bone marrow, spleen, and liver. It is also known as visceral leishmaniasis.
B. Oriental sore or Delhi Boil: This is a self-limiting paralyzed cutaneous lesion, developed at an exposed site of the body where the organisms are introduced by the bite of sand fly vector. Skin ulcers take more than a year to heal.
C. Mucocutaneous leishmaniasis: It is initiated like oriental sores but some patients develop metastatic lesions with various degrees of disfiguring and sometimes fatal tissue damages, localized primarily in the nasal and buccal cavities.

Vectors for Leishmaniasis

Sand flies of the genus Phlebotomus are of great importance as the transmitters of various types of leishmaniasis. *P. argenticus* is the vector transmitting *Leishmania donovani*, the causative agent of Kala-azar in India [5]. *Phlebotomous papatasi* and *P. sergenti* are the other two sand flies that transmit *Leishmania tropica* and *Leishmania donovani* [6].

These insects are small, about 3 mm long, slender, and buff coloured with a hairy body. They live in dark places and breed in sandy soil (hence the name sand fly), rubbish, and dump cracks. The female sand flies are hematophagous. Egg laying starts after 30-36 hrs of a blood meal. Female lays 30-35 eggs, which hatch in 6-12 days, undergo 4 moults in 25-35 days to become pupa, which further moults into adults in 6-14 days [7].

Life Cycle of Leishmania

Leishmania passes through two developmental stages; one in sand fly vector also known as the extracellular promastigote stage, and another in the macrophages of mammalian host also known as the intracellular amastigote form. The life cycle can be divided into following categories:

Life Cycle in the Sand Fly

The macrophages infected with amastigotes are introduced into the insect through the blood meal. Within the mid gut, up to 24 hrs after ingestion, the parasites remain immobile and then multiply and transform into slender promastigotes [8]. The promastigotes remain attached to the midgut by their long modified flagella interdigitated between microvilli and lining the midgut [9]. Promastigotes replicate by means of binary fission and give rise to the infectious metacyclic forms [10]. Metacyclic move anteriorly and are loaded in the biting apparatus of the insect for further transformation. During the blood meal, the infected fly injects the infectious metacyclic form into the blood stream of the native vertebrate host. The development of the infectious form takes place under nutrient depleted condition.

Life Cycle in the Vertebrate

After their introduction into the blood stream, within hours, infective promastigotes are phagocytosed into the acidic intracellular parasitophorus vacuoles of the macrophages, where they differentiate into amastigotes. There, the amastigotes replicate and eventually the parasitic burden lyses the host cell, releasing the amastigotes, which in turn infect fresh macrophages.

Morphology of Leishmania

Lesihmania sp. shows two different morphologies.

Promastigotes: (In greek, pro = in front, mastix = whip) Promastigote is a round to spindle shaped *Leishmania* of up to 20 µm length and 1.5-3.5 µm wide, with a long single flagellum. There is a centrally located nucleus and a rod shaped electron dense kinetoplast DNA in the cytoplasm [10]. Promastigotes divide by mitosis. Electron microscopy revealed three types of promastigotes in sand flies: nectonomads, haptomonads, and paramastigotes. In smears of the gut of sand flies, heavily infected with some *Leishmania* species, large rosettes of parasites are sometimes observed.

Amastogote: (In greek, a = without mastix = whip) Amastigote is a non-motile Leishmania of 2-5 µm in diameter, with no external flagellum, when observed under a light microscope. In electron microscopy, a flagellum protruding outside is observed. Amastigotes have a 1-1.2 µm diameter nucleus and a densely stained kinetoplast; 0.5-0.8 µm in length and 0.4-0.5 µm width.

Morphological and Molecular Changes during Transformation of Leishmania sp.

The following morphological and molecular changes are observed during Leishmania transformation:

Transformation from Amastigote to Promastigote

This transformation occurs within the peritrophic membrane of the insect gut within 12-24 hours after ingestion and is studied extensively *in vitro*. It is triggered by oxygen, as the amastigotes are predominantly anaerobic [11], while promastigotes are predominantly aerobic [12]. A shift in the ambient temperature from 22 °C to 35 °C is reported to hasten the process of transformation [13]. During transformation, the amastigotes first lengthen and the flagellar vacuole (lying near the flagellar pocket) increases in size. By 20 hrs, a stumpy flagellar rudiment is protruded and the body assumes an elongated promastigote form followed by flagellar vacuole contraction. Morphologically, a change in the surface coat occurs leading to an increasingly dense coat of glycocalyx composed of a variety of glycoconjugates bound to the parasitic surface by a glycophosphatidylinositol inositol anchor (GPI anchor) [14], specifically stage specific lipophosphoglycans (LPG), proteophosphoglycans (PPG), and low molecular weight glycoinositol phospholipids (GIPLs). Transformation from amastigote to promastigote is also accompanied by increase in respiratory rate, synthesis, or accumulation of cytochrome c, increase in cell and mitochondrial volume, synthesis of flagellum, and intra-flagellate bodies, acquisition of antigens, and changes in the respiratory stimulation by L-proline [15].

Leishmania sp. also demonstrates sequential development from a non-infective promastigote to a non-dividing infective 'metacyclic promastigote' form in insect vector and *in vitro* cultures. Progressive number of infective metacyclics appears when the cell population reaches stationary phase of their growth cycles [16]. *In vitro* development of metacyclic is associated with changes in the membrane carbohydrates [17], increased expression of gp63, increased resistance to lysis by normal human serum [18], altered mobility [19], enzyme activities, a long flagellum, and antigenicity [20].

Transformation from Promastigote to Amastigote Form

In mouse peritoneal macrophage culture, promastigotes transform into amastigotes within 12-24 hrs after its entry into the macrophage [21] at 37 °C and 25 °C [22]. This transformation requires glucose and amino acids [23]. There are several enzymes and metabolites which accumulate during this transformation. Phosphoenolpyruvate, carboxykinase, and malate dehydrogenase are the most important among them [24], along with cAMP [25] and polyamines [23] that have increased expression during the transformation. There is also a dramatic increase in expression in tubulin biosynthesis [24], oxidative [25], and glycolytic enzymes, glucose transporters [26] and nucleotides. However, there is down regulation of LPG and gp63 [26].

Pathogenesis and Inflammation of Leishmania

Leishmania major and *Leishmania tropica* cause cutaneous leishmaniasis in central Asia and Middle East whereas *Leishmania mexicana* and *Leishmania braziliensis* cause the disease in America. *Leishmania infantum, Leishmania chagasi, and Leishmania donovani* cause visceral leishmaniasis (VL, also called kala-azar disease). The various clinical manifestations of leishmaniasis are fever, wasting, compromised immunity, hepatospenomegaly, and anemia. Usually, leishmaniasis affects poverty stricken people living around East Africa, America, and South East Asia [27].

Induction of the T-helper 1 (Th1) cell cytokine interferon-γ (IFN-γ) generate immune responses against leishmaniasis. Also, neutrophils are important in inflammatory responses. Reports shows Th1 cells with IFN-γ and TNF-β secretion participate in immune responses against leishmania infection. Besides, neutrophils affect adaptive immune responses in leishmania infections by production of chemokine. Studies also showed interaction between dendritic cells and natural killer cells with parasite reservoirs results in host immune protection and destroying parasite by IFN-γ production while infection with *L. major* [28 - 34].

Various Anti Leishmania Drugs Available/ Clinical Trials (Table 1)

Pentavalent Antimonials

Sodium stibogluconate (SSG) and Pentavalent antimonials such as meglumine antimonate (MA) are used in treatment of VL and CL. Composition and chemical structure of sodium stibogluconate and meglumine antimonate have been confirmed by osmolarity experiments and electrospray ionization mass spectrometry (ESI-MS) [35]. Mixtures of SSG and MA in ratios 2:2, 2:3 and 2:1 exist as Sbv-ligand complexes in concentrated aqueous solutions. However, with increasing dilutions, increasing depolymerisation occurs resulting in conversion from aggregated state into antimonate and dissociated complexes form in human serum after administrating the drug. The final pharmacologically relevant form of the drug is 1:1 Sbv-ligand complexes, together with antimonate [35]. Pentavalent antimonials act as prodrugs requiring reduction to a trivalent form for their biological activity. The exact site of reduction whether in macrophage or amastigote as well as the mechanism (enzymatic and nonenzymatic) remain unclear. Studies implicate inhibition of macromolecular biosynthesis and energy metabolism. The inhibition targets glycolysis and fatty acid beta oxidation [36, 37].

Table 1. Currently available Major Drugs for treating *Visceral leishmaniasis.*

Drug	Trade Name	Efficiency	Dosage	Cost of Drug (US$)	Side Effects	References
Pentavalent Antimonials	Sodim Stibogluconate: Glaxosmithskline (Pentosam), Sanofi Aventis (Glucantime), Albert David (SSG)	30-95%	20-30 mg antimony per kg body weight for 25-30 days	53 (generic) to 198 (branded; SSG)	Toxicity, painful injection, drug resistanc-e	[35 - 41]
Amphotericin B	Bristol Meyers (Squibb; Fungizone), AmBisome (Liposomal Amphotericin B)	97%	1 mg/kg per day for 30 days; for AmBisome 5-20 mg/kg in 4-10 doses over 10-20 days, intravenous	20 per 50 mg vial of AmBisom-e	Nephortoxicity, hypokaleimia, myocarditis, heat instabilit-y,	[64 - 71]
Miltefosine	Paladin, Canada (Impavido)	90% (Asia). 60% (Africa)	50 mg for 28 days, oral	280 for 20 mg/kg dose	Nephrotoxicity, Cardiotoxicity, gastrointestinal effects, teratogenic, cannot be used in pregnancy	[45 - 54]
Paromo-mycin sulphate	Institute for One World Health; Gland Pharma, Hyderabad	94%	15 mg/kg daily for 21 days (India), intramuscular	15	Nephrotoxicity, ototoxicity, varied efficacy	[59 - 63]

Although response rates are over 95% in VL patients, but patients in Bihar, India showed acquired resistance to pentavalent antimony [38]. Antimony usage is now abandoned here [39]. Apart from this, issues which relate to effective treatment also include the side effects of various low-cost generic drugs, drug efficacy, and variation in one lot to another [40]. Cardiotoxicity has been reported as a side effect of drug usage [41, 42]. Sometimes, serious cardiotoxicity has been reported in 9-10% of treated patients [42]. The pharmacokinetics of pentavalent antimonials have been described in detail. This is termed as pharmacokinetic model. The model shows antimonials have an initial absorption phase, which successively follows a rapid elimination phase with a mean half-life of approximately 2 hr followed by a slow elimination with a mean half-life of 76 hrs [43].

Miltefosine

Chemically the drug is an alkylphosphocholine, which was actually developed as an anti-cancer drug. Miltefosine is the first oral anti-leishmanial drug that was registered for treatment of CL in Columbia and VL in India and Germany [44]. A plasma membrane P-type ATPase aminophospholipid translocase mediates uptake of miltefosine [45 - 47]. The various targets of miltefosine include perturbation of glycosyl phosphatidylinositol (GPI) anchor biosynthesis, ether-lipid metabolism, and signal transduction [48]. Besides the drug inhibits glycosomal located alkyl-specific acyl-Co-A acyltransferase, an enzyme which is specifically involved in lipid-remodeling [49]. Recent reports indicate mitochondria and cytochrome *c* oxidase are also potential targets of miltefosine in *L. donovani* promastigotes [50]. The drug also effect lipid metabolism as described in *L. donovani* promastigotes [51]. The pharmacokinetics of miltefosine can be explained by two-compartment disposition model. When CL patients were treated with 50 mg miltefosine for 28 days, the first elimination half-life happens after approximately 7.05 days and a terminal half-life happens at 30.9 days [52]. The common adverse effect in clinical trials is gastrointestinal symptoms [53]. Hepatic enzymes show slightly increased expression. However, miltefosine cannot be used in pregnancy and for women in child-bearing age as investigated on rats [54].

Pentamidine

Pentamidine, an aromatic diamidine, is used as first line drug for certain forms of CL. However, it is used as second line treatment in VL due to toxicity and efficacy [40]. It is reported to be inducing insulin-dependent diabetes mellitus and therefore in India its use has been abandoned [41]. In electron microscopy studies on *Leishmania* spp., swelling of mitochondria as well as fragmentation of kinetoplastid DNA were found [55, 56]. In *L. donovani* promastigotes, a collapse of mitochondrial membrane potential has been reported [57].

Paromomycin

The latest anti-leishmanial drug registered for VL in India is Paromomycin, an aminoglycoside antibiotic. Paromomycin was non-inferior to amphotericin B as observed in a controlled, randomized, phase 3 study in India with a cure rate of approximately 94.6% *versus* 98.8% [58]. It has also been formulated for topical use in CL [40, 59]. The topical formulations offer ease of fewer side effects, administration, and cost effectiveness when compared to systemic treatment [60]. However, in the phase 3 trial for VL in India, injection-site pain was reported to be major side effect [58]. Although nephrotoxicity and ototoxicity are known drug effects, however the frequency is low at therapeutic dosage for VL [59]. Pharmacokinetic data is obtained during the phase 3 trial from VL patients. Paromomycin got absorbed very fast after intramuscular injection and peak plasma levels reached within 1 hr. It ranged from 18.3 µg/mL to 20.5 µg/mL within 1 hr [58]. For absorption and elimination half-lives, population estimates were reported as 0.33 hrs and 2.62 hrs respectively [59]. The targets of the molecule involve ribosomes as well as mitochondrial membrane de-polarisation and respiratory dysfunction [61 - 63].

Amphotericin B

Amphotericin B, a crystalline polyene antibiotic was purified from *Streptomyces nodosus*. It is insoluble in water and various formulations are available. In case of unresponsiveness to anitmonials, Amphotericin B is used as first line treatment and it is used as a second line treatment elsewhere [40]. Lipid based formulations or liposomal amphotericin B (AmBisome®) have been approved by the U.S. Food and Drug Administration (FDA) for treatment of VL [64]. Amphotericin B lipid complex (ABLC) and Amphotericin B colloidal dispersion (ABCD) are other commercially available lipid formulations used for treatment of VL [65]. A different commercial product of amphotericin B deoxycholate premixed with lipid emulsion containing egg lecithin and soybean oil (ABLE) is licensed in India for usage in VL, however curing rate is very low in phase II clinical trials [66, 67]. However, various toxicities are reported for liposomal formulations such as nephrotoxicity, hypokalaemia, and myocarditis [41]. Liposomal amphotericin B is safer and of more efficacy than amphotericin B deoxycholate [40, 41]. A general, effective pricing was agreed in many countries that costs $20 per 50 mg vial of AmBisome® [68]. Preclinical pharmacokinetics of AmBisome® is reported in humans. The terminal elimination half-life after repeated administration is around 7 hrs [69]. Amphotericin B targets *Leishmania* specifically because it has high affinity for 24-substituted sterols, the predominant sterol in *Leishmania* membranes, over cholesterol. The drugs form aqueous pores, transmembrane amphotericin B channels, and leakage of cations [70, 71].

Sitamaquine

For oral treatment of VL, Glaxo Smith Kline is currently developing Sitamaquine (WR6026), an 8-aminoquinoline [72]. Two major metabolites of sitamaquine are desethyl and 4-CH_2OH derivatives as observed in rat and hamster liver microsomes [72, 73]. 5- hydroxylation and side chain oxidation are important steps in the metabolic pathway of 8-aminoquinolines [72, 74]. Sitamaquine also induced morphological changes in *L. tropica* amastigotes as well as in host macrophages. Mitochondrial membrane potential collapse in *L. donovani* promastigotes has also been reported [57] along with alkalisation of acidocalcisomes [75]. The interaction of Sitamaquine and membrane lipids of *L. donovani* promastigotes interact with each other as a two-step process [76]. Role of chemotherapy in treatment of leishmaniasis is reported recently [40].

8-aminoquinolines

Although developed as antimalarials, 8-aminoquinolines have also successfully used in treatment of leishmaniasis [77].

2-substituted Quinolines

Originally isolated from a Bolivian medicinal plant (*Galipea longiflora* Kr, Rutaceae), this substituted quinoline alkaloids were effective in treatment of experimental New World CL [78] and also reported in *L. donovani*- BALB/c mouse model after using 2-n-propylquinolinein oral administration and chimanine D after subcutaneous administration [79].

Buparvaquone

Buparvaquone, a hydroxynaphtoquinone, is marketed as Butalex® for treatment of theileriosis in cattle. It is highly active *in vitro* against intracellular *L. donovani* amastigotes in macrophages, however less active *in vivo* in BALB/c mouse [80 - 84]. Its potent *in vitro* activity against a range of *Leishmania* spp. was reported in the low micromolar to nanomolar range for EC_{50} values on the intracellular amastigote stage [85]. Buparvaquone oxime derivatives showed lower *in vitro* activity against *L. donovani* comparative to the parent compound [86]. The drug is also used for topical drug delivery. Formulations for topical delivery of buparvaquone was developed and characterized in *in vitro* mouse skin and human models [87]. Efficacy of topical formulations of buparvaquone in *in vivo* models of VL and CL were also observed [88].

Combination Chemotherapy

As multidrug therapy in other infectious diseases such malaria, tuberculosis, and leprosy, anti-leishmanial chemotherapy including involving new drugs are also being developed [85 - 88]. These drug combinations shorten the course of treatment, delay/prevent the emergence of resistance, and lower required doses [89]. A combination of drugs including sodium stibogluconate, and paromomycin is currently manufactured in Sudan by Médecins sans frontiers (MSF) [90]. Besides, the single dose liposomal amphotericin B is also included in this new treatment approach for VL. A single dose of liposomal amphotericin B, followed by treatment of miltefosine for approximately 7-14 days showed satisfactorily results with cure rates >95% in treatment groups in India [89].

CONCLUDING REMARKS

In modern era, various approaches are being used for anti-leishmanial drug discovery such as molecular-target based approaches and exploratory drug screening. These different approaches involving whole cell based approaches, molecular approaches, and a compromise approach between them is being formulated in antiparasitic drug discovery [90 - 92]. The standard criteria for target assessment and target validation methods have recently been developed [90]. An open access database for many tropical diseases has been established that merges data from genome sequencing as well as functional genomics projects and combines protein structural data. Together, this approach provides information on target essentiality and drug ability [92, 93].

The development process is guided by target product profiles (TPP), a list of standards for potential new drugs [90, 94]. Guidelines that define "hit" and "lead" along with hit-to-lead identification criteria leading to optimization and candidate selection have also been summarized. These can be used as complementary approach to TPP in making further synthesis of compounds [95]. Consortium of many new public-private partnerships, non-profit organizations and consortia have also been established that support drug discovery and for neglected parasitic/ tropical diseases. A few examples of such consortiums are Drugs for Neglected Diseases Initiative (DNDi) and The Consortium for Parasitic Drug Development (CPDD). Many philanthropic organizations such as Bill and Melinda Gates Foundation as well as governments are also putting up increased (financial) support [93, 96]. Programs such as TDR Screening Network have evolved to ease in various stages of drug discovery and development. The various aspects integrated are target selection, medicinal chemistry and drug metabolism and pharmacokinetics (DMPK) [94, 95].

Section B: Helminth Infections: Epidemiology and Anti-Helminthic Drugs (Special Emphasis on Elephantiasis)

INTRODUCTION

Elephantiasis

It is known medically as lymphatic filariasis. Elephantiasis includes symptoms such as swelling and enlargement of the arms and legs. The World Health Organization (WHO) reported 120 million people worldwide get affected by elephantiasis.

Elephantiasis is a major public health problem in tropical as well as subtropical regions of the world. The disease is characterized by thickened skin specially underlying subcutaneous tissues in the legs, male genitals, and female breasts, which finally lead to permanent disability. The disease is caused by filarial worms or non-filarial heavy metals [97].

Two forms of elephantiasis are commonly seen. In one form, patients develop massive edema in the lower extremities which are secondary to lymphatic obstruction. The pathogenesis is caused as the adult stage of the causative agents of filarial elephantiasis invades the lymph nodes of humans; the female worms produce microfilariae which could be found in blood [98]. Another same clinical picture is also reported in non-filarial elephantiasis, a non- communicable geochemical disease which is induced by absorption of ultrafine silica particles from soil through the skin in the feet; however, the swelling is involved below the knee [99, 100].

Elephantiasis, therefore, is classified into filarial elephantiasis and non-filarial elephantiasis (also known as Podoconiosis).

Filarial Elephantiasis

Filarial elephantiasis or lymphatic filariasis (LF) is caused by three different thread-like parasitic worms: *Wuchereria bancrofti*, *Brugiati mori* and *Brugia malayi* that damage human lymphatic system. The worms are transmitted by mosquitoes [99]. *Wuchereria bancrofti* (most common and causes 90% of cases), *Brugia malay* and *Brugiati mori* [101]. *Wuchereria bancrofti* lives in warm regions in all continents except North America [102]. On the other hand, *Brugiati mori* is found in Timor and *Brugia malayi* is primarily found in Southeast Asia, Indonesia, and India [103].

It is second most common vector-borne parasitic disease after malaria [103]. Globally, million men suffer with genital disease and approximately 15 million people are affected with lymphoedema [98]. It is one of the world's most disabling diseases. More than 40 million persons have severe chronic manifestations of the disease [102]. It has endemic nature in >39 countries in Africa [103]. The disease is poverty-related and affects the poor and marginalized people.

Podoconiosis (Non Filarial Elephantiasis)

Podoconiosis, coined by Ernest Price, is derived from Greek words *podos* and *konos*, meaning foot and dust implying disease is caused by exposure of feet to clay soil [104, 105]. It is non-filarial elephantiasis predominantly affecting barefoot farmers in areas having red volcanic soil [106]. However, in this chapter we will discuss on filarial elephantiasis.

Symptoms

The disease involves two stages; acute and chronic. During acute phase of the disease, the symptoms involve recurring fever and infections of the lymph vessels (nodes in the arms, legs or genitals) leading to severe and permanent swelling of the lymph vessels followed by secondary infections [107]. In the chronic stage, worms block the lymphatic areas of the limbs causing overgrowth of the limb and body parts as lymphatic system can't perform the function of draining fluid out of the area [108]. Males also find swelling in the scrotum. The limbs enlarge to resemble elephant limbs and the skin has a rough texture like elephant skin [109].

Etiology

The parasite shows following etiologies:

i. Incubation Period

The pathogenesis of the disease is not known and some people who get infected may not show any signs/symptoms for months/years [110]. The parasite infects only humans, not other animals. The parasite migrates to lymphatic vessels and stays there gradually maturing into an adult worm and in a few months to one year produce the microfilariae. Microfilariae cause the initial fevers and chills, the first symptoms of the disease [110]. When a person is infected, they may never actually develop any symptoms even although the worm is in their lymphatic system and circulating in their blood. Only when there is repeated exposure with multiple worms and blockage of lymphatic system, the disease progressed [110].

ii. Duration of Disease

Duration of Lymphatic Filariasis depend on the number of re-infections suffe red by the host. A person having Elephantiasis can live with the disease and death can result from complications and secondary infections from the living and dead worms. The disease can last lifelong and if untreated can worsen over time. The side effects include disfigured limbs and genitalia, permanent damage to lymphatic system and kidneys, and secondary infections. The disease is also associated with social stigma in various chronic stages. The adult worm lives three to five years and the microfilariae die after twelve months if the mosquito doesn't take up in the next life cycle [102].

iii. Transmission

The disease is caused when a person gets bitten by an infected mosquito of genera including Culex, Anopheles, or Aedes. Mosquitoes serve as intermediate hosts. As they bite someone, the third-stage larvae are injected into the blood of the host [107]. Once injected, larvae mature into worms moving into the lymphatic system. After one year, the worms produce embryo called microfilariae [108]. Life time of Adult worms is for about seven years. The build-up of adult worms in the lymphatic system over time causes lymph fluid to collect leading to severe swelling of the limbs. The microfilariae circulate in the blood stream and mosquito takes up in the next life cycle. The microfilariae are active in the blood at night when mosquitoes are also active. Therefore mosquito easily takes up the microfilaria as the mosquito bites the infected host. The larvae get matured into the second state in the mosquitoes. Thus, in the process of repeated exposures and repeated transmissions of larvae into mature adult, worms' symptoms appear [109].

Anti-Elephantiasis Drugs

WHO has been working for remedy of the disease from many angles. Persons having active parasite are treated with drug Diethylcarbamazine (DEC) that limit the number of microfilariae in the blood stream and gradually also kills the parasite. The drug causes nausea, vomiting and fever which depend on the number of microfilariae in blood [107]. As the drug DEC act as a deterrent and also a cure, DEC has been proposed to be distributed in the affected areas in the world by adding salt in the same manner as iodine is added to salt (Lammie, Milner &Houston, 2006). Successful trials with DEC fortified salt have been carried out in India, China, Brazil, Haiti, and Tanzania (Lammie, Milner & Houston, 2006).

Other types of drugs used in treatment of Elephantiasis include ivermectin, albendazole and doxycycline [111]. Albendazole kills the worms but it has no effect on the microfilaria in the blood. Therefore, the transmission cycle continues unless the intermediate host is reduced or eliminated [111]. Besides drug therapies, movement of the affected limbs is encouraged by treatment with antibiotics to control secondary infections that cause damage to lymphatic system If the lymphatic swelling has initiated, compression bandages can be used to force the lymph out [107].

Since the causative agent spends a sufficient portion of lifecycle within the mosquito, the preventative measures could be usage of insect repellent and protective clothes and water treatment to reduce the insect population transmitting the disease to humans [111]. The other measures include the usage of mosquito netting and window screens. Besides, the population near the affected area should be given DEC as a preventative drug for breaking the cycle of transmission [107].

In the past, antibiotics were effective in the past. However, antibiotics couldn't affect a nematode, so the usage of antibiotics was dropped until recently. A new investigation finds a new bacterial symbiont of the worm, which can be treated with antibiotics [110]. The hypothesis was killing the symbiont worm will kill the worm as well. It is suspected some forms of inflammation is actually caused due to the symbiont bacteria.

CONCLUDING REMARKS

To conclude, Lymphatic Filariasis, a preventable disease, affects poverty stricken tropical and sub-tropical countries. The disease is highly debilitating. The various prevention methods include controlling the mosquitos by using protective clothing, netting and sprays and treating the population with DEC laced salt /administration of DEC in tablet forms to break the cycle of infection.

CONSENT FOR PUBLICATION

Not applicable.

CONFLICT OF INTEREST

The authors confirm that this chapter contents have no conflict of interest.

ACKNOWLEDGEMENTS

The authors wish to thank Department of Biotechnology (DBT), Govt. of India for sponsoring the host laboratory under the scheme "Establishment of State Biotech Hubs" (BT/04/NE/2009).

REFERENCES

[1] Chang KP, Fong D, Bray RS. Biology of Leishmania and Leishmaniasis. 1988.

[2] "WHO at the cross roads" – Report of the Director General to 30th World Health Assembly on the work of WHO in 1976. WHO Chron 1977; 207.

[3] Sanyal RK. Leishmaniasis. Amsterdam: Elsevier 1985.

[4] Madson PD, Jones TC. Clinical manifestations, diagnosis, and treatment of leishmaniasis, Vol -1.

Amsterdam: Elsevier Biomedical Press 1985.

[5] Mani MS. In General Ezymology. 3rd ed., New Delhi: Oxford & IBM Publishing Co. 1982.

[6] Mukherjee S, Hassan MQ, Ghosh A, Ghosh KN, Bhattacharya A, Adhya S. Short report: Leishmania DNA in Phlebotomus and Sergentomyia species during a kala-azar epidemic. Am J Trop Med Hyg 1997; 57(4): 423-5. [http://dx.doi.org/10.4269/ajtmh.1997.57.423] [PMID: 9347957]

[7] Srivastava KP. The Text Book of Applied Enzymology, vol -III. India: Kalyani Publishers 1993.

[8] Strangways-Dixon J, Lainson R. The epidemiology of dermal leishmansiasis in British Honduras. 3. The transmission of Leishmania mexicana to man by Phlebotomus pessoanus, with observations on the development of the parasite in different species of Phlebotomus. Trans R Soc Trop Med Hyg 1966; 60(2): 192-207. [http://dx.doi.org/10.1016/0035-9203(66)90027-7] [PMID: 5922608]

[9] Sacks DL, Perkins PV. Identification of an infective stage of Leishmania promastigotes. Science 1984; 223(4643): 1417-9. [http://dx.doi.org/10.1126/science.6701528] [PMID: 6701528]

[10] Molyneux DH, Killick-Kendrick R. Morphology, Ultrastructure, and Life Cycle, the leishmania in biology and medicine.Academic Press: London 1987; 1.

[11] Grimstone AV. Structure and function in Protozoa. Annu Rev Microbiol 1966; 20: 131-50. [http://dx.doi.org/10.1146/annurev.mi.20.100166.001023] [PMID: 5330229]

[12] Salle AJ, Schmidt CA. The metabolism of *Leishmania tropica.* J Infect Dis 1928; 43(5): 378-84. [http://dx.doi.org/10.1093/infdis/43.5.378]

[13] Adler S. Leishmania. Adv Parasitol 1964; 2: 35-96. [http://dx.doi.org/10.1016/S0065-308X(08)60586-2]

[14] Turco SJ, Descoteaux A. The lipophosphoglycan of Leishmania parasites. Annu Rev Microbiol 1992; 46: 65-94. [http://dx.doi.org/10.1146/annurev.mi.46.100192.000433] [PMID: 1444269]

[15] Doran TI, Herman R. Characterization of populations of promastigotes of Leishmania donovani. J Protozool 1981; 28(3): 345-50. [http://dx.doi.org/10.1111/j.1550-7408.1981.tb02863.x] [PMID: 7031232]

[16] Grögl M, Oduola AMJ, Cordero LDC, Kyle DE. Leishmania spp.: development of pentostam-resistant clones *in vitro* by discontinuous drug exposure. Exp Parasitol 1989; 69(1): 78-90. [http://dx.doi.org/10.1016/0014-4894(89)90173-2] [PMID: 2543590]

[17] Howard MK, Sayers G, Miles MA. *Leishmania donovani* metacyclic promastigotes: transformation *in vitro*, lectin agglutination, complement resistance, and infectivity. Exp Parasitol 1987; 64(2): 147-56. [http://dx.doi.org/10.1016/0014-4894(87)90138-X] [PMID: 3653336]

[18] Sacks DL, Hieny S, Sher A. Identification of cell surface carbohydrate and antigenic changes between noninfective and infective developmental stages of *Leishmania major* promastigotes. J Immunol 1985; 135(1): 564-9. [PMID: 2582050]

[19] Mallinson DJ, Coombs GH. Interaction of leishmania metacyclics with macrophages. Int J Parasitol 1989; 19(6): 647-56. [http://dx.doi.org/10.1016/0020-7519(89)90043-X] [PMID: 2807719]

[20] Akiyama HJ, Taylor JC. Effect of macrophage engulfment and temperature on the transformation process of *Leishmania donovani.* Am J Trop Med Hyg 1970; 19(5): 747-54. [http://dx.doi.org/10.4269/ajtmh.1970.19.747] [PMID: 4195298]

[21] Alexander J. Effect of the antiphagocytic agent cytochalasin B on macrophage invasion by Leishmania mexicana promastigotes and Trypanosoma cruzi epimastigotes. J Protozool 1975; 22(2): 237-40.

[http://dx.doi.org/10.1111/j.1550-7408.1975.tb05858.x] [PMID: 1097661]

[22] Schleyer M, Schmidt B, Neupert W. Requirement of a membrane potential for the posttranslational transfer of proteins into mitochondria. Eur J Biochem 1982; 125(1): 109-16. [http://dx.doi.org/10.1111/j.1432-1033.1982.tb06657.x] [PMID: 6213410]

[23] Simpson L. The leishmania-leptomonad transformation of Leishmania donovani: nutritional requirements, respiration changes and antigenic changes. J Protozool 1968; 15(1): 201-7. [http://dx.doi.org/10.1111/j.1550-7408.1968.tb02112.x] [PMID: 4966877]

[24] Mottram JC, Coombs GH. Purification of particulate malate dehydrogenase and phosphoenolpyruvate carboxykinase from Leishmania mexicana mexicana. Biochim Biophys Acta 1985; 827(3): 310-9. [http://dx.doi.org/10.1016/0167-4838(85)90216-X] [PMID: 3970941]

[25] Walter RD, Buse E, Ebert F. Effect of cyclic AMP on transformation and proliferation of leishmania cells. Tropenmed Parasitol 1978; 29(4): 439-42. [PMID: 217133]

[26] Stack SP, Stein DA, Landfear SM. Structural isoforms of a membrane transport protein from Leishmania enriettii. Mol Cell Biol 1990; 10(12): 6785-90. [http://dx.doi.org/10.1128/MCB.10.12.6785] [PMID: 1701025]

[27] Savoia D. Recent updates and perspectives on leishmaniasis. J Infect Dev Ctries 2015; 9(6): 588-96. [http://dx.doi.org/10.3855/jidc.6833] [PMID: 26142667]

[28] Peters NC, Egen JG, Secundino N, *et al. In vivo* imaging reveals an essential role for neutrophils in leishmaniasis transmitted by sand flies. Science 2008; 321(5891): 970-4. [http://dx.doi.org/10.1126/science.1159194] [PMID: 18703742]

[29] Amulic B, Cazalet C, Hayes GL, Metzler KD, Zychlinsky A. Neutrophil function: from mechanisms to disease. Annu Rev Immunol 2012; 30: 459-89. [http://dx.doi.org/10.1146/annurev-immunol-020711-074942] [PMID: 22224774]

[30] Antonelli LR, Dutra WO, Almeida RP, Bacellar O, Carvalho EM, Gollob KJ. Activated inflammatory T cells correlate with lesion size in human cutaneous leishmaniasis. Immunol Lett 2005; 101(2): 226-30. [http://dx.doi.org/10.1016/j.imlet.2005.06.004] [PMID: 16083969]

[31] Bacellar O, Lessa H, Schriefer A, *et al.* Up-regulation of Th1-type responses in mucosal leishmaniasis patients. Infect Immun 2002; 70(12): 6734-40. [http://dx.doi.org/10.1128/IAI.70.12.6734-6740.2002] [PMID: 12438348]

[32] Conceição J, Davis R, Carneiro PP, *et al.* Characterization of neutrophil function in human cutaneous leishmaniasis caused by *Leishmania braziliensis.* PLoS Negl Trop Dis 2016; 10(5)e0004715 [http://dx.doi.org/10.1371/journal.pntd.0004715] [PMID: 27167379]

[33] Müller K, van Zandbergen G, Hansen B, *et al.* Chemokines, natural killer cells and granulocytes in the early course of *Leishmania major* infection in mice. Med Microbiol Immunol (Berl) 2001; 190(1-2): 73-6. [http://dx.doi.org/10.1007/s004300100084] [PMID: 11770115]

[34] Ribeiro-de-Jesus A, Almeida RP, Lessa H, Bacellar O, Carvalho EM. Cytokine profile and pathology in human leishmaniasis. Braz J Med Biol Res 1998; 31(1): 143-8. [http://dx.doi.org/10.1590/S0100-879X1998000100020] [PMID: 9686192]

[35] Frézard F, Martins PS, Barbosa MC, *et al.* New insights into the chemical structure and composition of the pentavalent antimonial drugs, meglumine antimonate and sodium stibogluconate. J Inorg Biochem 2008; 102(4): 656-65. [http://dx.doi.org/10.1016/j.jinorgbio.2007.10.010] [PMID: 18061680]

[36] Berman JD, Waddell D, Hanson BD. Biochemical mechanisms of the antileishmanial activity of sodium stibogluconate. Antimicrob Agents Chemother 1985; 27(6): 916-20. [http://dx.doi.org/10.1128/AAC.27.6.916] [PMID: 2411217]

[37] Berman JD, Gallalee JV, Best JM. Sodium stibogluconate (Pentostam) inhibition of glucose catabolism *via* the glycolytic pathway, and fatty acid beta-oxidation in *Leishmania mexicana* amastigotes. Biochem Pharmacol 1987; 36(2): 197-201.
[http://dx.doi.org/10.1016/0006-2952(87)90689-7] [PMID: 3028425]

[38] Croft SL, Sundar S, Fairlamb AH. Drug resistance in leishmaniasis. Clin Microbiol Rev 2006; 19(1): 111-26.
[http://dx.doi.org/10.1128/CMR.19.1.111-126.2006] [PMID: 16418526]

[39] Sundar S, More DK, Singh MK, *et al.* Failure of pentavalent antimony in visceral leishmaniasis in India: report from the center of the Indian epidemic. Clin Infect Dis 2000; 31(4): 1104-7.
[http://dx.doi.org/10.1086/318121] [PMID: 11049798]

[40] Alvar J, Croft S, Olliaro P. Chemotherapy in the treatment and control of leishmaniasis. Adv Parasitol 2006; 61: 223-74.
[http://dx.doi.org/10.1016/S0065-308X(05)61006-8] [PMID: 16735166]

[41] Olliaro PL, Guerin PJ, Gerstl S, Haaskjold AA, Rottingen JA, Sundar S. Treatment options for visceral leishmaniasis: a systematic review of clinical studies done in India, 1980-2004. Lancet Infect Dis 2005; 5(12): 763-74.
[http://dx.doi.org/10.1016/S1473-3099(05)70296-6] [PMID: 16310148]

[42] Sundar S, Sinha PR, Agrawal NK, *et al.* A cluster of cases of severe cardiotoxicity among kala-azar patients treated with a high-osmolarity lot of sodium antimony gluconate. Am J Trop Med Hyg 1998; 59(1): 139-43.
[http://dx.doi.org/10.4269/ajtmh.1998.59.139] [PMID: 9684642]

[43] Chulay JD, Fleckenstein L, Smith DH. Pharmacokinetics of antimony during treatment of visceral leishmaniasis with sodium stibogluconate or meglumine antimoniate. Trans R Soc Trop Med Hyg 1988; 82(1): 69-72.
[http://dx.doi.org/10.1016/0035-9203(88)90267-2] [PMID: 2845611]

[44] Seifert K, Pérez-Victoria FJ, Stettler M, *et al.* Inactivation of the miltefosine transporter, LdMT, causes miltefosine resistance that is conferred to the amastigote stage of *Leishmania donovani* and persists *in vivo.* Int J Antimicrob Agents 2007; 30(3): 229-35.
[http://dx.doi.org/10.1016/j.ijantimicag.2007.05.007] [PMID: 17628445]

[45] Pérez-Victoria FJ, Gamarro F, Ouellette M, Castanys S. Functional cloning of the miltefosine transporter. A novel P-type phospholipid translocase from Leishmania involved in drug resistance. J Biol Chem 2003; 278(50): 49965-71.
[http://dx.doi.org/10.1074/jbc.M308352200] [PMID: 14514670]

[46] Pérez-Victoria FJ, Sánchez-Cañete MP, Castanys S, Gamarro F. Phospholipid translocation and miltefosine potency require both *L. donovani miltefosine* transporter and the new protein LdRos3 in Leishmania parasites. J Biol Chem 2006; 281(33): 23766-75.
[http://dx.doi.org/10.1074/jbc.M605214200] [PMID: 16785229]

[47] Pérez-Victoria FJ, Sánchez-Cañete MP, Seifert K, *et al.* Mechanisms of experimental resistance of Leishmania to miltefosine: Implications for clinical use. Drug Resist Updat 2006; 9(1-2): 26-39.
[http://dx.doi.org/10.1016/j.drup.2006.04.001] [PMID: 16814199]

[48] Lux H, Hart DT, Parker PJ, Klenner T. Ether lipid metabolism, GPI anchor biosynthesis, and signal transduction are putative targets for anti-leishmanial alkyl phospholipid analogues. Adv Exp Med Biol 1996; 416: 201-11.
[http://dx.doi.org/10.1007/978-1-4899-0179-8_33] [PMID: 9131149]

[49] Lux H, Heise N, Klenner T, Hart D, Opperdoes FR. Ether--lipid (alkyl-phospholipid) metabolism and the mechanism of action of ether--lipid analogues in Leishmania. Mol Biochem Parasitol 2000; 111(1): 1-14.
[http://dx.doi.org/10.1016/S0166-6851(00)00278-4] [PMID: 11087912]

[50] Luque-Ortega JR, Rivas L. Miltefosine (hexadecylphosphocholine) inhibits cytochrome c oxidase in *Leishmania donovani* promastigotes. Antimicrob Agents Chemother 2007; 51(4): 1327-32. [http://dx.doi.org/10.1128/AAC.01415-06] [PMID: 17283192]

[51] Rakotomanga M, Blanc S, Gaudin K, Chaminade P, Loiseau PM. Miltefosine affects lipid metabolism in *Leishmania donovani* promastigotes. Antimicrob Agents Chemother 2007; 51(4): 1425-30. [http://dx.doi.org/10.1128/AAC.01123-06] [PMID: 17242145]

[52] Dorlo TP, van Thiel PP, Huitema AD, *et al.* Pharmacokinetics of miltefosine in Old World cutaneous leishmaniasis patients. Antimicrob Agents Chemother 2008; 52(8): 2855-60. [http://dx.doi.org/10.1128/AAC.00014-08] [PMID: 18519729]

[53] Bhattacharya SK, Sinha PK, Sundar S, *et al.* Phase 4 trial of miltefosine for the treatment of Indian visceral leishmaniasis. J Infect Dis 2007; 196(4): 591-8. [http://dx.doi.org/10.1086/519690] [PMID: 17624846]

[54] Sindermann H, Engel J. Development of miltefosine as an oral treatment for leishmaniasis. Trans R Soc Trop Med Hyg 2006; 100(100) (Suppl. 1): S17-20. [http://dx.doi.org/10.1016/j.trstmh.2006.02.010] [PMID: 16730362]

[55] Langreth SG, Berman JD, Riordan GP, Lee LS. Fine-structural alterations in *Leishmania tropica* within human macrophages exposed to antileishmanial drugs *in vitro.* J Protozool 1983; 30(3): 555-61. [http://dx.doi.org/10.1111/j.1550-7408.1983.tb01421.x] [PMID: 6315928]

[56] Croft SL, Brazil RP. Effect of pentamidine isethionate on the ultrastructure and morphology of *Leishmania mexicana* amazonensis *in vitro.* Ann Trop Med Parasitol 1982; 76(1): 37-43. [http://dx.doi.org/10.1080/00034983.1982.11687502] [PMID: 7082077]

[57] Vercesi AE, Docampo R. Ca2+ transport by digitonin-permeabilized *Leishmania donovani.* Effects of Ca2+, pentamidine and WR-6026 on mitochondrial membrane potential *in situ.* Biochem J 1992; 284(Pt 2): 463-7. [http://dx.doi.org/10.1042/bj2840463] [PMID: 1376113]

[58] Sundar S, Jha TK, Thakur CP, Sinha PK, Bhattacharya SK. Injectable paromomycin for Visceral leishmaniasis in India. N Engl J Med 2007; 356(25): 2571-81. [http://dx.doi.org/10.1056/NEJMoa066536] [PMID: 17582067]

[59] Davidson RN, den Boer M, Ritmeijer K. Paromomycin. Trans R Soc Trop Med Hyg 2009; 103(7): 653-60. [http://dx.doi.org/10.1016/j.trstmh.2008.09.008] [PMID: 18947845]

[60] Garnier T, Croft SL. Topical treatment for cutaneous leishmaniasis. Curr Opin Investig Drugs 2002; 3(4): 538-44. [PMID: 12090720]

[61] Maarouf M, Lawrence F, Croft SL, Robert-Gero M. Ribosomes of Leishmania are a target for the aminoglycosides. Parasitol Res 1995; 81(5): 421-5. [http://dx.doi.org/10.1007/BF00931504] [PMID: 7501642]

[62] Maarouf M, de Kouchkovsky Y, Brown S, Petit PX, Robert-Gero M. *In vivo* interference of paromomycin with mitochondrial activity of Leishmania. Exp Cell Res 1997; 232(2): 339-48. [http://dx.doi.org/10.1006/excr.1997.3500] [PMID: 9168810]

[63] Maarouf M, Lawrence F, Brown S, Robert-Gero M. Biochemical alterations in paromomycin-treated *Leishmania donovani* promastigotes. Parasitol Res 1997; 83(2): 198-202. [http://dx.doi.org/10.1007/s004360050232] [PMID: 9039704]

[64] Meyerhoff A. U.S. Food and Drug Administration approval of AmBisome (liposomal amphotericin B) for treatment of visceral leishmaniasis. Clin Infect Dis 1999; 28(1): 42-8. [http://dx.doi.org/10.1086/515085] [PMID: 10028069]

[65] Sundar S, Mehta H, Chhabra A, *et al.* Amphotericin B colloidal dispersion for the treatment of Indian

visceral leishmaniasis. Clin Infect Dis 2006; 42(5): 608-13.
[http://dx.doi.org/10.1086/500138] [PMID: 16447104]

[66] Sundar S, Singh A, Agarwal D, Rai M, Agrawal N, Chakravarty J. Safety and efficacy of high-dose infusions of a preformed amphotericin B fat emulsion for treatment of Indian visceral leishmaniasis. Am J Trop Med Hyg 2009; 80(5): 700-3.
[http://dx.doi.org/10.4269/ajtmh.2009.80.700] [PMID: 19407109]

[67] Sundar S, Chakravarty J, Agarwal D, Shah A, Agrawal N, Rai M. Safety of a pre-formulated amphotericin B lipid emulsion for the treatment of Indian Kala-azar. Trop Med Int Health 2008; 13(9): 1208-12.
[http://dx.doi.org/10.1111/j.1365-3156.2008.02128.x] [PMID: 18664241]

[68] Olliaro P, Darley S, Laxminarayan R, Sundar S. Cost-effectiveness projections of single and combination therapies for visceral leishmaniasis in Bihar, India. Trop Med Int Health 2009; 14(8): 918-25.
[http://dx.doi.org/10.1111/j.1365-3156.2009.02306.x] [PMID: 19563434]

[69] WHO, Report of a WHO informal consultation on liposomal amphotericin B in the treatment of visceral leishmaniasis.WHO/CDS/NTD/IDM/2007.4 2007.

[70] Pourshafie M, Morand S, Virion A, Rakotomanga M, Dupuy C, Loiseau PM. Cloning of S-adenosy--L-methionine:C-24-Delta-sterol-methyltransferase (ERG6) from *Leishmania donovani* and characterization of mRNAs in wild-type and amphotericin B-Resistant promastigotes. Antimicrob Agents Chemother 2004; 48(7): 2409-14.
[http://dx.doi.org/10.1128/AAC.48.7.2409-2414.2004] [PMID: 15215088]

[71] Brajtburg J, Bolard J. Carrier effects on biological activity of amphotericin B. Clin Microbiol Rev 1996; 9(4): 512-31.
[http://dx.doi.org/10.1128/CMR.9.4.512] [PMID: 8894350]

[72] Yeates C. Sitamaquine (GlaxoSmithKline/Walter Reed Army Institute). Curr Opin Investig Drugs 2002; 3(10): 1446-52.
[PMID: 12431016]

[73] Theoharides AD, Chung H, Velazquez H. Metabolism of a potential 8-aminoquinoline antileishmanial drug in rat liver microsomes. Biochem Pharmacol 1985; 34(2): 181-8.
[http://dx.doi.org/10.1016/0006-2952(85)90122-4] [PMID: 3917669]

[74] Idowu OR, Peggins JO, Brewer TG. Side-chain hydroxylation in the metabolism of 8-aminoquinoline antiparasitic agents. Drug Metab Dispos 1995; 23(1): 18-27.
[PMID: 7720521]

[75] Vercesi AE, Rodrigues CO, Catisti R, Docampo R. Presence of a Na(+)/H(+) exchanger in acidocalcisomes of *Leishmania donovani* and their alkalization by anti-leishmanial drugs. FEBS Lett 2000; 473(2): 203-6.
[http://dx.doi.org/10.1016/S0014-5793(00)01531-3] [PMID: 10812075]

[76] Dueñas-Romero AM, Loiseau PM, Saint-Pierre-Chazalet M. Interaction of sitamaquine with membrane lipids of *Leishmania donovani* promastigotes. Biochim Biophys Acta 2007; 1768(2): 246-52.
[http://dx.doi.org/10.1016/j.bbamem.2006.07.003] [PMID: 16945323]

[77] Nanayakkara NP, Ager AL Jr, Bartlett MS, *et al.* Antiparasitic activities and toxicities of individual enantiomers of the 8-aminoquinoline 8-[(4-amino-1-methylbutyl)amino]-6-methoxy-4-met-yl-5-[3,4-dichlorophenoxy]quinoline succinate. Antimicrob Agents Chemother 2008; 52(6): 2130-7.
[http://dx.doi.org/10.1128/AAC.00645-07] [PMID: 18378716]

[78] Fournet A, Barrios AA, Muñoz V, Hocquemiller R, Cavé A, Bruneton J. 2-substituted quinoline alkaloids as potential antileishmanial drugs. Antimicrob Agents Chemother 1993; 37(4): 859-63.
[http://dx.doi.org/10.1128/AAC.37.4.859] [PMID: 8494383]

[79] Fournet A, Gantier JC, Gautheret A, *et al.* The activity of 2-substituted quinoline alkaloids in BALB/c mice infected with *Leishmania donovani.* J Antimicrob Chemother 1994; 33(3): 537-44. [http://dx.doi.org/10.1093/jac/33.3.537] [PMID: 8040117]

[80] Croft SL, Hogg J, Gutteridge WE, Hudson AT, Randall AW. The activity of hydroxynaphthoquinones against *Leishmania donovani.* J Antimicrob Chemother 1992; 30(6): 827-32. [http://dx.doi.org/10.1093/jac/30.6.827] [PMID: 1289357]

[81] Mäntylä A, Garnier T, Rautio J, *et al.* Synthesis, *in vitro* evaluation, and antileishmanial activity of water-soluble prodrugs of buparvaquone. J Med Chem 2004; 47(1): 188-95. [http://dx.doi.org/10.1021/jm030868a] [PMID: 14695832]

[82] Mäntylä A, Rautio J, Nevalainen T, *et al.* Synthesis and antileishmanial activity of novel buparvaquone oxime derivatives. Bioorg Med Chem 2004; 12(13): 3497-502. [http://dx.doi.org/10.1016/j.bmc.2004.04.032] [PMID: 15186834]

[83] Garnier T, Mäntylä A, Järvinen T, Lawrence MJ, Brown MB, Croft SL. Topical buparvaquone formulations for the treatment of cutaneous leishmaniasis. J Pharm Pharmacol 2007; 59(1): 41-9. [http://dx.doi.org/10.1211/jpp.59.1.0006] [PMID: 17227619]

[84] Garnier T, Mäntylä A, Järvinen T, Lawrence J, Brown M, Croft S. *In vivo* studies on the antileishmanial activity of buparvaquone and its prodrugs. J Antimicrob Chemother 2007; 60(4): 802-10. [http://dx.doi.org/10.1093/jac/dkm303] [PMID: 17715126]

[85] Jawahar MS. Current trends in chemotherapy of tuberculosis. Indian J Med Res 2004; 120(4): 398-417. [PMID: 15520489]

[86] Ellard GA. Rationale of the multidrug regimens recommended by a World Health Organization Study Group on Chemotherapy of Leprosy for Control Programs. Int J Lepr Other Mycobact Dis 1984; 52(3): 395-401. [PMID: 6541207]

[87] Walker SL, Lockwood DN. Leprosy. Clin Dermatol 2007; 25(2): 165-72. [http://dx.doi.org/10.1016/j.clindermatol.2006.05.012] [PMID: 17350495]

[88] Kremsner PG, Krishna S. Antimalarial combinations. Lancet 2004; 364(9430): 285-94. [http://dx.doi.org/10.1016/S0140-6736(04)16680-4] [PMID: 15262108]

[89] Sundar S, Rai M, Chakravarty J, *et al.* New treatment approach in Indian visceral leishmaniasis: single-dose liposomal amphotericin B followed by short-course oral miltefosine. Clin Infect Dis 2008; 47(8): 1000-6. [http://dx.doi.org/10.1086/591972] [PMID: 18781879]

[90] Melaku Y, Collin SM, Keus K, Gatluak F, Ritmeijer K, Davidson RN. Treatment of kala-azar in southern Sudan using a 17-day regimen of sodium stibogluconate combined with paromomycin: a retrospective comparison with 30-day sodium stibogluconate monotherapy. Am J Trop Med Hyg 2007; 77(1): 89-94. [http://dx.doi.org/10.4269/ajtmh.2007.77.89] [PMID: 17620635]

[91] Frearson JA, Wyatt PG, Gilbert IH, Fairlamb AH. Target assessment for antiparasitic drug discovery. Trends Parasitol 2007; 23(12): 589-95. [http://dx.doi.org/10.1016/j.pt.2007.08.019] [PMID: 17962072]

[92] Renslo AR, McKerrow JH. Drug discovery and development for neglected parasitic diseases. Nat Chem Biol 2006; 2(12): 701-10. [http://dx.doi.org/10.1038/nchembio837] [PMID: 17108988]

[93] Hopkins AL, Witty MJ, Nwaka S. Mission possible. Nature 2007; 449(7159): 166-9. [http://dx.doi.org/10.1038/449166a] [PMID: 17851512]

[94] Agüero F, Al-Lazikani B, Aslett M, *et al.* Genomic-scale prioritization of drug targets: the TDR Targets database. Nat Rev Drug Discov 2008; 7(11): 900-7. [http://dx.doi.org/10.1038/nrd2684] [PMID: 18927591]

[95] Nwaka S, Hudson A. Innovative lead discovery strategies for tropical diseases. Nat Rev Drug Discov 2006; 5(11): 941-55. [http://dx.doi.org/10.1038/nrd2144] [PMID: 17080030]

[96] Nwaka S, Ramirez B, Brun R, Maes L, Douglas F, Ridley R. Advancing drug innovation for neglected diseases-criteria for lead progression. PLoS Negl Trop Dis 2009; 3(8) e440. [http://dx.doi.org/10.1371/journal.pntd.0000440] [PMID: 19707561]

[97] Erko B, Ye-Ebiyo Y, Seyoum A, Desta H, Tekilehymanot A. An overview of neglected tropical diseases in Ethiopia. Ethiop Med J 2007; 6(2): 173-91.

[98] Lymphatic filariasis. Fact sheet No. 102, May 2015. Available from: factsheets/fs102/en [Accessed on May 18, 2015].

[99] Gail D. Podoconiosis: Let Ethiopia to lead the way. Ethiop J Health Dev 2008; 22(1): 1-2.

[100] John E. Surgical treatment of incapacitating lymphedema or elephantiasis 2010. Available from: www.woundsinternational.com/media/issues/210/files/content-175.pdf [Accessed on May 2018].

[101] Callahan HL, Portal IF, Bensinger SJ, Grogl M. Leishmania spp: temperature sensitivity of promastigotes *in vitro* as a model for tropism *in vivo*. Exp Parasitol 1996; 84(3): 400-9. [http://dx.doi.org/10.1006/expr.1996.0128] [PMID: 8948329]

[102] McCall LI, Zhang WW, Matlashewski G. Determinants for the development of visceral leishmaniasis disease. PLoS Pathog 2013; 9(1) e1003053. [http://dx.doi.org/10.1371/journal.ppat.1003053] [PMID: 23300451]

[103] Wynd S, Melrose WD, Durrheim DN, Carron J, Gyapong M. Understanding the community impact of lymphatic filariasis: a review of the sociocultural literature. Bull World Health Organ 2007; 85(6): 493-8. [http://dx.doi.org/10.2471/BLT.06.031047] [PMID: 17639248]

[104] Destas K, Ashine M, Davey G. Prevalence of podoconiosis (endemic non-filarial elephantiasis) in Wolaitta, Southern Ethiopia. Trop Doct 2003; 33(4): 217-20. [http://dx.doi.org/10.1177/004947550303300410] [PMID: 14620426]

[105] Alemu G, Tekola Ayele F, Daniel T, Ahrens C, Davey G. Burden of podoconiosis in poor rural communities in Gulliso woreda, West Ethiopia. PLoS Negl Trop Dis 2011; 5(6) e1184. [http://dx.doi.org/10.1371/journal.pntd.0001184] [PMID: 21666795]

[106] Mousley E, Deribe K, Tamiru A, Davey G. The impact of podoconiosis on quality of life in Northern Ethiopia. Health Qual Life Outcomes 2013; 11: 122. [http://dx.doi.org/10.1186/1477-7525-11-122] [PMID: 23866905]

[107] Gordon CA, Jones MK, McManus DP. The History of Bancroftian Lymphatic Filariasis in Australasia and Oceania: Is There a Threat of Re-Occurrence in Mainland Australia? Trop Med Infect Dis 2018; 3(2): 58. [http://dx.doi.org/10.3390/tropicalmed3020058] [PMID: 30274454]

[108] Shenoy RK. Clinical and pathological aspects of filarial lymphedema and its management. Korean J Parasitol 2008; 46(3): 119-25. [http://dx.doi.org/10.3347/kjp.2008.46.3.119] [PMID: 18830049]

[109] Joseph H, Speare R, Melrose W. Laboratory diagnosis of lymphatic filariasis in Australia: Available laboratory diagnostic tools and interpretation. Aust J Med Sci 2012; 33(1): 2-9.

[110] Rajan TV. Natural course of lymphatic filariasis: insights from epidemiology, experimental human infections, and clinical observations. Am J Trop Med Hyg 2005; 73(6): 995-8. [http://dx.doi.org/10.4269/ajtmh.2005.73.995] [PMID: 16354800]

[111] Wallace RB, Kohatsu N. Wallace/Maxcy-Rosenau-Last public health & preventive medicine. 15th ed., New York: McGraw-Hill Medical 2008.

CHAPTER 3

Therapeutic Drugs Used for Effective Lifelong Control of HIV and AIDS

Elangbam Shanta Singh[1,*], **Debananda S. Ningthoujam**[1], **Laishram Jaya Devi**[1], **Rakhi Khunjamayum**[1], **Dollyca Ningombam**[2] and **Laishram Somenkumar Singh**[3]

[1] *Microbial Biotechnology Research Laboratory (MBRL), Department of Biochemistry, Manipur University, Canchipur-795003, India*

[2] *Department of Life Science, Manipur University, Canchipur-795003, India*

[3] *Department of Obstetrics and Gynaecology, Regional Institute of Medical Science (RIMS), Imphal, Manipur-795004, India*

Abstract: AIDS (Acquired immune deficiency syndrome) is caused by the retrovirus HIV (Human immune deficiency virus). HIV destroys T-cells which provide cell-mediated immunity (CMI) to human beings. Like other viruses, HIV has a protein capsid and a core RNA genome. HIV infection causes severe damage to the immune system making it vulnerable to various infectious pathogens when the damaged immune system fails to fight the infection, resulting in the advanced stage called AIDS. Two types of HIV exist. HIV-1 is the causative organism of HIV infection worldwide with around 90% of infection. HIV-2 has been reported in a small group of people in western Africa. Both HIV-1 and HIV-2 lead to AIDS in their advance stages. The treatment of HIV infection and AIDS is a big challenge to medical sciences. Many drugs are available that can be used against HIV infection and AIDS. These drugs are known as antiretrovirals (ARVs). ARVs prevent replication of HIV inside the host cell gradually slowing down the progress of HIV infection. Therefore, antiretroviral drugs can prevent AIDS-related complicated diseases and prolong longevity. However, it does not fully restore health. The potential effect of HIV on our health is clearly exhibited by many immunologic abnormalities that occur despite effective suppression of HIV replication by ARVs. The cure for AIDS is still a distant future.

Keywords: AIDS, Antiretroviral, Cell-mediated immunity, HIV, T-cells, Vaccine.

* **Corresponding author: Elangbam Shanta Singh:** Microbial Biotechnology Research Lab (MBRL), Department of Biochemistry, Manipur University, Canchipur, Imphal, Manipur 795003, Inida; Tel: +91 961 2426 886; E-mail: e.shanta96@gmail.com

K. Tamreihao, Saikat Mukherjee and Debananda S. Ningthoujam (Eds.)
All rights reserved-© 2019 Bentham Science Publishers

INTRODUCTION

Human immunodeficiency virus HIV is a *Lentivirus* which constitutes a separate genus of the *Retroviridae* family [1] and class *Retrovirus*. Retroviruses store their genetic information as ribonucleic acid (RNA), unlike other viruses which have deoxyribonucleic acid (DNA) as genetic material [2]. RNA present as genetic material in retroviruses form DNA before replication take place. The process is called reverse transcription (Latin term *Retro*, meaning "returned back") [3]. HIV infects vital organs and cells of the human immune system. It spreads throughout all the tissues of the body of an infected person. The transmission takes place through the body fluids such as semen, vaginal fluids, blood, and breast milk of the infected individuals. HIV infection leads to AIDS which does not have a cure or treatment.

Types of HIV

There are two types of Human immunodeficiency virus (HIV): HIV-1 and HIV-2 [4]. They are different from each other, but infection with both lead to AIDS [5]. HIV-1 is a common type and causes over 90% of human infections in the world. In the USA, the total individuals infected with HIV-1 are reported to be 1.1 million, and around 56,000 individuals are newly infected every year. HIV-2 has been reported only in a small group of people in West Africa. Both HIV-1 and HIV-2 have multiple groups that can branch out further into subtypes or strains. HIV-1 give rises to three different subtypes or strains, M (Major), N (New) and O (Outlier) [4]. The M strain has a wide geographical distribution. The World Health Organization (WHO) estimated that each year around 4.3 million individuals are newly infected by HIV. It has been estimated that over 95% of infections occur in the developing countries and Sub-Saharan Africa.

Brief History of HIV and AIDS

Various theories and myths about the origin of HIV exist. The most accepted theory explains that HIV infection was transmitted into human beings from non-human primates like monkeys. Researchers believe that HIV was originated from the monkeys in sub-Saharan Africa and transferred to humans when hunters became exposed to infected blood in the late 19th or in the early 20th century [6 - 8]. Simian immunodeficiency virus (SIV) is another virus found in monkeys which is similar to HIV. There is strong evidence that SIV found in the equatorial Africa is closely related to HIV [9]. The SIV was found in nine different classes of monkeys and chimpanzees. The genetic sequencing strongly suggests that SIV transferred to Robust chimpanzee (*Pan troglodytes troglodytes*) [10], and then gradually transmitted to other species by crossing the species barrier. Between 1955 and 1972, the population of sooty mangabey monkey found in Gabon and

Cameroon were infected by SIV [11, 12]. This virus is an ancestor of HIV-1 [13]. SIV crossed the species barrier from monkeys through several ways and ultimately infected human beings. The genome of this virus differs from HIV-1 by 30% to 40%, but is similar to HIV-2. Subsequent studies link HIV with the destruction of immune system and the development of acquired immune deficiency syndrome (AIDS). The syndrome is characterized by the development of opportunistic infections (OI) by different microorganisms such as bacteria, protozoa, fungi, and other viruses. The earliest well documented case of Human Immunodeficiency Virus (HIV) infection in humans is found in 1959 [9]. The virus may have been present in the United States as early as 1966 [14], but the majority of infections occurring outside sub-Saharan Africa (including the U.S.) can be traced with the help of a single unknown individual who got infected with HIV in Haiti. The virus was then brought to the United States in around 1969. Further, the epidemic rapidly spread among high risk groups such as gay males. It was estimated that among the gays of New York and San Francisco, 5% were infected in 1978. The first cases of acquired immune deficiency syndrome (AIDS) were reported in the United States in between late 1980 and early 1981 [15]. HIV is the causative agent of AIDS and was isolated in 1983. Early in the U.S., the routes of HIV infections were well known due to spreading of AIDS in a specific group of people. The direct route of HIV infection occurred among drug users by injection drug use (IDU). Early cases of HIV infection were recognized among homosexual men in the United States and majority of the cases occurred in urban, educated peoples who were addicted to alcohol and drugs. The injection drug users and gay men showed symptoms of *Pneumocystis carinii pneumonia* (PCP) infection with an unknown cause of impaired immunity, a rare opportunistic infection found in people with compromised immune systems [16, 17]. Soon after, other gay men developed a previously known rare skin cancer called *Kaposi's sarcoma* (KS) [18, 19]. Many cases of PCP and KS quietly emerged.

Structure of HIV

HIV is round or ball shaped, 100 nm in diameter, which is different from other retroviruses (Fig. **1**). HIV membrane consists of an outer envelope of lipid bilayers with spikes of glycoprotein's (gp); gp41 and gp120 [20, 21]. These glycoproteins are linked in a way that gp120 protrudes from the surface of the virus, while gp41 invades inside the lipid bilayers. Inside, there is a nucleocapsid (p17), which surrounds a central core of protein (p24). Within this core protein, there are two copies of single stranded RNA (ssRNA) serving as the genome of the virus. Two proteins namely, p7 and p9, are found bounded to the RNA and are believed to be involved in regulating gene expression. Multiple enzymes, including proteases, integrases and two reverse transcriptase enzymes are also found within the core. These two reverse transcriptase enzymes are responsible for converting viral RNA into proviral DNA by reverse transcription [3].

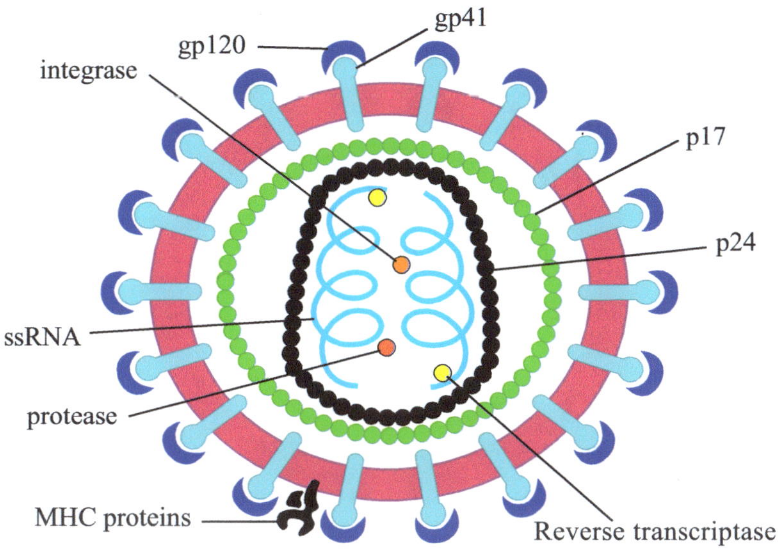

Fig. (1). Structure of the HIV.

HIV Genome and Functions of Genes

A long strand of RNA encodes the genome of HIV. The size of viral genome is around 10 Kb which encodes 16 distinct proteins [22]. There are two separate strands of RNA in HIV, but they are exactly similar to each other. The organization of the HIV genome and the function of individual genes are shown in Fig. (**2**) [23, 24].

HIV genome has a "Long Terminal Repeat" (LTR) at each end of its genome. LTR has two main functions:

1. They are "sticky ends" which makes it easy for HIV genome to insert into host DNA by the integrase protein.
2. They act as promoters or enhancers after being integrated into the host genome. They also influence the cellular machinery to transcribe the DNA. They alter the transcription level with the help of Protein binding sites present in the LTR that are involved in the initiation of RNA formation.

There are many genes between the LTRs of the two ends which consist of the structural genes *(gag, pol*, and *env)*, regulatory genes *(tat* and r*ev)* and accessory genes *(nef, vif, vpr* and *vpu* in HIV-1 or *vpx* in HIV-2) [25].

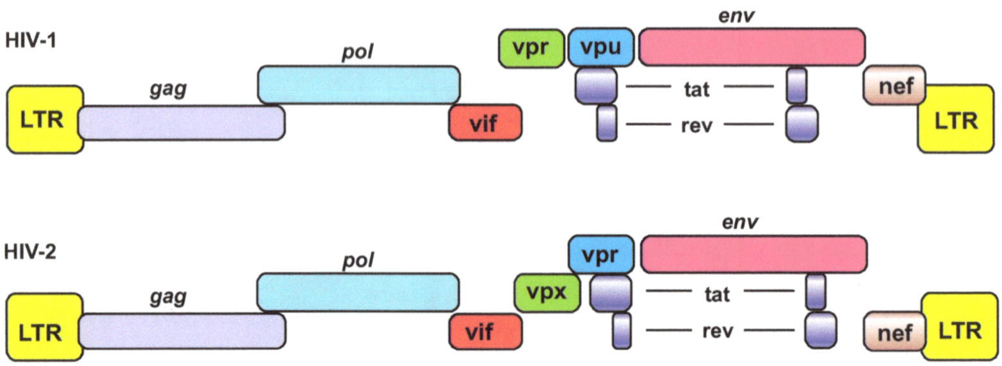

Fig. (2). Structure of the genome of HIV-1 and HIV-2.

Structural Genes

HIV genome contains *gag, pol*, and *env* as structural genes.

gag (Group Specific Antigen) Gene

gag is one of the three "main" genes found in all retroviruses (along with *pol* and *env*). It contains around 1500 nucleotides encoding four separate proteins forming the viral core, namely *Capsid protein* (p24), *Matrix protein* (p17), and *Nucleocapsid proteins* (p9 and p6).The most significant role of *gag* gene is encoding majority of the proteins which builds the viral core.

pol (Polymerase) Gene

pol is an important retroviral gene. It encodes four proteins such as *Reverse transcriptase*, *Protease*, *RNAse H* and *Integrase etc.* which are important in the life cycle of HIV. *Reverse transcriptase* helps to undergo reverse transcription.

env (Envelop Protein) Gene

env in HIV encodes a single protein which produces a glycoprotein (gp160) after binding with carbohydrate. When new virus particles bud off from the host cell, gp160 travels to the cell surface which undergoes chopping into two pieces, gp120, and gp41, by cellular enzymes. These two pieces lie on opposite sides of the virus membrane in such a way that gp120 protrudes outside the membrane of virus particle forming the virus's spikes, while gp41 protrudes inside the membrane in such a way that each gp41 gets anchored to a gp120 through the membrane. HIV particles may have a varying number of spikes but normally they have around 72 spikes.

Regulatory Genes

Genome of HIV contains *tat* and *rev* as regulatory genes.

tat (Transcriptional Transactivator) Gene

tat is a regulatory gene which produces *Tat protein* (Tat-transactivator). Tat accelerates the production of HIV virus progeny. Large amount of tat protein is released into the blood by HIV infected cells cause toxicity.

rev Gene

rev is another regulatory gene which stimulates the production of HIV proteins, but suppresses the expression of other regulatory genes present in HIV.

Accessory Genes

The genome of HIV also has accessory genes like *nef, vif*, *vpr* and *vpu* or *vpx, etc.*

nef (Negative Factor) Gene

nef encodes a protein called *"negative replication factor"*, which hangs around the cytoplasm of the cell and retards HIV replication. This protein modifies cellular proteins which regulate the initiation of transcription therefore are unable to form mRNA from DNA.

vif (Viral Infectivity Factor) Gene

vif encodes a protein called *"virion infectivity factor"* that increases the infectivity of the HIV particle. This protein is found inside HIV infected cells which interferes with cellular antiviral proteins called APOBEC3G and APOBEC3F that help in immunity. Vif sticks to both APOBEC3G and APOBEC3F proteins to encourage cell degradation. Vif protein also helps in the packaging of the nucleoprotein core at the final stage [26 - 30].

vpr (Viral Protein R) Gene

vpr encodes a protein called *"Viral protein R"* which enhances the production of HIV proteins. Another cellular protein called *cyclophilin A* is necessary for the production of Vpr. The Vpr carries "nuclear localisation signals" that mimics the signal of a protein called *importin-beta.* The principle function of Vpr protein is to stop the cell cycle undergo by the host cell. Vpr stops the cell cycle in G2 phase [31].

vpu (Viral Protein U) Gene

vpu is found only in HIV-1. It encodes a protein known as *"Viral protein U". Vpu* protein enhances the assembly of new virus particles, degrades CD4 in the endoplasmic reticulum and finally budding out from the host cell [32 - 34].

vpx (Viral Protein X) Gene

vpx is found in HIV-2 and SIV, but not in HIV-1. It is closely related to *vpr* gene. Its role in the life of HIV is not entirely clear as the HIV-2 without a functioning *vpx* gene still seems to be able to replicate and infect cells [35, 36].

Life Cycle and Mechanisms of HIV Infection

HIV infects certain types of the cells. Generally, they infect T4 Lymphocytes or T-helper cells which have CD4 receptors in the cell surface. These cells are also known as CD4 cells or T4 cells. Other cells carrying CD4 receptors are white blood cells (monocytes and macrophages), glial cells in brain, chromaffin cells in intestine, and Langerhans cells in the skin [32]. All cells having CD4 receptors have been shown to be infected with HIV.

When HIV comes in contact with T-lymphocyte (CD4 cells), the spikes of gp120 in the virus binds with CD4 receptors present in the host cell like a lock and key. The virus loses its outer envelope once it enters the host cell. Then, viral RNA and reverse transcriptase enzymes are released into the cytoplasm of the host cell. A complementary strand of the DNA is synthesized by reverse transcriptase with viral RNA acting as a template within the host cell [3]. This single strand DNA act as a template for the synthesis of another strand of DNA resulting in the formation of a double-stranded DNA. This step is mediated by *reverse transcriptase*. The virus particle with double stranded DNA is known as proviral DNA [3]. This double stranded DNA incorporates into the host cell by integrase enzyme. This integration of the viral genetic material into the host cell takes place without damaging the genetic material of the host cell. Finally, the assembled viral particles are released from the infected cells infecting other cells in the body (Fig. **3**).

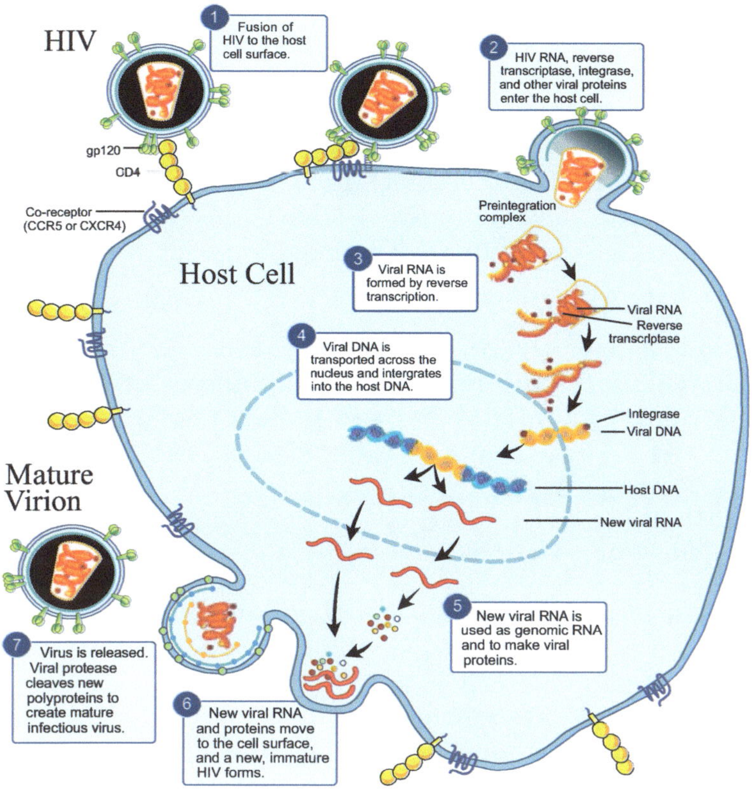

Fig. (3). Life cycle of HIV (Courtesy: National Institute of Allergy and Infectious Diseases).

Routes of HIV Transmission

There are several routes of HIV infections [37]. HIV is a sexually transmitted disease (STD) and is transmitted through homosexual, bisexual or heterosexual contact with the infected person [38]. HIV is also transmitted during blood, organ or tissue transplantation. Besides, HIV is transmitted with the sharing of contaminated needles used for intravenous drug injection or for general medical purposes in countries where disposable needles or sterilising equipment may be scarce. HIV is also transmitted during injuries in healthcare settings, *e.g.,* in people working at blood banks.

Stages of HIV Infections and Symptoms

There are 3 advanced stages of HIV infections, regardless of the number of CD4 cells in the blood of the infected person. The stages are:

First Stage: Acute HIV Infection

Most people do not know right away when they have been infected with HIV, but after a short time, symptoms start to appear. This is when our body's immune system puts up a fight, typically within 2 to 6 weeks after infection with the virus. It is called acute retroviral syndrome or primary HIV infection. The symptoms shown in this stage are similar to those of other viral illnesses such as flu, rash, muscle aches, headache, and fatigue. The symptoms last for 1-2 weeks before completely disappearing.

HIV infection in this stage can be prevented by doctors, if they act quickly. For example, people who may have been infected by unprotected sex with an HIV-positive patient can take anti-HIV drugs to protect themselves. This protection method is called PEP (Post exposure prophylaxis). The effective PEP should undergo within 72 hours of exposure.

Second Stage: Chronic HIV Infection

This stage is characterised by flu like symptom but disappears after some days. This stage is known as asymptomatic or clinical latency period. Most people do not realize their infection and can pass HIV to uninfected people in this stage. This stage can take around 10 years or more. In this stage, HIV kills CD4 T-cells and destroys the immune system. The HIV infection can be detected by CD4 T-cell count with blood tests. Normal people have CD4 count between 450 and 1,400 cells/mm^3, while the HIV infected person has less than 200 cells/mm^3 [39]. As the number drops, infected person becomes vulnerable to other infections.

Third Stage: AIDS (Acquired Immunodeficiency Syndrome)

The final stage of the HIV infection is known as Acquired Immuno deficiency Syndrome (AIDS). AIDS causes alteration of the immune system, making people more vulnerable to other infections and diseases. These diseases include a number of unusual infectious diseases, cancers, and debilitating illnesses which result in severe weight loss or wasting away as well as diseases affecting the brain and central nervous system. There is no cure for AIDS nor a vaccine to prevent HIV infection.

Categories of AIDS

The Centre for disease control (CDC) in Atlanta, Georgia has developed a widely used system to monitor AIDS by which the status of HIV infected adolescents and adults is categorised according to the different stages of HIV infection and their CD4 cell counts. There are 3 categories of AIDS which are divided on the basis

CD4 cell counts:

Category A: It consists of one or more of the conditions of initial HIV infection.

Category B: It consists of symptomatic conditions.

Category C: It is the clinical condition which must meet at least one of the following criteria,

1. The conditions are attributed to HIV infection or indicative of a defect in cell-mediated immunity.
2. The conditions are considered by physicians to have a clinical course or to require management that is complicated by HIV infection (CDC).

A patient with any disease included in Category C is considered to have AIDS. The person with AIDS can be recognised by the symptoms like extreme fatigue, persistent diarrhoea, rapid loss of weight from an unknown cause, appearance of swollen or tender glands in the neck, armpits or groin, intermittent high fever or soaking night sweats of unknown origin. Other symptoms include unexplained shortness of breath, frequently accompanied by a dry cough not due to allergies or smoking, whitish coating on the tongue, throat or vagina, a marked change in the illness pattern either in frequency, severity, or length of sickness, appearance of one or more purple spots on the surface of the skin, inside the mouth, anus or nasal passages and forgetfulness, confusion and other signs of mental deterioration. It can take as short as a year to as long as 10 to 15 years to go from being infected with HIV to "full-blown" AIDS [38].

Opportunistic Infections of AIDS

The weakening of immune system by HIV increases vulnerability to a number of opportunistic infections, cancers, and other conditions. The opportunistic infections (OIs) are caused by pathogenic organisms like bacteria, viruses and fungi etc. that the immune system can normally fight off. According to CDC, the condition of OIs is known as "AIDS-defining" conditions [40]. AIDS-defining conditions are of different types:

Skin and Mouth Infections and Symptoms

The skin and mouth diseases related to opportunistic infections of AIDS were explained in a study [41].

a. Seborrhoeic dermatitis is caused by yeast. It is characterised by red patches, greasy skin, scaly rash on the face, and scalp.

b. Tinea is a group of fungal infections which, although not serious, are uncomfortable. It includes ring worm, athlete's foot and jock itching.
c. Candidiasis is a fungal disease caused by *Candida albicans.* This infection occurs as thrush in the mouth, oesophagus and vagina.
d. Oral hairy leukoplakia is caused by Epstein Barr virus. It is characterised by a white, warty like growth on the side of the tongue and cheek that is usually painless.
e. Impetigo is a bacterial disease caused by *Streptococcus aureus.* It is characterised by an irritating and contagious bacterial skin infection.
f. Genital herpes is a sexually transmitted disease (STD) caused by Herpes simplex virus (HSV-2). The common symptoms may range from mild irritation in genital and anal areas to painful, deep ulcers.
g. Shingles or Herpes zoster is a viral disease caused by Varicella zoster virus. It is the same virus that causes chickenpox, which can be fatal if it spreads throughout the body.
h. Kaposi's sarcoma is a cancer which is often found in people with AIDS. It frequently occurs as raised purplish patches on the skin. A herpes-like virus has been implicated in the development of Kaposi sarcoma.

Effect on Nervous System and Symptoms

The effects on the nervous system related to opportunistic infections of AIDS were explained in a study [15].

a. AIDS dementia complex (ADC) is an AIDS defining illness characterised by the symptoms; slowed thinking, impaired concentration, memory deficit, confusion, clumsiness, loss of coordination, tremor, inability to walk, incontinence, social withdrawal, noticeable change in personality and irrational behaviour. It is also known as HIV-Associated dementia (HAD).
b. Peripheral neuropathy is a disorder that occurs when the peripheral nerves malfunction due to the destruction of nerve tissues. It occurs in 10 to 15 percent of individuals with AIDS. It shows symptoms such as severe pain in the legs, feet and extremities.
c. Meningitis is a common fungal disease caused by *Cryptococcus neoformans,* a fungus found in soil. It is recognised as the cause of generalised infection in the body which is life threatening in approximately 10 percent of individuals with AIDS.
d. Toxoplasmosis is a neurodegenerative disease caused by *Toxoplasma gondii,* a parasitic protozoan. Toxoplasmosis of the brain is associated with headache, confusion, personality changes, and seizures which can result in coma and death.
e. Retinitis is a viral disease caused by Cytomegalovirus. It is associated with the

symptoms, such as blindness and may also be associated with neurological illnesses, including encephalitis (inflammation of the brain).

f. Lymphoma (a tumour of the lymphoid tissue) can occur in the brain causing headaches, confusion, seizures and problems with vision.

Effect of Respiratory System and Symptoms

The effects on respiratory system related to opportunistic infections of AIDS were explained in a study [42].

a. Pneumocystis carinii pneumonia (PCP) is a life-threatening lung infection. It is the most common opportunistic infection (OI) in people with AIDS. The symptoms of PCP include dry cough, shortness of breath, and sometimes, pneumonitis, causing painful breathing.
b. Tuberculosis (TB) is caused by the bacterium *Mycobacterium tuberculosis.* Many developing countries have seen a rise in the number of cases of TB, with the increasing incidence of HIV infection. The antibiotic resistant *Mycobacterium tuberculosis* strain is becoming a problem worldwide if proper therapy is not adopted. This infection spreads due to poverty and overcrowding, and it is endemic in many developing countries.
c. Mycobacterium avium intracellulare (MAI) is a disease caused by *Mycobacterium.* It occurs in approximately 50 per cent of individuals who have low CD4 counts. The symptoms are generally non-specific which include fever, weight loss, anaemia, enlarged liver, and chronic diarrhoea.
d. Bronchitis and pneumonia are lung disorders caused by a variety of bacteria. HIV infected people are more prone to these lungs disorders.
e. Kaposi sarcoma and other types of cancer are often the cause of lung complications in people with AIDS.

Effect on Gastrointestinal Tract (GI) and Symptoms

The effects on gastrointestinal tract related to opportunistic infections of AIDS were explained in a study [43].

a. Candidiasis caused by *Candida albicans* is the early infection stage with signs of faltering immune system. It often affects the oesophagus which leads to pain and difficulty to swallow.
b. The inflammation and ulceration of gastrointestinal tract (GI) is caused by Herpes simplex virus (HSV-1). The infection causes inflammation and ulceration from mouth to the anus.
c. *Cryptosporidium muris* and *Microsporidium* are protozoa which damage the gastrointestinal tract (GI) causing severe diarrhoea frequently.

d. Kaposi sarcoma of the gastrointestinal tract (GI) is found in many people suffering from AIDS.

Cancers

Cancers related to opportunistic infections of AIDS were explained in a study [44].

a. Kaposi sarcoma (KS) is a malignant cancer of the blood vessels which can affect any part of the body. It is characterised by flat, purplish patches on the skin. Young, male homosexuals appear to be the most vulnerable to this cancer. Herpes like virus are implicated in the development of Karposi sarcoma.
b. Non-Hodgkin's lymphoma (NHL) is a life-threatening cancer affecting people with advanced HIV infection. Around 30 per cent of HIV-infected individuals with NHL have some involvement of the brain.
c. Cervical cancer is caused by a virus called Human papilloma virus (HPV), which occur mainly in the cell lining of uterus and vagina. It can spread outside the cervix and affect other body organs also. The treatment methods for this cancer are surgery, radiation therapy, or chemotherapy.
d. Other cancers have also been found in people with HIV and AIDS, including rectal cancer, head and neck cancer and melanoma.

According to the Centre for Disease Control and Prevention (CDC), such syndromes may also develop to the disease in people who are not infected with HIV. Therefore, the presence of such syndrome does not mean that the person has AIDS. If a person is infected with HIV then the person will be diagnosed with AIDS.

HIV infected people can develop a disease that may be less serious than AIDS. Such a diseased condition is known as AIDS Related Complex (ARC). ARC is a condition caused by HIV virus in which the patient shows positive test due to the development of AIDS and its clinical symptoms. However, the symptoms of ARC patients are less severe than those patients with classical AIDS because the degree of the destruction of the immune system is not progressed so far compared with classical AIDS [45].

The symptoms of ARC may include loss of appetite, weight loss, fever, night sweats, skin rashes, diarrhoea, tiredness, and lack of resistance to infection or swollen lymph nodes. People suffering from AIDS can survive only about 3 years without medication; even if they are suffering from a less infectious disease. If the patient has the right treatment and a healthy lifestyle, then they can live for a longer time [46].

Diagnosis of HIV Infection (AIDS)

The first line of HIV infection is diagnosed by the Enzyme-Linked Immune Sorbent Assay (ELISA) technique. ELISA detects the presence of antibodies to HIV in blood samples, although kits are now available to test urine and saliva samples [47]. If any sample is found to be positive in the ELISA test, then further confirmatory tests are required to ensure that the initial results are not inaccurate, therefore termed as 'false positives'. Western Blot (antibody reaction to viral proteins and glycoproteins) is a confirmatory test for HIV infection or AIDS. In Western Blotting, a positive result is indicated by the presence of bands correlating to p24, p31, gp41, and gp120 or gp160 [48].

A number of techniques are also have been developed in the recent years to enable accurate monitoring of HIV infection. These techniques include:

Polymerase Chain Reaction (PCR)

This technique has the ability to detect the presence of viral genetic material (RNA or DNA) PCR by undergoing three distinct steps: denaturation, annealing and polymerisation. Repeated cycles of these processes produce microgram quantities of viral RNA or DNA to enable the detection by agarose gel electrophoresis [49].

Branched-chain DNA (b-DNA)

This technique differs from other assays. It is mainly based on signal amplification rather than target amplification [50].

Nucleic Acid Sequence-based Amplification (NASBA)

This technique involves the isolation and lysis of nucleic acid. In this technique, nucleic acids undergo isothermal amplification after binding with silicon dioxide particles and are then detected by enzyme-linked gel assay or electro chemiluminescence [47].

Misconceptions and Facts about HIV Infection (AIDS)

There are many misconceptions about HIV infection (AIDS). The HIV cannot be transmitted from infected individuals to other people by activities like shaking hands, hugging, casual kissing, sneezing, touching undamaged skin, using same toilet, sharing towels, sharing cutlery, mouth to mouth resuscitation, any other forms of casual contact, *etc*.

Drugs Available for the Treatment of HIV Infection or AIDS

AIDS is the last stage in the progression of diseases resulting from HIV infection. However, new medications can slow the progression of the infection and can also markedly suppress the virus, thereby restoring the body's immune function and permitting many HIV infected individuals to lead a normal healthy life.

The treatment of HIV infection requires several antiretroviral drugs. The use of single antiretroviral drug does not show much effectiveness as it can resist the drug. Therefore, a new therapy method by combining three or more antiretroviral drugs has been introduced to prevent HIV infection. This therapy is known as highly active antiretroviral therapy (HAART). The drugs do not cure HIV/AIDS or do not eliminate the risk of passing HIV to uninfected people. The treatment of HIV is different from persons to persons because the antiretroviral drugs work by different mechanisms to combat HIV (Table **1**) [51]. The drugs vary from one individual to another. There are six different classes of antiretroviral drugs and pharmacokinetic enhancers for effective treatment of HIV/AIDS.

Table 1. Currently available antiretroviral drugs.

S. No.	Generic Name	Trade Name	Company
A. Fusion inhibitors			
1	Enfuvirtide (T-20)	Fuzeon	Genentech
B. CCR5 Antagonists			
1	Maraviroc	Selzentry, Celsentri	ViiV Healthcare
C. Nucleoside reverse transcriptase inhibitors (NRTIs)			
1	Abacavir (ABC)	Ziagen	ViiV Healthcare & generic
2	Tenofovir disoproxil fumarate (TDF)	Viread	Gilead Sciences & generic
3	Emtricitabine (FTC)	Emtriva	Gilead Sciences
4	Zidovudine (AZT or ZDV)	Retrovir	ViiV Healthcare & generic
5	Lamivudine (3TC)	Epivir	ViiV Healthcare & generic
6	Tenofovir alafenamide (TAF)	Biktarvy and Vemlidy	Gilead Sciences
D. Non-Nucleoside reverse transcriptase inhibitors (NNRTIs)			
1	Efavirenz (EFV)	Sustiva	Bristol-Myers Squibb & generic
2	Etravirine	Intelence	Tibotec
3	Nevirapine (NVP)	Viramune and Viramune XR	Boehringer Ingelheim & generic
4	Rilpivirine	Edurant	Tibotec & generic
E. Protease inhibitors (PIs)			

(Table 1) cont.....

S. No.	Generic Name	Trade Name	Company
1	Atazanavir	Reyataz	Bristol-Myers Squibb
2	Nelfinevir	Viracept	ViiV Healthcare
3	Darunavir	Prezista	Tibotec
4	Ritonavir	Norvir	Abbott & generic
5	Saquinavir	Envirase	Roche
6	Fosamprenavir	Lexiva	ViiV Healthcare
7	Tipranavir	Aptivus	Boehringer Ingelheim
8	Lopinavir/Ritonavir	Kaletra	Abbott & generic
F. Integrase strand transfer inhibitors (INSTIs)			
1	Dolutegravir	Tivicay	ViiV Healthcare
2	Elvitegravir	Vitekta	Gilead Sciences
3	Raltegravir	Isentress	Merck
G. Pharmacokinetic (PK) Enhancer			
1	Cobicistat	Tybost	Gilead Sciences

Fusion Inhibitors

The fusion inhibitors block HIV from entering inside the CD4 cells of the immune system.

i) CCR5 Antagonists

CCR5 antagonists block CCR5, a protein present in CD4 receptor of T-cells which is recognised by gp120 of the HIV.

ii) Nucleoside reverse transcriptase inhibitors (NRTIs)

NRTIs mainly block the reverse transcriptase enzyme and do not allow the formation of DNA from RNA molecule.

Non-Nucleoside Reverse Transcriptase Inhibitors (NNRTIs)

NNRTIs bind to reverse transcriptase enzyme and alter its functions, thereby inhibiting the reverse transcription.

Protease Inhibitors (PIs)

PIs block the enzyme protease which is present inside the core of HIV. Therefore, it blocks the synthesis of DNA from RNA by reverse transcription.

Integrase Strand Transfer Inhibitors (INSTIs)

INSTIs block HIV integrase enzyme which is needed for the synthesis of DNA from RNA by reverse transcription process.

Pharmacokinetic (PK) Enhancer

Pharmacokinetic (PK) Enhancers can be used as booster in the HIV treatment to increase the effectiveness of antiretroviral medication; however, they are not antiretroviral drugs.

Moreover, CDC has recommended the guidelines of the combination therapies for the individuals who have previously been on antiretroviral medications regarding the optimal response to treatment which is shown in Table **2** [51]. The general guidelines for combination therapies are

Fixed-dose Combination (FDC) Antiretroviral Drugs

Fixed-dose combination antiretroviral drugs contain two or more medicines of different classes of drugs. These drugs have more effectiveness as compared to single drugs.

Nucleoside Reverse Transcriptase Inhibitor (NRTI) Combinations

NRTI Combinations contain two or more NRTI Drugs.

PK-Enhanced PI Formulations

It is the combination of both the PI drugs which are boosted by PK Enhancers.

Table 2. Combined antiretroviral drugs.

S. No.	Components of Generic Drugs	Trade Name	Company
A. Fixed-dose combination (FDC) antiretroviral drugs			
1	Abacavir, Dolutegravir and Lamivudine	Triumeq	ViiV Healthcare
2	Elvitegravir, Cobicistat, Emtricitabine and Tenofovir DF	Stribild	Gilead Sciences
3	Emtricitabine, Rilpivirine, and Tenofovir Alafenamide	Odefsey	Gilead Sciences
4	Efavirenz, Emtricitabine and Tenofovir DF	Atripla	Gilead Sciences
5	Elvitegravir, Cobicistat, Emtricitabine and Tenofovir Alafenamide	Genvoya	Gilead Sciences
6	Emtricitabine, Rilpivirine and Tenofovir DF	Complera	Gilead Sciences
B. Nucleoside reverse transcriptase inhibitor (NRTI) Combinations			
1	Abacavir and Lamivudine	Epzicom	ViiV Healthcare

(Table 2) cont.....

S. No.	Components of Generic Drugs	Trade Name	Company
2	Abacavir, Lamivudine and Zidovudine	Trizivir	Generic & Cipla
3	Emtricitabine and Tenofovir DF	Truvada	Gilead Science & Cipla
4	Emtricitabine and Tenofovir Alafenamide	Descovy	Generic Drug
5	Lamivudine and Zidovudine	Combivir	ViiV Healthcare & Generic
C. PK-Enhanced PI Formulations			
1	Atazanavir and Cobicistat	Evotaz	Bristol-Myers Squibb
2	Darunavir and Cobicistat	Prezcobix	Johnson & Johnson
3	Lopinavir and Ritonavir	Kaletra	AbbVie

Future Therapies

Research for the prevention of HIV has come a long way since the disease was discovered. Antiretroviral therapy is the major treatment method that can change the lives of millions of people who are HIV infected. But the goal is to search a proper cure method.

Ten years ago, an HIV patient was cured for the first time in the world. This patient was from Berlin, named Timothy Ray Brown, who received a bone marrow from a donor naturally resistance against HIV. He has not taken antiretroviral drugs from the day of transplantation [52]. But till today we could not have a proper treatment method. The future treatment methods for HIV could be:

Stopping Replication of HIV

Inhibiting the replication of RNA genome of HIV could be an advanced HIV treatment method. A French company, Abivax, is undertaking clinical trials for the production of a drug that has the potential for functional cure of HIV by stopping the replication of RNA genome. The drug called AVX464 was produced by Abivax that binds to a specific sequence in the RNA of HIV and inhibits the replication process. In phase 2a clinical trials, several patients were given the drug along with antiretroviral therapy. 8 out of 15 patients treated with the drug showed a 25% - 50% reduction in their HIV reservoir after 28 days, but there was no reduction in those undergoing only antiretroviral therapy. Now, this company is planning for a Phase 2b clinical trial to observe the long term effects of the drug [52].

Shock and Kill or Kick and Kill

Another approach to treat HIV is to fight against HIV present in the HIV reservoir. In this method, latency reversing agents (LRAs) are used to activate or kick the latent HIV reservoir Which makes HIV possible to be killed by antiretroviral drugs. In 2016, a group of UK universities have reported that a patient was treated with this approach. Now, Gilead Company also carries out clinical trials for the medicines with similar approach [52].

Immunotherapy

HIV attack the immune system leaving the patient unprotected against infections. In this approach, the immune system become super charged to fight back. This approach is totally different from other vaccines of HIV which boost a specific response. The most advanced immunotherapy vaccine is being developed by the French company InnaVirVax. The vaccine, called VAC-3S was produced by this company that stimulates the production of antibodies against the HIV protein 3S enabling T cells to attack HIV virus. Now, this company is carrying out testing of VAC-3S in combination with a DNA based vaccine from the Finnish FIT Biotech, which could lead to a functional cure for HIV [52].

Gene Therapy

Around 1% people in this world are naturally immune against HIV because of gene mutation on the gene encoding CCR5, a surface protein of immune cells bound by HIV. The mutant CCR5 protein cannot bind to HIV. By using gene therapy, we can modify the gene that encoded the protein CCR5, so that HIV did not bind to the the immune cells. One of the most advanced developers of this approach are US based Sangamo Therapeutics company. This company isolated the immune cells HIV patient, and used zinc finger nucleases to edit the CCR5 gene to make it resistant against HIV. In 2016, 4 out of 9 patients treated with gene therapy in Phase 2 clinical trial were found with undetectable levels of HIV [52].

CRISPR, a gene editing tool could be the gene therapy approach for HIV treatment in the future. The use of CRISPR will be much easier and faster than other gene editing tools.

CONCLUDING REMARKS

The development of HIV vaccine is a scientific challenge due to extreme genetic variability of the HIV virus. The lack of good animal models and limitations of the technology to understand the mechanisms involved in the immunity are the main reasons of inability to produce a proper drug to cure this disease. More than 543 clinical trials were performed in the field of HIV vaccines, according to the clinicaltrials.gov database.

We should focus mainly on the controlling methods till we find a proper way to end the HIV and AIDS pandemic. Scientifically challenging research and clinical trials should be well planned to produce a cure mechanism. An aggressive scientific research is needed to develop an effective approach by using modern technologies for ending the HIV and AIDS epidemic.

CONSENT FOR PUBLICATION

Not applicable.

CONFLICT OF INTEREST

The authors confirm that this chapter contents have no conflict of interest.

ACKNOWLEDGEMENTS

The authors wish to thank Department of Biotechnology (DBT), Govt. of India for sponsoring the host laboratory under the scheme "Establishment of State Biotech Hubs" (BT/04/NE/2009).

REFERENCES

[1] Barré-Sinoussi F, Chermann JC, Rey F, *et al.* Isolation of a T-lymphotropic retrovirus from a patient at risk for acquired immune deficiency syndrome (AIDS). Science 1983; 220(4599): 868-71. [http://dx.doi.org/10.1126/science.6189183] [PMID: 6189183]

[2] Yamashita M, Emerman M. Retroviral infection of non-dividing cells: old and new perspectives. Virology 2006; 344(1): 88-93. [http://dx.doi.org/10.1016/j.virol.2005.09.012] [PMID: 16364740]

[3] Abbas A, Lichtman A, Pober J. Cellular and Molecular Immunology. Philadelphia: W.B. Saunders 2000.

[4] Clavel F, Guétard D, Brun-Vézinet F, *et al.* Isolation of a new human retrovirus from West African patients with AIDS. Science 1986; 233(4761): 343-6. [http://dx.doi.org/10.1126/science.2425430] [PMID: 2425430]

[5] Eckstein DA, Sherman MP, Penn ML, *et al.* HIV-1 Vpr enhances viral burden by facilitating infection of tissue macrophages but not nondividing CD4+ T cells. J Exp Med 2001; 194(10): 1407-19. [http://dx.doi.org/10.1084/jem.194.10.1407] [PMID: 11714748]

[6] Salemi M, Strimmer K, Hall WW, *et al.* Dating the common ancestor of SIVcpz and HIV-1 group M and the origin of HIV-1 subtypes using a new method to uncover clock-like molecular evolution. FASEB J 2001; 15(2): 276-8. [http://dx.doi.org/10.1096/fj.00-0449fje] [PMID: 11156935]

[7] Korber B, Muldoon M, Theiler J, *et al.* Timing the ancestor of the HIV-1 pandemic strains. Science 2000; 288(5472): 1789-96. [http://dx.doi.org/10.1126/science.288.5472.1789] [PMID: 10846155]

[8] Worobey M, Gemmel M, Teuwen DE, *et al.* Direct evidence of extensive diversity of HIV-1 in Kinshasa by 1960. Nature 2008; 455(7213): 661-4.

[http://dx.doi.org/10.1038/nature07390] [PMID: 18833279]

[9] Zhu T, Korber BT, Nahmias AJ, Hooper E, Sharp PM, Ho DD. An African HIV-1 sequence from 1959 and implications for the origin of the epidemic. Nature 1998; 391(6667): 594-7. [http://dx.doi.org/10.1038/35400] [PMID: 9468138]

[10] Gao F, Bailes E, Robertson DL, *et al.* Origin of HIV-1 in the chimpanzee Pan troglodytes troglodytes. Nature 1999; 397(6718): 436-41. [http://dx.doi.org/10.1038/17130] [PMID: 9989410]

[11] Sharp PM, Bailes E, Chaudhuri RR, Rodenburg CM, Santiago MO, Hahn BH. The origins of acquired immune deficiency syndrome viruses: where and when? Philos Trans R Soc Lond B Biol Sci 2001; 356(1410): 867-76. [http://dx.doi.org/10.1098/rstb.2001.0863] [PMID: 11405934]

[12] Hirsch VM, Olmsted RA, Murphey-Corb M, Purcell RH, Johnson PR. An African primate *Lentivirus* (SIVsm) closely related to HIV-2. Nature 1989; 339(6223): 389-92. [http://dx.doi.org/10.1038/339389a0] [PMID: 2786147]

[13] Gao K, Gorelick RJ, Johnson DG, Bushman F. Cofactors for human immunodeficiency virus type 1 cDNA integration in vitro. J Virol 2003; 77(2): 1598-603. [http://dx.doi.org/10.1128/JVI.77.2.1598-1603.2003] [PMID: 12502875]

[14] Kolata Gina. Boy's 1969 Death Suggests AIDS Invaded U.S. Several Times. The NewYork Times 1987 Oct. 28; Retrieved, 11 February. 2009.

[15] Tardieu M. HIV-1-related central nervous system diseases. Curr Opin Neurol 1999; 12(4): 377-81. [http://dx.doi.org/10.1097/00019052-199908000-00002] [PMID: 10555824]

[16] Masur H, Michelis MA, Greene JB, *et al.* An outbreak of community-acquired Pneumocystis carinii pneumonia: initial manifestation of cellular immune dysfunction. N Engl J Med 1981; 305(24): 1431-8. [http://dx.doi.org/10.1056/NEJM198112103052402] [PMID: 6975437]

[17] Gottlieb MS, Schroff R, Schanker HM, *et al.* Pneumocystis carinii pneumonia and mucosal candidiasis in previously healthy homosexual men: evidence of a new acquired cellular immunodeficiency. N Engl J Med 1981; 305(24): 1425-31. [http://dx.doi.org/10.1056/NEJM198112103052401] [PMID: 6272109]

[18] Friedman-Kien AE. Disseminated Kaposi's sarcoma syndrome in young homosexual men. J Am Acad Dermatol 1981; 5(4): 468-71. [http://dx.doi.org/10.1016/S0190-9622(81)80010-2] [PMID: 7287964]

[19] Hymes KB, Cheung T, Greene JB, *et al.* Kaposi's sarcoma in homosexual men-a report of eight cases. Lancet 1981; 2(8247): 598-600. [http://dx.doi.org/10.1016/S0140-6736(81)92740-9] [PMID: 6116083]

[20] Gramberg T, Sunseri N, Landau NR. Accessories to the crime: recent advances in HIV accessory protein biology. Curr HIV/AIDS Rep 2009; 6(1): 36-42. [http://dx.doi.org/10.1007/s11904-009-0006-z] [PMID: 19149995]

[21] Malim MH, Emerman M. HIV-1 accessory proteins-ensuring viral survival in a hostile environment. Cell Host Microbe 2008; 3(6): 388-98. [http://dx.doi.org/10.1016/j.chom.2008.04.008] [PMID: 18541215]

[22] Sodroski J, Rosen C, Wong-Staal F, *et al.* Trans-acting transcriptional regulation of human T-cell leukemia virus type III long terminal repeat. Science 1985; 227(4683): 171-3. [http://dx.doi.org/10.1126/science.2981427] [PMID: 2981427]

[23] Cohen EA, Terwilliger EF, Jalinoos Y, Proulx J, Sodroski JG, Haseltine WA. Identification of HIV-1 vpr product and function. J Acquir Immune Defic Syndr 1990; 3(1): 11-8. [PMID: 2136707]

[24] Kappes JC, Morrow CD, Lee SW, *et al.* Identification of a novel retroviral gene unique to human immunodeficiency virus type 2 and simian immunodeficiency virus SIVMAC. J Virol 1988; 62(9): 3501-5.
[PMID: 3136256]

[25] Emerman M, Malim MH. HIV-1 regulatory/accessory genes: keys to unraveling viral and host cell biology. Science 1998; 280(5371): 1880-4.
[http://dx.doi.org/10.1126/science.280.5371.1880] [PMID: 9632380]

[26] Peterlin BM, Trono D. Hide, shield and strike back: how HIV-infected cells avoid immune eradication. Nat Rev Immunol 2003; 3(2): 97-107.
[http://dx.doi.org/10.1038/nri998] [PMID: 12563294]

[27] Yu X, Yu Y, Liu B, *et al.* Induction of APOBEC3G ubiquitination and degradation by an HIV-1 Vif-Cul5-SCF complex. Science 2003; 302(5647): 1056-60.
[http://dx.doi.org/10.1126/science.1089591] [PMID: 14564014]

[28] Mehle A, Strack B, Ancuta P, Zhang C, McPike M, Gabuzda D. Vif overcomes the innate antiviral activity of APOBEC3G by promoting its degradation in the ubiquitin-proteasome pathway. J Biol Chem 2004; 279(9): 7792-8.
[http://dx.doi.org/10.1074/jbc.M313093200] [PMID: 14672928]

[29] Wiegand HL, Doehle BP, Bogerd HP, Cullen BR. A second human antiretroviral factor, APOBEC3F, is suppressed by the HIV-1 and HIV-2 Vif proteins. EMBO J 2004; 23(12): 2451-8.
[http://dx.doi.org/10.1038/sj.emboj.7600246] [PMID: 15152192]

[30] Yu Y, Xiao Z, Ehrlich ES, Yu X, Yu XF. Selective assembly of HIV-1 Vif-Cul5-ElonginB-ElonginC E3 ubiquitin ligase complex through a novel SOCS box and upstream cysteines. Genes Dev 2004; 18(23): 2867-72.
[http://dx.doi.org/10.1101/gad.1250204] [PMID: 15574593]

[31] Jowett JB, Planelles V, Poon B, Shah NP, Chen ML, Chen IS. The human immunodeficiency virus type 1 vpr gene arrests infected T cells in the G2 + M phase of the cell cycle. J Virol 1995; 69(10): 6304-13.
[PMID: 7666531]

[32] Höglund S, Ohagen A, Lawrence K, Gabuzda D. Role of vif during packing of the core of HIV-1. Virology 1994; 201(2): 349-55.
[http://dx.doi.org/10.1006/viro.1994.1300] [PMID: 8184544]

[33] Bour S, Strebel K. The HIV-1 Vpu protein: a multifunctional enhancer of viral particle release Microb Infect 5(11): 1029-39.

[34] Terwilliger EF, Cohen EA, Lu YC, Sodroski JG, Haseltine WA. Functional role of human immunodeficiency virus type 1 vpu. Proc Natl Acad Sci USA 1989; 86(13): 5163-7.
[http://dx.doi.org/10.1073/pnas.86.13.5163] [PMID: 2472639]

[35] Marcon L, Michaels F, Hattori N, Fargnoli K, Gallo RC, Franchini G. Dispensable role of the human immunodeficiency virus type 2 Vpx protein in viral replication. J Virol 1991; 65(7): 3938-42.
[PMID: 2041103]

[36] Ueno F, Shiota H, Miyaura M, *et al.* Vpx and Vpr proteins of HIV-2 up-regulate the viral infectivity by a distinct mechanism in lymphocytic cells. Microbes Infect 2003; 5(5): 387-95.
[http://dx.doi.org/10.1016/S1286-4579(03)00042-X] [PMID: 12737994]

[37] Negishi M. Preventive methods against HIV transmission. Nippon Rinsho 1993; 51(Supp): 509-11.

[38] Marr L. Sexually Transmitted Diseases: A Physician Tells You What You Need to Know. Batimore, MD: Johns Hopkins University Press 1998.

[39] Chibatamoto PP, Chandiwana SK, Sabeta CT, Gomo E. Retrospective study on the criteria for diagnosis of HIV infection in adults in Zimbabwe. Cent Afr J Med 1996; 42(5): 141-4.

[PMID: 8771933]

[40] Centers for Disease Control (CDC). A cluster of Kaposi's sarcoma and Pneumocystis cariniipneumonia among homosexual male residents of Los Angeles and Orange Counties, California. MMWRMorb Mortal Wkly 1982; Rep.. 31(23): 305-7.

[41] Schneider MM. Change in natural history of opportunistic infections in HIV infected patients. Neth J Med 2000; 57(1): 1-3.
[http://dx.doi.org/10.1016/S0300-2977(00)00034-6]

[42] de Leon FC, Britt EJ. The noninfectious respiratory complications of infection with HIV. Curr Opin Pulm Med 1995; 1(3): 223-33.
[PMID: 9363057]

[43] Knox TA, Spiegelman D, Skinner SC, Gorbach S. Diarrhea and abnormalities of gastrointestinal function in a cohort of men and women with HIV infection. Am J Gastroenterol 2000; 95(12): 3482-9.
[http://dx.doi.org/10.1111/j.1572-0241.2000.03365.x] [PMID: 11151881]

[44] Clarke CA, Glaser SL. Epidemiologic trends in HIV-associated lymphomas. Curr Opin Oncol 2001; 13(5): 354-9.
[http://dx.doi.org/10.1097/00001622-200109000-00007] [PMID: 11555712]

[45] www. clinicaltrials.gov/ct2/show/NCT00002063 Treatment of AIDS and AIDS Related Complex. Part-1- Treatment of Patients with ARC (AZT Vs. Placebo).

[46] Centers for Disease Control (CDC). Pneumocystis pneumonia - Los Angeles. MMWRMorb. Mortal Wkly 1981; Rep.. 30(21): 250-52.

[47] Kosko DA, Becker KL. HIV counseling, testing, and prevention in primary care. Lippincotts Prim Care Pract 2000; 4(1): 29-39.
[PMID: 11022518]

[48] Roberts BD. HIV antibody testing methods: 1985-1988. J Insur Med 1994; 26(1): 13-4.
[PMID: 10147063]

[49] Lakshmi V, Sudha T, Dandona R, Kumar GA, Dandona L. Application of Polymerase Chain Reaction to Detect HIV-1 DNA in Pools of Dried Blood Spots. Indian J Microbiol 2011; 51(2): 147-52.
[http://dx.doi.org/10.1007/s12088-011-0135-0] [PMID: 22654156]

[50] Baumeister MA, Zhang N, Beas H, *et al.* A sensitive branched DNA HIV-1 signal amplification viral load assay with single day turnaround. PLoS One 2012; 7(3) e33295.
[http://dx.doi.org/10.1371/journal.pone.0033295] [PMID: 22479381]

[51] www.healthline.com/health/hiv-aids/medications-list by Danirel Murrell, MD 02/01/2018.

[52] www.labiotech.eu/features/hiv-cure-2020-research-review An HIV cure by 2020? A review of the future of HIV therapy- by Clara Rodriguez Fernandez on 07/05/2018.

CHAPTER 4

Bioactive Peptides and Their Therapeutic Potential as Antimicrobial Drugs

Pintubala Kshetri*, **Thangjam Surchandra Singh** and **Subhra Saikat Roy***

ICAR Complex for NEH region, Manipur Centre, Lamphelpat 795004, India

Abstract: Peptides are short chain amino acids having low molecular weight usually less than 20 kDa. Peptides having health beneficial biological activity are known as bioactive peptides (BP). BP may be free or encrypted within the protein sequence and encrypted peptides are active only when released from the parent protein. Enzymatic hydrolysis and microbial fermentation are the most common methods for the production of BP from the parent protein. BP have numerous beneficial biomedical functions. They can act as antihypertensive, antioxidant, angiotensin converting enzyme inhibitors, and antimicrobial agents. With the emergence of new infectious diseases and multidrug resistant pathogenic bacterial strains, there is an urgent need for the discovery of new antimicrobial agents having a broad spectrum of activity. In this context, BP having antimicrobial activity (antimicrobial peptides) can be a potential candidate for the development of new antimicrobial drugs. Antimicrobial peptides (AMPs) have played an important role in the innate immune system of plants and animals. Hence, various AMPs have been isolated from microbes, plants, and animals. AMPs can directly or indirectly kill the pathogen and their mechanism of action is different from conventional antibiotics. They also have immunomodulatory functions. Moreover, AMPs have lower pathogen resistance as compared to conventional antibiotics. These properties attract researchers and pharmaceutical industries toward the development of AMPs as new anti-infective drugs against the multi-drug resistant pathogens. The present chapter highlights the production and application of BP as well as their potential use as antimicrobial drugs.

Keywords: Antimicrobial peptides, Bioactive peptides, Encrypted peptides, Immunomodulatory, Multi-drug resistant.

INTRODUCTION

Bioactive Peptides (BPs) are defined as specific protein fragments that have a positive impact on body functions. They differ widely in their amino acid composition, sequence, chemical structure and therefore, in their biological fun-

* **Corresponding author Pintubala Kshetri and Subhra Saikat Roy:** ICAR Complex for NEH region, Manipur Centre, Lamphelpat 795004, India; Tel: +91 977 494 1355 and +91 9436891040; E-mails: pintuksh@gmail.com and subhrasaikat@gmail.com, respectively

K. Tamreihao, Saikat Mukherjee and Debananda S. Ningthoujam (Eds.)
All rights reserved-© 2019 Bentham Science Publishers

ction. BP are also known for their ability to inhibit protein-protein interactions due to their small size and specificity. Nature remains the largest source of BP since plants, animals, fungi, microbes and their products contain various proteins. Currently, more than 3600 different BPs have been reported in 'BIOPEP-UWM Database'. BPs have also been considered the new generation of biologically active regulators that can prevent oxidation and microbial degradation in foods. BPs may be free or encrypted within the protein sequence [1]. Encrypted peptides become active when released from the protein sequence by enzymatic hydrolysis (gastrointestinal digestion or *in vitro* hydrolysis by proteases) of proteinaceous food and also during food processing (cooking, fermentation, ripening). However, the most widely used techniques for production of BP in food and pharmaceutical applications are microbial fermentation and enzymatic hydrolysis of proteins. Many BPs have been reported for their cholesterol-lowering effects, antiprotozoal, antiviral, antithrombotic, antityrosinase, antioxidant, antihypertensive and antimicrobial activities which made them attractive for applications in functional foods and pharmaceuticals [2].

The rapid increase in multiple drug resistance in bacteria and the failure of the most potent antibiotics to kill "superbugs" have become serious challenges to current antimicrobial therapies and this led to the development of various strategies for the production of new antimicrobial drugs. Recently, BP having antimicrobial activity (or antimicrobial peptides) are becoming an attractive option for the development of a new class of antimicrobial drugs that are effective against antibiotic-resistant bacteria because the mode of action of antimicrobial peptides (AMPs) is markedly different from that of traditional antibiotics. AMPs are evolutionarily ancient molecules that have been identified from diverse sources such as microorganisms, plants and animals. They also play an important role in the innate immune system and are the first line of defence to protect internal and external surfaces of the host [3]. Structurally, AMPs are oligopeptides with a varying number (from five to over a hundred) of amino acids. They have a broad spectrum of target organisms ranging from viruses to parasites. Some AMPs are already available in the market and some are in the advanced phase of clinical trial.

The increasing health care costs have prompted researchers to discover novel BPs or compounds from new sources. The past few decades have seen an exponential increase in bioactive peptide research and the therapeutic peptide market value is projected to reach USD 25 billion by 2018 [1]. However, the research and development sector is facing challenges in developing new antimicrobial peptides as their market is at the initial stage. Keeping this in view, the U.S. and European Union have taken the initiatives and launched a Transatlantic Task Force and the Infectious Diseases Society of America in 2012 for the development of novel antimicrobial peptides by the end of 2020. Moreover, in the Asia-Pacific region, Australian and New Zealand Biotechnology Organisations are funding together for the synthesis of new peptides. In 2007, Mimotopes Pty Ltd. and GlycoSyn were funded with USD 519.85 million to manufacture new peptides and specialized small molecules under the conditions of Good Manufacturing Practices (GMP) [4]. Hence, the production and development of novel BPs having a wide range of antimicrobial activities are becoming a focal area of interest for many researchers. In order to achieve this goal, researchers are adopting a variety of approaches for the production of BPs from new or unusual sources (*e.g.* marine organisms, insects, *etc.*), chemical synthesis and mining of BPs from food using bioinformatics tools. With this background, the present chapter will discuss the production and application of BPs. In addition, it will also highlight the potential of BPs as antimicrobial agents and their mechanisms of action.

Processing and Production of BPs

BPs can be produced using different methods from the parent protein. However, the most common methods reported in literature is microbial fermentation and enzymatic hydrolysis [5]. Microbial fermentation involves the cultivation of bacteria or fungi on protein rich substrates. Bacteria and fungi are well known for the secretion of proteases. These proteases hydrolyse protein to small peptides. The extent of hydrolysis depends on the type of bacterial or fungal strain used, the nature of protein substrate and the fermentation conditions. Based on the type of microbe used for protein hydrolysation, the fermentation conditions such as pH, temperature, incubation time and substrate concentration have to be optimised accordingly. Bacteria of the same species may also differ in their proteolytic capacities which may result in the production of peptides having different bioactivities. For example, Chen *et al.* [6] reported that skim milk fermented with 37 different *Lactobacillus helveticus* strains showed different extents of bioactivity. Sanjukta *et al.* [7] also observed that fermentation of soybean protein with two different strains of *Bacillus subtilis* resulted in difference in the degree of hydrolysis and content of free amino acids. From the literature available, soybean and milk are the major substrates used in microbial fermentation for BP production. However, some other substrates such as wheat, rye and meat [8 - 11] are also reported. Many BPs are derived from milk fermentation [12 - 14]. The industrially used dairy starter cultures are highly proteolytic in nature. These proteases produce peptides and amino acids from milk proteins during fermentation which contribute to the typical flavour, aroma and texture of the products and this property is traditionally exploited by the dairy industry [15]. Lactic acid bacteria are well known for the production of BPs from milk fermentation. For instance, *Lactobacillus helveticus* produces an angiotensin I converting enzyme (ACE) inhibitory peptide (Val-Pro-Pro Ile-Pro-Pro) from milk

[16]. Kunda *et al.* [17] identified fifty BPs from yogurt which is available as an antihypertensive functional food in the market. Fermentation of soybean with bacteria or fungi produces many BPs. Soybean fermentation may be either alkaline nature using *Bacillus* sp. or acidic using lactic acid bacteria. Some traditional fermented soybean foods such as natto, chungkookjang, and tempeh were found to be good sources of BPs having ACE inhibitory, anti-thrombotic and anti-inflammatory activities [18, 19]. Other than bacteria, yeast and filamentous fungi also produce BPs [20 - 23]. Fermentation of protein substrate is also performed by the co-culturing of bacteria and fungi. For example, Chaves-López [24] observed that the co-culturing of yeast (*Pichia kudriavzevii* KL84A) and lactic acid bacteria (*Lactobacillus plantarum* LAT3 and *Enterococcus faecalis* KL06) exhibited more ACEI inhibitory activity than the single culture.

In enzymatic hydrolysis, the protein substrate is treated with enzyme at a particular temperature, pH and incubation time. The optimal reaction conditions such as enzyme and substrate concentration, pH, temperature and incubation time depends on the nature of the enzyme use. Peptide sequences and their biological activities may differ depending on the types of enzyme used. In many cases, the digestive enzyme trypsin, chymotrypsin and pepsin are used for producing protein hydrolysates and peptides. For instance, a peptide having anti-oxidant, anti-tyrosinase and anti-biofilm activities have been derived from *Vicia faba* seeds protein by tryptic digestion [25]. El-Fattah *et al.* [26] used a combination of enzymes such as trypsin, pepsin and papain for the production of peptides from milk. However, trypsin has been a preferred choice for the production of peptides since it has exceptional cleavage specificity. It cleaves proteins into peptides with an average size of 700 to 1500 Da and only hydrolyses the peptide bonds on the carboxyl terminal side of arginine and lysine amino acid residue. Moreover, it has a high proteolytic activity and is very aggressive and stable under a wide range of conditions. Hence, trypsin digestion has been used for the chemical characterisation and identification of many known BPs [15]. Other than digestive enzymes, many bacterial, fungal and plant derived proteolytic enzymes have also been used in production of BPs from protein rich substrates [27 - 30]. Among them, bacterial enzymes are most commonly used. The use of microbial enzymes has certain advantages over the animal derived proteolytic enzymes. For instance, microbial enzymes can be produced anywhere, are amenable to mass scale production under short duration and occupy little space for cultivation. Moreover, enzyme yield can be enhanced by optimizing the fermentation parameters [31]. Some examples of microbial proteases are thermolysin and proteinase K. Subtilisin Carlsberg, an alkaline protease from *Bacillus licheniformis,* has been used for the production of low molecular weight BP from food derived peptides. This enzyme is commercially available as “Alcalase”. Subtilisin hydrolysed protein hydrolysates were reported to have higher number of low molecular weight peptides than samples hydrolysed by using digestive enzymes [32, 33]. Low molecular weight BPs (<10 kDa) have been found to be more effective as drugs since they are more easily absorbed in the intestine. Production of BP by enzymatic hydrolysis is preferred than microbial fermentation due to the short reaction time, ease of scalability and predictability. Other than these two methods, chemical hydrolysis, solvent extraction and microwave assisted extraction have also been reported for the production of BPs from the parent protein [34]. Once the structure of the BP is known, it is also possible to synthesize peptides. Three main approaches for BP synthesis available at present are chemical synthesis, recombinant DNA technology and enzymatic synthesis. Chemical synthesis is the pioneer one, and had been initiated more than 30 years back [35]. On the other hand, enzymatic synthesis of peptides involves formation of peptide bonds by proteases such as chymotrypsin, papain, pepsin, subtilisin, thermolysin and, trypsin in the presence of organic solvents as catalysts [36, 37]. Recently, synthesis of peptides using modern recombinant technology has also been reported. For example, Feng *et al.* [38] reported production of a novel hybrid antimicrobial peptide LFT33 as fusion protein. The fusion protein was expressed in *Escherichia coli* and was cleaved successfully by enterokinase releasing the peptide LFT33.

Application of BP

Since, BPs have numerous functions; they find wide applications in food, cosmetic and pharmaceutical industries. Peptides are naturally suited for biomedical applications because of their general biocompatibility with the human body [39]. The most common biomedical applications of peptides are as antihypertensive, antioxidant, immunomodulatory and antimicrobial agents [2]. Antihypertensive peptides can also inhibit ACE which is closely linked with high blood pressure [40]. The antihypertensive peptides were identified in protein hydrolysates of soybean, garlic, cereals, milk, pork sarcoplasmic and, chicken proteins [41 - 43]. A potent ACE inhibitory lactoferrin-derived peptide DPYKLRP was extracted from the fermentation of *Kluyveromyces marxianus* [44]. Besides the common ones, several novel functions of BPs such as antityrosinase, anticancer, anti-obesity and antidiabetic activities have also been discovered [40 - 47]. BPs also find applications in clinical therapy and early diagnosis of neurodegenerative diseases such as Alzheimer's disease. A peptide (KLPGF) derived from albumin showed inhibitory activity against acetylcholinesterase (AChE). AChE inhibitors are currently the most prescribed drug class for treatment of Alzheimer's disease [48]. Small peptides have cell penetrating property and these cell-penetrating peptides (CPP) have been used to deliver various molecules and particles into cells. In addition to the medical and pharmaceutical arena, CPPs have also found applications in biochemistry, molecular biology and immunology. Synthetic peptides are extremely useful in studies regarding polypeptides as well as peptide hormones, hormone analogues, cross-reacting antibody preparation and design of novel enzymes [49].

BPs having potent antimicrobial activities finds major potential application in pharmaceutical industries as AMPs that have unique characteristic in combating the pathogens as compared to conventional antibiotics. For instance, the general mechanism of conventional antibiotics falls within one of four mechanisms; three of which involves the inhibition or regulation of enzymes involved in cell wall biosynthesis, nucleic acid metabolism and repair or protein synthesis. The fourth mechanism involves the disruption of the membrane structure. On the other hand, AMPs combat pathogens through direct killing or inmmunomodulation. Moreover, AMPs are also active against biofilm forming pathogens. Currently, the rise of drug resistant bacteria (superbugs) and opportunistic fungal infections is becoming the major issue for human health and world economy. This dictates the search for a new class of antimicrobial drugs having good activity against multi-drug resistant pathogenic strains. Hence, researchers are targeting AMPs for the development of new antibiotics in the pharmaceutical industries as novel antimicrobial drugs. The following section will discuss the structure, classification, mechanism of action and current status and, challenges of AMPs.

Antimicrobial Peptides (AMPs)

AMPs are oligopeptides having a varying number of amino acids usually 10-50. They are potent, broad spectrum antibiotics which can kill not only bacteria (both gram positive and negative bacteria) and fungi but also viruses and transformed cells. They display an overall positive charge ranging from +2 to +13, and contain a substantial proportion of hydrophobic amino acids [50]. Short antimicrobial peptides (SAMPs) composed of 2-10 amino acid residues are also reported. Generally SAMPs are synthetic compounds. Ahn *et al.* [51] reported that short peptides (<10 amino acid residues) have antibacterial activity against *Escherichia coli, Micrococcus luteus, Pseudomonas aeruginosa* and *Staphylococcus aureus.* Naturally occurring AMPs have longer sequences as compared to synthetic AMPs. The AMPs having longer sequence of 84 amino acid residues have been reported from hemolymph of *Holotrichia diomphalia* larvae [52]. The shortest naturally occurring antimicrobial dipeptide EL (APD ID-AP02381) has been identified from marine bacterium *Bacillus subtilis* [53].

The discovery of AMPs dates back to 1939 when Dubos [54] extracted a peptide antibiotic "gramicidin" from a *Bacillus brevis* strain. Gramicidin is the first AMP for which the primary structure was characterized and the first antibiotic to be commercially manufactured [55]. After this many AMPs have been isolated from plants, animals and microbes. For example, purothionins, an AMP isolated from wheat endosperm, had inhibitory effect on growth of *Pseudomonas solanacearum*, *Xanthomonas campestris, Erwinia* and *Corynebacterium* spp [56]. The first animal originated AMP is defensin which display broad spectrum of antimicrobial activity [57]. Extractions of defensins from plants have also been reported [58]. In 1987, Zasloff and his co-workers isolated and characterised an AMP known as magainin from African clawed frog (*Xenopus laevis)* skin. Magainin is a 23-residue cationic peptide having bactericidal, fungicidal and tumoricidal activities [59]. Discovery of magainin became a landmark in the history of AMPs research. More than 1000 AMPs have been isolated from amphibians. AMPs are also reported from animal products such as milk protein, egg, meat *etc* [60 - 62]. Lactoferricin is the first and most studied AMP derived from milk protein. It is produced by enzymatic digestion of lactoferrin, an iron binding protein present in milk [60]. Till date, 3027 AMPs are available in Antimicrobial Peptide Database (APD). These AMPs were reported from six kingdoms; 336 bacteriocins/peptide antibiotics from bacteria, 4 from archaea, 8 from protists, 18 from fungi, 344 from plants and 2236 from animals, including some synthetic peptides (Fig. **1**). Table **1** summarises the AMPs extracted from different sources.

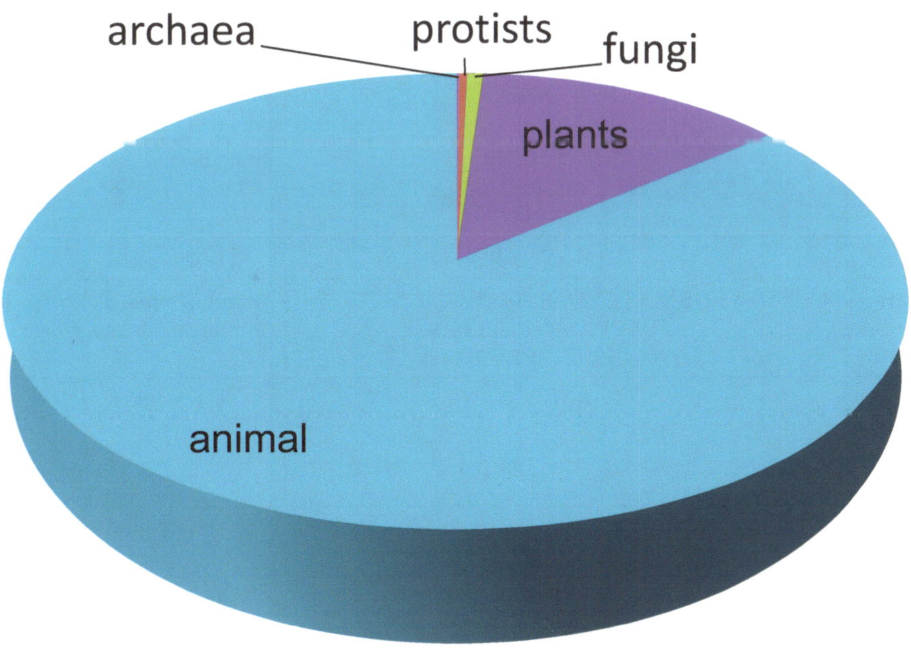

Fig. (1). Sources of 3017 antimicrobial peptides as of November 2018 from the antimicrobial peptide database. Numbers obtained from http://aps.unmc.edu/AP/, last accessed on 5 October, 2018.

Table 1. Antimicrobial peptides from various sources.

Source	Peptide Sequence	Activity	References
Milk	LKKISQ, LKKISQYYQKFAWPQYL, ATKCFQWQRNMRKVRGPPVSCIKRD, QPEATKCFQWQRNMRKVRGPPVSCIKRDS	Antibacterial	[63 - 65]
Egg lysozyme	IVSAGAGMAAT	Antimicrobial	[66]
Phaseolus vulgaris and Wheat Bread	DPVAPLQRSGPEIP, PRSGNVGESGLID, ESVSLVA,PHAVAAVPPVLR, LLGWGHKGSSIID, HCNDPEKKNL, PILQSLIRFDGGACSSF, RSQIKREQYTPQDVEMLFSSF	Antifungal	[10]
oyster (*Crassostrea gigas)*	Cystine rich AMP	Antibacterial and antifungal	[67]
Yellow Catfish Skin Mucus	GKLNLFLSRLE ILKLFVGAL	Antimicrobial	[68]
Marine Snail (*Cenchritis muricatus)*	SRSELIVHQR	Antifungal	[69]
Fruits of *Capsicum annuum*	Thionin-like peptides	Antibacterial and antifungal	[70]
Barley	EVSLNSGYY	Antibacterial and antifungal	[71]
Fermented milk	QEPVL, QEPV, WMHQPHQPLPPTVMFPPQ, LYQQPVLGPVR, SCDKFLDD	Immunomodul-ating	[72, 73]
casein	LRLKKYKVPQL	Antibacterial	[74]
Kefir	VLNENLLR, YQEPVLGPVRGPFPIIV YQEPVLGPVRGPFPIIV, LYQEPVLGPVRGPFPIIV	Antimicrobial and Immunomodulatory	[75]
Anchovy cooking waste water hydrolysate	ACWWP	Antibacterial	[76]
Soy-protein	PGTAVFK, IKAFKEATKVDKVVVLWTA	Antibacterial	[77]
Bacillus subtilis E20-fermented soybean meal	HTSKALLDMLKRLGK	Antibacterial	[78]

Classification of AMPs

Classification of AMPs is difficult because of its complex diversity. There are numerous approaches for classifying AMPs based on source, function, properties, structure and molecular targets of the peptides. For example, based on secondary structure, AMPs have been classified into four major groups [79]:

i. α-helical (*e.g.*, cecropin, dermcidin, LL-37, magainin)
ii. β-sheet (*e.g.*, human alpha defensin)
iii. αβ structure (*e.g.*, drosomycin, human beta defensins)
iv. Non αβ structure (*e.g.*, indolicidin, tritrpticin).

Among these α-helical and β-sheet are most commonly found in nature [80]. Based on net charge, AMPs can be classified into cationic, neutral and anionic peptides. Majority of AMPs have a net positive charge.

Universal classification of AMPs was proposed by Wang [79], which is based on the linking mode of polypeptide chains. In these, AMPs are categorized into four classes:

i. Linear one-chain peptides (*e.g.*, LL-37 and magainins) or two linear peptides not connected *via* a covalent bond (*e.g.* enterocin L50)
ii. Class II, sidechain-sidechain linked peptides. A sidechain-sidechain connection can occur within a single peptide chain (*e.g.*, defensin-like, lantibiotics) or between two different peptide chains (*e.g.*, distinctin, halocidin, centrocin)
iii. Polypeptide chains with a sidechain to backbone connection (*e.g.*, microcin J25, lariatins)
iv. Circular polypeptides with a peptide bond between the N- and C-termini (i.e., backbone-backbone connection). Circular peptides are found in bacteria (*e.g.*, AS-48), plants (*e.g.*, cyclotides) and animals (*e.g.*, theta-defensins).

Although AMPs are a diverse group of molecules, there are several characteristics that are common to almost all AMPs. Firstly, AMPs are cationic because of the presence of basic amino acids such as lysine and arginine (and sometimes histidine). Secondly, AMPs are hydrophobic in nature. Typically, 50% of peptide sequence of AMPs is constituted by hydrophobic amino acid residues such as valine, leucine, isoleucine, alanine, methionine, phenylalanine, tyrosine and, tryptophan. Lastly, amphipathicity is another property which is shared by all AMPs. Amphipathicity refers to the relative abundance of hydrophilic and hydrophobic residues or domains within the AMPs [81].

Mechanism of AMPs

Mechanism of action of AMPs is different from conventional antibiotics. Their mechanism of action has been studied extensively. Mechanism of action can be broadly divided into two; direct killing and indirect killing (or immune modulation). Direct killing mechanism can be further divided into membrane disruption (or membrane targeting) and non-membrane disruption (non-membrane targeting). The general mechanism of membrane disruption model is as follows:

i. AMP-membrane attraction
ii. Attachment of the AMP onto the membrane
iii. Insertion of the AMP into the membrane causing disruption leading to the leakage of ions and metabolites from cell.

Membrane disruption mechanism of AMPs may be either receptor-mediated or nonreceptor-mediated. The receptor mediated pathway mostly includes AMPs produced by bacteria such as mesentericin and nisin. Mesentericin Y 105^{37} is a 37 residue cationic peptide produced by bacterium *Leuconostoc mesenteroides.* Secondary structure reveals that it has 30-40% α-helical conformation, the amphipathic helix spanning over residues 17-31. The amphipathic helical domain of the peptide interacts with lipid bilayers, leading to disruption of membrane, whereas, residues 1-14 forms part of a recognition structure for a membrane-bound receptor [82].

The most abundant nonreceptor-mediated peptides are the small cationic peptides that target negatively-charged bacterial membranes. Cationic AMPs bind to the surface of the membrane until a critical threshold concentration is reached after which they self-organize to form a permeation pathway. Three membrane disruption models have been proposed *viz*., toroidal-pore, barrel-stave and carpet models. In the toroidal-pore model, peptide initially binds the membrane followed by aggregation of monomer units perpendicularly in the lipid bilayer. However, specific peptide-peptide interaction is absent. This alters the membrane structure and the lipid moieties of outer and inner membranes fold inward forming a continuous channel lined by multiple peptide units. In the barrel stave model, the AMPs are initially oriented parallel to the membrane and then insert perpendicularly in the lipid bilayer. Unlike toroidal-pore model, it requires specific peptide-peptide interaction. Moreover, the peptide has to be amphipathic in nature so that hydrophobic regions can interact with the membrane lipids and hydrophilic residues lined the lumen of the channels. In this way, the protein complex is inserted into the membrane forming a channel which in turn ruptures the cells. In contrast to the above two models, carpet model do not involve the pore formation. Instead it has detergent like effects on membrane disruption. At first the AMPs adsorb parallel to the lipid bilayer and reach a threshold concentration to cover the surface of the membrane thereby forming a "carpet" like structure leading to unfavorable interactions on the membrane surface. Consequently, the membrane integrity is lost which eventually disintegrates the membrane by forming micelles [83].

The membrane disruption activity of the AMPs is influenced by the property of the peptides. Many studies have established the correlation between charge and antimicrobial activity of AMPs. For example, increasing the charge of magainin 2 from +3 to +5 improved the antibacterial activity against both Gram-positive and Gram-negative bacteria. However, further increase in charge to +6 or +7 lead to loss of antimicrobial activity [84]. Another important factor is hydrophobicity. This feature is required for membrane permeabilization; however, excessive levels of hydrophobicity can lead to mammalian cell toxicity and loss of antimicrobial selectivity [85]. For a good antimicrobial activity an optimal hydrophobicity of the peptide is required. AMPs also exhibits no-membrane disruption activity. In this mechanism of action, the AMPs target the intracellular activities such as nucleic acid and protein biosynthesis, protein-folding, protease, cell division and, cell wall biosynthesis. For example, buforins inhibits DNA synthesis, Bac7 AMP inhibits protein biosynthesis and Histatin 5 inhibits host matrix metalloproteases [86].

In addition to the direct killing of microbes, AMPs can also kill microbes indirectly by activating the immune cells. Host defence peptides are the most common AMPs which have immunomodulatory activity. Defensins and cathelicidins are the two major families of naturally occurring AMPs. Some AMPs can modulate immune responses in other ways. For example, human cathelicidin LL-37 attracts neutrophils, monocytes, T cells and mast cells [87]. They can also stimulate angiogenesis, or reduce inflammation by lowering the expression of pro-inflammatory chemokines.

Some of the pathogens have the ability to form stable biofilm which is the common cause of both persistent and device-associated infections [88]. Biofilm forming pathogens are less susceptible to antimicrobial agents creating a significant burden on public health. However, AMPs are effective in combating biofilm forming pathogens. They can either penetrate the biofilm or inhibit the formation of biofilm. Hence, AMPs represent a novel and promising approach for the eradication of biofilm forming pathogenic bacteria which are the main features of chronic and long-term infections [89].

Current Status and Challenges of AMPs

With the emergence of new diseases and bacterial resistance to conventional antibiotics, development of novel anti-infective agents is becoming a challenge for pharmaceutical companies. Nevertheless, they have overcome these challenges by developing new antibiotics from different sources and modifying existing antibiotics. However, the rapid rise in resistance of life-threatening infections creates a major burden in the development of anti-infective agents. The best example is HIV where the rapid emergence of resistance to single drugs posed daunting clinical problems. So researchers are searching for new class of antibiotics having broad spectrum activity and different mechanism of action for combating the pathogens. Since AMPs have broad spectrum antimicrobial activity and most of them also showed immunomodulatory activity, they can be employed as ideal candidates for generation of new class of antibiotics. AMPs have some advantages over conventional antibiotics as they have broad spectrum of activity, rapid onset of killing, diverse mechanism of action, anti-inflammatory activity and are less prone to resistance.

On the other hand, AMPs possess some limitations that hinder their clinical and commercial development. The major limiting factor includes high production cost, potential toxicity, susceptibility to proteases and unknown pharmacokinetics. In fact, very few AMPs have reached the market. Some of the AMPs (*e.g.*, Pexiganan, Omiganan, Iseganan) reached the advanced stage of clinical trial but failed at phase III. To reduce the high production costs, researchers are looking for alternative source of BP having antimicrobial activity. For example, BP have been reported from by-products of food protein and agro-industrial wastes. However, there are two major limitations of AMPs:

i. AMPs are sensitive to proteolytic digestion in the digestive tract when they are orally administrated [90].
ii. Due to cationic and hydrophobic nature, there is limitation in their solubility and membrane permeability.

To overcome these issues, many strategies have been developed and investigated which includes chemical modification of AMPs and the use of specialized delivery strategies such as peptide encapsulation with micro- and nano-sized coordination polymers or liposome. Encapsulation not only delivers the AMPs at target tissues but also protects them from proteolytic digestion and reduces their toxicity [91].

CONCLUDING REMARKS

BP are well known for their multi-functional activities which makes them a potential therapeutic drugs. BP having antimicrobial activities attracts researchers and pharmaceutical industry for development of new antimicrobial drugs because

AMPs are well known for their wide range of antimicrobial activity, less proneness to resistance and effective action against biofilm forming pathogens. Moreover, the ability of AMPs to disrupt the bacterial membrane makes them interesting compounds for use in synergistic combinations with other antimicrobial agents. Till date, therapeutic applications of commercially available and clinically trial AMPs as anti-infective agents are limited due to their toxic properties to human cells. So the use of innovative technologies such as entrapment with liposome or nanostructures for delivery of peptides to target tissues is required for application as effective anti-infective agents. Nevertheless, further studies on BP are still needed in order to reduce the costs of production and downstream processes.

CONSENT FOR PUBLICATION

Not applicable.

CONFLICT OF INTEREST

The author confirms that this chapter contents have no conflict of interest.

ACKNOWLEDGEMENTS

Declare none.

REFERENCES

[1] Daliri EB-M, Oh DH, Lee BH. Bioactive Peptides. Foods 2017; 6(5): 32. [http://dx.doi.org/10.3390/foods6050032] [PMID: 28445415]

[2] Korhonen H, Pihlanto A. Technological options for the production of health-promoting proteins and peptides derived from milk and colostrum. Curr Pharm Des 2007; 13(8): 829-43. [http://dx.doi.org/10.2174/138161207780363112] [PMID: 17430184]

[3] Gordon YJ, Romanowski EG, McDermott AM. A review of antimicrobial peptides and their therapeutic potential as anti-infective drugs. Curr Eye Res 2005; 30(7): 505-15. [http://dx.doi.org/10.1080/02713680590968637] [PMID: 16020284]

[4] http://www.insightpharmareports.com/Affiliated-Reports/Goldstein-Research/Global-Anti-Microbial-Peptides-Market/ last assessed on 15 October, 2018.

[5] Korhonen H, Pihlanto A. Bioactive peptides: Production and functionality. Int Dairy J 2006; 16(9): 945-60. [http://dx.doi.org/10.1016/j.idairyj.2005.10.012]

[6] Chen Y, Liu W, Xue J, *et al.* Angiotensin-converting enzyme inhibitory activity of *Lactobacillus helveticus* strains from traditional fermented dairy foods and antihypertensive effect of fermented milk of strain H9. J Dairy Sci 2014; 97(11): 6680-92. [http://dx.doi.org/10.3168/jds.2014-7962] [PMID: 25151888]

[7] Sanjukta S, Rai AK, Muhammed A, Jeyaram K, Talukdar NC. Enhancement of antioxidant properties of two soybean varieties of sikkim himalayan region by proteolytic *Bacillus subtilis* fermentation. J Funct Foods 2015; 14: 650-8. [http://dx.doi.org/10.1016/j.jff.2015.02.033]

[8] Rizzello CG, Cassone A, Coda R, Gobbetti M. Antifungal activity of sourdough fermented wheat germ used as an ingredient for bread making. Food Chem 2011; 127(3): 952-9. [http://dx.doi.org/10.1016/j.foodchem.2011.01.063] [PMID: 25214083]

[9] Coda R, Cassone A, Rizzello CG, Nionelli L, Cardinali G, Gobbetti M. Antifungal activity of *Wickerhamomyces anomalus* and *Lactobacillus plantarum* during sourdough fermentation: identification of novel compounds and long-term effect during storage of wheat bread. Appl Environ Microbiol 2011; 77(10): 3484-92. [http://dx.doi.org/10.1128/AEM.02669-10] [PMID: 21441340]

[10] Coda R, Rizzello CG, Nigro F, De Angelis M, Arnault P, Gobbetti M. Long-term fungal inhibitory activity of water-soluble extracts of Phaseolus vulgaris cv. Pinto and sourdough lactic acid bacteria during bread storage. Appl Environ Microbiol 2008; 74(23): 7391-8. [http://dx.doi.org/10.1128/AEM.01420-08] [PMID: 18849463]

[11] Broncano JM, Otte J, Petrón MJ, Parra V, Timón ML. Isolation and identification of low molecular weight antioxidant compounds from fermented "chorizo" sausages. Meat Sci 2012; 90(2): 494-501. [http://dx.doi.org/10.1016/j.meatsci.2011.09.015] [PMID: 22000499]

[12] Regazzo D, Da-Dalt L, Lombardi A, Andrighetto C, Negro A, Gabai G. Fermented milks from *Enterococcus faecalis* TH563 and *Lactobacillus delbrueckii* subsp. *bulgaricus* LA2 manifest different degrees of ACE-inhibitory and immunomodulatory activities. Dairy Sci Technol 2010; 90(4): 469-76. [http://dx.doi.org/10.1051/dst/2010009]

[13] Pihlanto A, Virtanen T, Korhonen H. Angiotensin I converting enzyme (ACE) inhibitory activity and antihypertensive effect of fermented milk. Int Dairy J 2010; 20(1): 3-10. [http://dx.doi.org/10.1016/j.idairyj.2009.07.003]

[14] Pan D, Guo Y. Optimization of sour milk fermentation for the production of ACE-inhibitory peptides and purification of a novel peptide from whey protein hydrolysate. Int Dairy J 2010; 20(7): 472-9. [http://dx.doi.org/10.1016/j.idairyj.2010.01.007]

[15] Korhonen H, Pihlanto A. Food-derived bioactive peptides-opportunities for designing future foods. Curr Pharm Des 2003; 9(16): 1297-308. [http://dx.doi.org/10.2174/1381612033454892] [PMID: 12769738]

[16] Wakai T, Yamaguchi N, Hatanaka M, Nakamura Y, Yamamoto N. Repressive processing of antihypertensive peptides, Val-Pro-Pro and Ile-Pro-Pro, in *Lactobacillus helveticus* fermented milk by added peptides. J Biosci Bioeng 2012; 114(2): 133-7. [http://dx.doi.org/10.1016/j.jbiosc.2012.03.015] [PMID: 22591842]

[17] Kunda PB, Benavente F, Catalá-Clariana S, Giménez E, Barbosa J, Sanz-Nebot V. Identification of bioactive peptides in a functional yogurt by micro liquid chromatography time-of-flight mass spectrometry assisted by retention time prediction. J Chromatogr A 2012; 1229: 121-8. [http://dx.doi.org/10.1016/j.chroma.2011.12.093] [PMID: 22305364]

[18] Gibbs BF, Zougman A, Masse R, Mulligan C. Production and characterization of bioactive peptides from soy hydrolysate and soy-fermented food. Food Res Int 2004; 37(2): 123-31. [http://dx.doi.org/10.1016/j.foodres.2003.09.010]

[19] Huang YL, Ma MF, Chow CJ, Tsai YH. Angiotensin I-converting enzyme inhibitory and hypocholesterolemic activities: Effects of protein hydrolysates prepared from *Achatina fulica* snail foot muscle. Int J Food Prop 2017; 20(12): 3102-11. [http://dx.doi.org/10.1080/10942912.2016.1274904]

[20] García-Tejedor A, Sánchez-Rivera L, Castelló-Ruiz M, Recio I, Salom JB, Manzanares P. Novel antihypertensive lactoferrin-derived peptides produced by *Kluyveromyces marxianus*: gastrointestinal stability profile and *in vivo* angiotensin I-converting enzyme (ACE) inhibition. J Agric Food Chem 2014; 62(7): 1609-16. [http://dx.doi.org/10.1021/jf4053868] [PMID: 24476136]

[21] García-Tejedor A, Sánchez-Rivera L, Recio I, Salom JB, Manzanares P. Dairy *Debaryomyces hansenii* strains produce the antihypertensive casein-derived peptides LHLPLP and HLPLP. Food Sci Technol 2015; 61: 550-6. [http://dx.doi.org/10.1016/j.lwt.2014.12.019]

[22] Lima CA, Campos JF, Filho JL, Converti A, da Cunha MGC, Porto AL. Antimicrobial and radical scavenging properties of bovine collagen hydrolysates produced by *Penicillium aurantiogriseum* URM 4622 collagenase. J Food Sci Technol 2015; 52(7): 4459-66. [http://dx.doi.org/10.1007/s13197-014-1463-y] [PMID: 26139912]

[23] Giri A, Nasu M, Ohshima T. Bioactive properties of Japanese fermented fish paste, fish miso, using koji inoculated with *Aspergillus oryzae.* Int J Nutr Food Sci 2012; 1(1): 13-22. [http://dx.doi.org/10.11648/j.ijnfs.20120101.12]

[24] Chaves-López C, Serio A, Paparella A, *et al.* Impact of microbial cultures on proteolysis and release of bioactive peptides in fermented milk. Food Microbiol 2014; 42: 117-21. [http://dx.doi.org/10.1016/j.fm.2014.03.005] [PMID: 24929726]

[25] Karkouch I, Tabbene O, Gharbi D, *et al.* Antioxidant, antityrosinase and antibiofilm activities of synthesized peptides derived from *Vicia faba* protein hydrolysate: A powerful agents in cosmetic application. Ind Crops Prod 2017; 109: 310-9. [http://dx.doi.org/10.1016/j.indcrop.2017.08.025]

[26] El-Fattah AMA, Sakr SS, El-Dieb SM, Elkashe HAS. Bioactive peptides with ACE-I and antioxidant activity produced from milk proteolysis. Int J Food Prop 2017; 20(12): 3033-42. [http://dx.doi.org/10.1080/10942912.2016.1270963]

[27] Cian RE, Alaiz M, Vioque J, Drago SR. Enzyme proteolysis enhanced extraction of ACE inhibitory and antioxidant compounds (peptides and polyphenols) from *Porphyra columbina* cake. J Appl Phycol 2013; 25(4): 1197-206. [http://dx.doi.org/10.1007/s10811-012-9913-2]

[28] Cian RE, Garz'on AG, Ancona DB, Guerrero LC, Drago SR. Hydrolyzates from *Pyropia columbina* seaweed have antiplatelet aggregation, antioxidant and ACE I inhibitory peptides which maintain bioactivity after simulated gastrointestinal digestion. Lebensm Wiss Technol 2015; 64(2): 881-8. [http://dx.doi.org/10.1016/j.lwt.2015.06.043]

[29] Fitzgerald C, Mora-Soler L, Gallagher E, *et al.* Isolation and characterization of bioactive pro-peptides with *in vivo* renin inhibitory activities from the macroalga *Palmaria palmata.* J Agric Food Chem 2012; 60(30): 7421-7. [http://dx.doi.org/10.1021/jf301361c] [PMID: 22747312]

[30] Furuta T, Miyabe Y, Yasui H, Kinoshita Y, Kishimura H. Angiotensin I converting enzyme inhibitory peptides derived from phycobiliproteins of *Dulse Palmaria palmata.* Mar Drugs 2016; 14(2) E32. [http://dx.doi.org/10.3390/md14020032] [PMID: 26861357]

[31] Paola A, Chao O, Jauregi P. Enzymatic production of bioactive peptides from milk and whey proteins. Novel Enzyme Technology for Food Applications Woodhead Publishing Series in Food Science, Technology and Nutrition 2007; pp. 160-82.

[32] Zhang H, Yokoyama WH, Zhang H. Concentration-dependent displacement of cholesterol in micelles by hydrophobic rice bran protein hydrolysates. J Sci Food Agric 2012; 92(7): 1395-401. [http://dx.doi.org/10.1002/jsfa.4713] [PMID: 22083811]

[33] Hwang JS, Yoo HJ, Song HJ, *et al.* Inflammation-related signaling pathways implicating TGFβ are revealed in the expression profiling of MCF7 cell treated with fermented soybean, chungkookjang. Nutr Cancer 2011; 63(4): 645-52. [http://dx.doi.org/10.1080/01635581.2011.551987] [PMID: 21547849]

[34] Wang X, Yu H, Xing R, Li P. Characterization, preparation, and purification of marine bioactive peptides. BioMed Res Int 2017; 2017 9746720.

[http://dx.doi.org/10.1155/2017/9746720] [PMID: 28761878]

[35] Espitia PJP, Soares NDFF, Coimbra JSDR, Andrade NJD, Cruz RS, Medeiros EAA. Bioactive peptides: synthesis, properties, and applications in the packaging and preservation of food. Compr Rev Food Sci Food Saf 2012; 11(2): 187-204.
[http://dx.doi.org/10.1111/j.1541-4337.2011.00179.x]

[36] So JE, Kang SH, Kim BG. Lipase-catalyzed synthesis of peptides containing D-amino acid: facts and artifacts. Enzyme Microb Technol 1998; 23: 211-5.
[http://dx.doi.org/10.1016/S0141-0229(98)00051-9]

[37] Ogino H, Yamada M, Watanabe F, Ichinose H, Yasuda M, Ishikawa H. Peptide synthesis catalyzed by organic solvent-stable protease from *Pseudomonas aeruginosa* PST-01 in monophasic aqueous-organic solvent systems. J Biosci Bioeng 1999; 88(5): 513-8.
[http://dx.doi.org/10.1016/S1389-1723(00)87668-9] [PMID: 16232654]

[38] Feng X, Liu C, Guo J, *et al.* Recombinant expression, purification, and antimicrobial activity of a novel hybrid antimicrobial peptide LFT33. Appl Microbiol Biotechnol 2012; 95(5): 1191-8.
[http://dx.doi.org/10.1007/s00253-011-3816-z] [PMID: 22189867]

[39] Chan KH, Lee WH, Zhuo S, Ni M. Harnessing supramolecular peptide nanotechnology in biomedical applications. Int J Nanomedicine 2017; 12: 1171-82.
[http://dx.doi.org/10.2147/IJN.S126154] [PMID: 28223805]

[40] Erdmann K, Cheung BWY, Schröder H. The possible roles of food-derived bioactive peptides in reducing the risk of cardiovascular disease. J Nutr Biochem 2008; 19(10): 643-54.
[http://dx.doi.org/10.1016/j.jnutbio.2007.11.010] [PMID: 18495464]

[41] Castellano P, Aristoy MC, Sentandreu MÁ, Vignolo G, Toldrá F. Peptides with angiotensin I converting enzyme (ACE) inhibitory activity generated from porcine skeletal muscle proteins by the action of meat-borne *Lactobacillus.* J Proteomics 2013; 89: 183-90.
[http://dx.doi.org/10.1016/j.jprot.2013.06.023] [PMID: 23806758]

[42] García MC, Puchalska P, Esteve C, Marina ML. Vegetable foods: a cheap source of proteins and peptides with antihypertensive, antioxidant, and other less occurrence bioactivities. Talanta 2013; 106: 328-49.
[http://dx.doi.org/10.1016/j.talanta.2012.12.041] [PMID: 23598136]

[43] Iwaniak A, Dziuba J. Animal and plant proteins as precursors of peptides with ACE inhibitory activity - An in silico strategy of protein evaluation. Food Technol Biotechnol 2009; 47(4): 441-9.

[44] García-Tejedor A, Sánchez-Rivera L, Castelló-Ruiz M, Recio I, Salom JB, Manzanares P. Novel antihypertensive lactoferrin-derived peptides produced by Kluyveromyces marxianus: gastrointestinal stability profile and *in vivo* angiotensin I-converting enzyme (ACE) inhibition. J Agric Food Chem 2014; 62(7): 1609-16.
[http://dx.doi.org/10.1021/jf4053868] [PMID: 24476136]

[45] Karkouch I, Tabbene O, Gharbi D, *et al.* Antioxidant, antityrosinase and antibiofilm activities of synthesized peptides derived from *Vicia faba* protein hydrolysate: A powerful agents in cosmetic application. Ind Crops Prod 2017; 109: 310-9.
[http://dx.doi.org/10.1016/j.indcrop.2017.08.025]

[46] Kim SK, Mendis E. Bioactive compounds from marine processing byproducts - A review. Food Res Int 2006; 2(4): 383-96.
[http://dx.doi.org/10.1016/j.foodres.2005.10.010]

[47] Shahidi F, Zhong Y. Bioactive peptides. J AOAC Int 2008; 91(4): 914-31.
[PMID: 18727554]

[48] Yu Z, Wu S, Zhao W, *et al.* Anti-Alzheimers activity and molecular mechanism of albumin-derived peptides against AChE and BChE. Food Funct 2018; 9(2): 1173-8.
[http://dx.doi.org/10.1039/C7FO01462G] [PMID: 29363710]

[49] http://www.peptidesguide.com/peptides-application.html.

[50] Hancock REW, Lehrer R. Cationic peptides: a new source of antibiotics. Trends Biotechnol 1998; 16(2): 82-8.
[http://dx.doi.org/10.1016/S0167-7799(97)01156-6] [PMID: 9487736]

[51] Ahn HS, Cho W, Kang SH, *et al.* Design and synthesis of novel antimicrobial peptides on the basis of α helical domain of Tenecin 1, an insect defensin protein, and structure-activity relationship study. Peptides 2006; 27(4): 640-8.
[http://dx.doi.org/10.1016/j.peptides.2005.08.016] [PMID: 16226345]

[52] Lee SY, Moon HJ, Kurata S, Natori S, Lee BL. Purification and cDNA cloning of an antifungal protein from the hemolymph of Holotrichia diomphalia larvae. Biol Pharm Bull 1995; 18(8): 1049-52.
[http://dx.doi.org/10.1248/bpb.18.1049] [PMID: 8535393]

[53] Tareq FS, Lee MA, Lee HS, *et al.* Gageotetrins A-C, noncytotoxic antimicrobial linear lipopeptides from a marine bacterium *Bacillus subtilis.* Org Lett 2014; 16(3): 928-31.
[http://dx.doi.org/10.1021/ol403657r] [PMID: 24502521]

[54] Dubos RJ. Studies on a bactericidal agent extracted from a soil bacillus I. Preparation of the agent. Its activity *in vivo.* J Exp Med 1939; 70(1): 1-10.
[http://dx.doi.org/10.1084/jem.70.1.1] [PMID: 19870884]

[55] Nakatsuji T, Gallo RL. Antimicrobial peptides: old molecules with new ideas. J Invest Dermatol 2012; 132(3 Pt 2): 887-95.
[http://dx.doi.org/10.1038/jid.2011.387] [PMID: 22158560]

[56] Fernandez de Caleya R, Gonzalez-Pascual B, García-Olmedo F, Carbonero P. Susceptibility of phytopathogenic bacteria to wheat purothionins *in vivo.* Appl Microbiol 1972; 23(5): 998-1000.
[PMID: 5031563]

[57] Bahar AA, Ren D. Antimicrobial peptides. Pharmaceuticals (Basel) 2013; 6(12): 1543-75.
[http://dx.doi.org/10.3390/ph6121543] [PMID: 24287494]

[58] Hayes BME, Bleackley MR, Wiltshire JL, Anderson MA, Traven A, van der Weerden NL. Identification and mechanism of action of the plant defensin NaD1 as a new member of the antifungal drug arsenal against *Candida albicans.* Antimicrob Agents Chemother 2013; 57(8): 3667-75.
[http://dx.doi.org/10.1128/AAC.00365-13] [PMID: 23689717]

[59] Zasloff M, Martin B, Chen HC. Antimicrobial activity of synthetic magainin peptides and several analogues. Proc Natl Acad Sci USA 1988; 85(3): 910-3.
[http://dx.doi.org/10.1073/pnas.85.3.910] [PMID: 3277183]

[60] Wakabayashi H, Takase M, Tomita M. Lactoferricin derived from milk protein lactoferrin. Curr Pharm Des 2003; 9(16): 1277-87.
[http://dx.doi.org/10.2174/1381612033454829] [PMID: 12769736]

[61] Kovacs-Nolan J, Phillips M, Mine Y. Advances in the value of eggs and egg components for human health. J Agric Food Chem 2005; 53(22): 8421-31.
[http://dx.doi.org/10.1021/jf050964f] [PMID: 16248532]

[62] Jang A, Jo C, Kang KS, Lee M. Antimicrobial and human cancer cell cytotoxic effect of synthetic angiotensin-converting enzyme (ACE) inhibitory peptides. Food Chem 2008; 107(1): 327-36.
[http://dx.doi.org/10.1016/j.foodchem.2007.08.036]

[63] López-Expósito I, Gómez-Ruiz JÁ, Amigo L, Recio I. Identification of antibacterial peptides from ovine α S2-casein. Int Dairy J 2006; 16(9): 1072-80.
[http://dx.doi.org/10.1016/j.idairyj.2005.10.006]

[64] Vorland LH, Ulvatne H, Andersen J, *et al.* Lactoferricin of bovine origin is more active than lactoferricins of human, murine and caprine origin. Scand J Infect Dis 1998; 30(5): 513-7.
[http://dx.doi.org/10.1080/00365549850161557] [PMID: 10066056]

[65] Recio I, Visser S. Two ion-exchange chromatographic methods for the isolation of antibacterial peptides from lactoferrin. In situ enzymatic hydrolysis on an ion-exchange membrane. J Chromatogr A 1999; 831(2): 191-201.
[http://dx.doi.org/10.1016/S0021-9673(98)00950-9] [PMID: 10070763]

[66] Mine Y, Ma F, Lauriau S. Antimicrobial peptides released by enzymatic hydrolysis of hen egg white lysozyme. J Agric Food Chem 2004; 52(5): 1088-94.
[http://dx.doi.org/10.1021/jf0345752] [PMID: 14995103]

[67] Liu Z, Dong S, Xu J, Zeng M, Song H, Zhao Y. Production of cysteine-rich antimicrobial peptide by digestion of oyster (*Crassostrea gigas*) with alcalase and bromelin. Food Control 2008; 19(3): 231-5.
[http://dx.doi.org/10.1016/j.foodcont.2007.03.004]

[68] Su Y. Isolation and identification of pelteobagrin, a novel antimicrobial peptide from the skin mucus of yellow catfish *(Pelteobagrus fulvidraco).* Comp Biochem Physiol B Biochem Mol Biol 2011; 158(2): 149-54.
[http://dx.doi.org/10.1016/j.cbpb.2010.11.002] [PMID: 21073979]

[69] López-Abarrategui C, Alba A, Silva ON, *et al.* Functional characterization of a synthetic hydrophilic antifungal peptide derived from the marine snail *Cenchritis muricatus.* Biochimie 2012; 94(4): 968-74.
[http://dx.doi.org/10.1016/j.biochi.2011.12.016] [PMID: 22210491]

[70] Taveira GB, Mathias LS, da Motta OV, *et al.* Thionin-like peptides from Capsicum annuum fruits with high activity against human pathogenic bacteria and yeasts. Biopolymers 2014; 102(1): 30-9.
[http://dx.doi.org/10.1002/bip.22351] [PMID: 23896704]

[71] McClean S, Beggs LB, Welch RW. Antimicrobial activity of antihypertensive food-derived peptides and selected alanine analogues. Food Chem 2014; 146: 443-7.
[http://dx.doi.org/10.1016/j.foodchem.2013.09.094] [PMID: 24176365]

[72] Jiehui Z, Liuliu M, Haihong X, *et al.* Immunomodulating effects of casein-derived peptides QEPVL and QEPV on lymphocytes *in vitro* and *in vivo.* Food Funct 2014; 5(9): 2061-9.
[http://dx.doi.org/10.1039/C3FO60657K] [PMID: 24983024]

[73] Tellez A, Corredig M, Brovko LY, Griffiths MW. Characterization of immune-active peptides obtained from milk fermented by *Lactobacillus helveticus.* J Dairy Res 2010; 77(2): 129-36.
[http://dx.doi.org/10.1017/S002202990999046X] [PMID: 20078905]

[74] Tang W, Yuan H, Zhang H, Wang L, Qian H, Qi X. An antimicrobial peptide screened from casein hydrolyzate by *Saccharomyces cerevisiae* cell membrane affinity method. Food Control 2015; 50: 413-22.
[http://dx.doi.org/10.1016/j.foodcont.2014.09.030]

[75] Ryan JT, Ross RP, Bolton D, Fitzgerald GF, Stanton C. Bioactive peptides from muscle sources: meat and fish. Nutrients 2011; 3(9): 765-91.
[http://dx.doi.org/10.3390/nu3090765] [PMID: 22254123]

[76] Tang W, Zhang H, Wang L, Qian H, Qi X. Targeted separation of antibacterial peptide from protein hydrolysate of anchovy cooking wastewater by equilibrium dialysis. Food Chem 2015; 168: 115-23.
[http://dx.doi.org/10.1016/j.foodchem.2014.07.027] [PMID: 25172690]

[77] Dhayakaran R, Neethirajan S, Weng X. Investigation of the antimicrobial activity of soy peptides by developing a high throughput drug screening assay. Biochem Biophys Rep 2016; 6: 149-57.
[http://dx.doi.org/10.1016/j.bbrep.2016.04.001] [PMID: 28955872]

[78] Cheng AC, Lin HL, Shiu YL, Tyan YC, Liu CH. Isolation and characterization of antimicrobial peptides derived from *Bacillus subtilis* E20-fermented soybean meal and its use for preventing *Vibrio* infection in shrimp aquaculture. Fish Shellfish Immunol 2017; 67: 270-9.
[http://dx.doi.org/10.1016/j.fsi.2017.06.006] [PMID: 28602685]

[79] Wang G. Improved methods for classification, prediction, and design of antimicrobial peptides. Methods Mol Biol 2015; 1268: 43-66.

[http://dx.doi.org/10.1007/978-1-4939-2285-7_3] [PMID: 25555720]

[80] Ramesh S, Govender T, Kruger HG, de la Torre BG, Albericio F. Short AntiMicrobial Peptides (SAMPs) as a class of extraordinary promising therapeutic agents. J Pept Sci 2016; 22(7): 438-51. [http://dx.doi.org/10.1002/psc.2894] [PMID: 27352996]

[81] Kumar P, Kizhakkedathu JN, Straus SK. Antimicrobial peptides: diversity, mechanism of action and strategies to improve the activity and biocompatibility *in vivo*. Biomolecules 2018; 8(1) E4. [http://dx.doi.org/10.3390/biom8010004] [PMID: 29351202]

[82] Fleury Y, Dayem MA, Montagne JJ, *et al.* Covalent structure, synthesis, and structure-function studies of mesentericin Y 105(37), a defensive peptide from gram-positive bacteria Leuconostoc mesenteroides. J Biol Chem 1996; 271(24): 14421-9. [http://dx.doi.org/10.1074/jbc.271.24.14421] [PMID: 8662868]

[83] Yeaman MR, Yount NY. Mechanisms of antimicrobial peptide action and resistance. Pharmacol Rev 2003; 55(1): 27-55. [http://dx.doi.org/10.1124/pr.55.1.2] [PMID: 12615953]

[84] Dathe M, Nikolenko H, Meyer J, Beyermann M, Bienert M. Optimization of the antimicrobial activity of magainin peptides by modification of charge. FEBS Lett 2001; 501(2-3): 146-50. [http://dx.doi.org/10.1016/S0014-5793(01)02648-5] [PMID: 11470274]

[85] Edwards IA, Elliott AG, Kavanagh AM, Zuegg J, Blaskovich MAT, Cooper MA. Contribution of amphipathicity and hydrophobicity to the antimicrobial activity and cytotoxicity of β-hairpin peptides. ACS Infect Dis 2016; 2(6): 442-50. [http://dx.doi.org/10.1021/acsinfecdis.6b00045] [PMID: 27331141]

[86] Le CF, Fang CM, Sekaran SD. Intracellular targeting mechanisms by antimicrobial peptides. Antimicrob Agents Chemother 2017; 61(4): e02340-16. [http://dx.doi.org/10.1128/AAC.02340-16] [PMID: 28167546]

[87] Nijnik A, Hancock R. Host defence peptides: antimicrobial and immunomodulatory activity and potential applications for tackling antibiotic-resistant infections. Emerg Health Threats J 2009; 2 e1. [http://dx.doi.org/10.3402/ehtj.v2i0.7078] [PMID: 22460279]

[88] Donlan RM. Biofilm formation: a clinically relevant microbiological process. Clin Infect Dis 2001; 33(8): 1387-92. [http://dx.doi.org/10.1086/322972] [PMID: 11565080]

[89] Sierra JM, Fusté E, Rabanal F, Vinuesa T, Viñas M. An overview of antimicrobial peptides and the latest advances in their development. Expert Opin Biol Ther 2017; 17(6): 663-76. [http://dx.doi.org/10.1080/14712598.2017.1315402] [PMID: 28368216]

[90] Mahlapuu M, Håkansson J, Ringstad L, Björn C. Antimicrobial peptides: an emerging category of therapeutic agents. Front Cell Infect Microbiol 2016; 6: 194. [http://dx.doi.org/10.3389/fcimb.2016.00194] [PMID: 28083516]

[91] Brandelli A. Nanostructures as promising tools for delivery of antimicrobial peptides. Mini Rev Med Chem 2012; 12(8): 731-41. [http://dx.doi.org/10.2174/138955712801264774] [PMID: 22512554]

CHAPTER 5

Drugs for Superbugs: Strategies and Methods to Discover New Antibiotics against Drug Resistant Pathogens

Debananda S. Ningthoujam[*] and **Khullakpam Shaheen**

Advanced Level State Biotech Hub, Microbial Biotechnology Research Laboratory (MBRL), Department of Biochemistry, Manipur University, Canchipur, Imphal, Manipur795003, India

Abstract: The emergence of drug resistance in many bacterial pathogens and the rise of fungal infections have caused a resurgence of interest in finding new reserves of bioactive compounds. The increase in resistance to conventional antibiotics by many bacterial pathogens may be due to the decline in the discovery and development of novel antibiotics. Superbugs are those microorganisms (pathogens) that are resistant to the commonly used antibiotics. The World Health Organisation (WHO) has published a list of twelve potentially most dangerous priority pathogens with antibiotic resistance in 2017 and emphasized on discovering new antibiotics to tackle these pathogens. ESKAPE pathogens comprising *Enterococcus faecium*, *Staphylococcus aureus*, *Klebsiella pneumoniae*, *Acinetobacter baumanii*, *Pseudomonas aeruginosa* and, *Enterobacter* species can productively escape the antagonistic effects of the current antimicrobial agents. Urgent discovery of new drugs to tackle these resistant pathogens is required. This chapter mainly focuses on the strategies and methods on discovering novel antibiotics against drug resistant pathogens.

Keywords: Antibiotic Resistance, ESKAPE Pathogens, Superbugs, Strategies and Methods, World Health Organisation (WHO).

INTRODUCTION

Antibiotic Apocalypse and the Rise of Superbugs

Antibiotics have saved millions of lives in the 20th century and early 21st century but we will soon be running out of our antibiotic arsenal. Due to overuse, over prescription, under dosing and misuse of antibiotics, bacterial pathogens are now

[*] **Corresponding Author Debananda Singh Ningthoujam:** Advanced Level State Biotech Hub, Microbial Biotechnology Research Laboratory (MBRL), Department of Biochemistry, Manipur University, Canchipur, Imphal, Manipur 795003, India; Tel: +91 986 2027 271; E-mail: debananda.ningthoujam@gmail.com

K. Tamreihao, Saikat Mukherjee and Debananda S. Ningthoujam (Eds.)
All rights reserved-© 2019 Bentham Science Publishers

developing resistance to most of the clinically used antibiotics. Hence, there is an urgent need to develop new and novel forms of antibiotics.

Our antibiotic arsenal is now nearly exhausted. More than 7,00,000 people die of infections by drug-resistant pathogens across the world per year. This number is projected to rise to 10 million deaths by the year 2050 [1].

Superbugs are microorganisms that are resistant to commonly used antibiotics and can pass the trait along to other bacteria causing those strains to become resistant as well [2]. However, not all superbugs are created equally. *Staphylococcus aureus,* a harmless organism in the human body, was the first bug that became resistant to penicillin. It can cause severe illness such as pneumonia or toxic shock syndrome, when it becomes resistant. In 1967, another type of penicillin-resistant pneumonia, caused by *Streptococcus pneumonia* (pneumococcus) was reported in a remote village in Papua New Guinea. In 1983, a hospital acquired intestinal infection caused by *Enterococcus faecium* became resistant to penicillin. A large number of antibiotics classes have been discovered that inhibit cell-wall synthesis in the past half century [3].

Why We Need to Worry?

ESKAPE pathogens comprising *Enterococcus faecium*, *Staphylococcus aureus*, *Klebsiella pneumoniae*, *Acinetobacter baumanii*, *Pseudomonas aeruginosa* and, *Enterobacter* species have the capacity to escape the antagonistic effects of the current antimicrobial agents [4]. Rice reported that ESKAPE pathogens cause a greater number of infections in US hospitals as they can productively escape the effects of antibiotics [5].

The WHO has published a list of super-pathogens known by the acronym ESKAPE pathogens by using ten criteria to assess priority: mortality, health-care burden, community burden, and prevalence of resistance, 10-year trend of resistance, transmissibility, and preventability in the community setting, preventability in the health-care setting, treatability, and pipeline [6].

Types of Superbugs

As the threat of dangerous superbugs rise, the WHO has published a list of the twelve potentially most dangerous priority pathogens with antibiotic resistance in 2017 and pressed for urgent steps for discovering new antibiotics to tackle these pathogens [7, 8]. They used four criteria such as prevalence of the pathogen in the general community, overall mortality rates, burden on the health care system, and level of resistance to treatment [9]. The superbugs are classified into three categories which require prompt attention to keep them under control. They are classified as follows:

Critical (Priority 1)

The following bacteria are categorized under critical priority as they are multi drug resistant and often cause death in hospitals and nursing homes.

Carbapenem-Resistant Acinetobacter Baumannii

The superbug *Acinetobacter baumannii* develops resistance to antibiotics more quickly than other bacteria which can be found in soil and water and on the skin. It is most common in hospitals as it mainly affects people with compromised immune systems. It leads to pneumonia and deadly blood infections in hospitals. The incidence of infections by these deadly bacteria is projected to rise globally [10, 11].

Carbapenem-Resistant Pseudomonas Aeruginosa

Pseudomonas aeruginosa causes skin rashes, ear infections, blood infections, and often deadly bouts of pneumonia in hospital patients. It is highly amendable to developing antibiotic resistance. It mainly affects patients in intensive care units especially those who are ventilator dependent and those suffering from cystic fibrosis [12 - 14].

Carbapenem-Resistant Enterobacteriaceae (CRE)

CRE, 3rd generation cephalosporin-resistant, are typically found in human stomach (so, they are termed as "nightmare bacteria") [15], but some can cause life threatening blood infections, pneumonia and urinary tract infections. These superbugs are resistant to almost all kinds of conventional antibiotics. Hospitals are the source for enterobacteriaceae infection. Infection due to these bacteria is associated with significant morbidity and mortality [16].

High (Priority 2)

This category includes a variety of multi-drug resistant microbes that spread quickly and are dangerous to tackle such as Staphylococcus infections, Salmonella and gonorrhoea.

Vancomycin-Resistant Enterococcus Faecium (VRE)

They are often found harmless in the human intestine but can also cause serious diseases such as meningitis and endocarditis. Vancomycin resistance tends to rise among these isolates, with rate of 60% approximately [17].

Methicillin-Resistant Staphylococcus Aureus (MRSA)

It is difficult to treat MRSA infections, but some antibiotics exist to which it responds to and the frequency of life threatening MRSA has declined. It causes skin and respiratory infections and food poisoning. Hospitals are the main source of transmission of this superbug. Novel classes of antibiotics are clearly in need for MRSA. Non-drug therapies including vaccines and antibodies are also used to achieve some preventive measures for MRSA [18 - 20].

Clarithrocin-Resistant Helicobacter Pylori

They are often present in the stomachs of gastric ulcer patients. Moreover, it has been linked to stomach cancer patients [21] with no symptoms. Strains of antibiotic-resistant *Helicobacter pylori* are becoming more common, making effective treatments very difficult.

Fluoroquinolone-Resistant Campylobacter Spp.

They are found in poultry and spread to people who eat contaminated meat [22]. This microorganism causes blood diseases, diarrhoea, and food poisoning especially in developing countries that do not have access to proper antibiotics [23].

Fluoroquinolone-Resistant Salmonella Spp.

They are found worldwide and cause a variety of illnesses including typhoid fever and food poisoning. Infants, young children, and the elderly are at major risk.

3rd Generation Cephalosporin-Resistant, Fluoroquinolone Resistant Neisseria Gonorrhoeae

It is an antibiotic-resistant superbug causing the sexually transmitted disease gonorrhea. Most forms of this superbug are resistant to every drug used.

Medium (Priority 3)

Many childhood infections are caused by this category of the WHO priority pathogens which are most likely to become more widespread.

Penicillin-non-susceptible Streptococcus Pneumonia

It causes pneumonia and meningitis in people with compromised immune systems (such as children and the elderly) even though *Streptococcus pneumoniae* is relatively common in the lungs of healthy people.

Ampicillin-Resistant Haemophilus Influenzae

It is responsible for infections such as bacterial meningitis, pneumonia, and infectious arthritis. It is resistant to penicillin group of antibiotics.

Fluoroquinolone-Resistant Shigella Spp.

This superbug is naturally found in humans and gorillas and is the main cause of diarrhea globally. The organism is resistant to most antibiotics now.

Need to Discover New Antibiotics

Discovery of new drugs is urgently warranted to tackle these resistant pathogens.

Strategies and Methods

Several strategies have been reported such as the discovery of new drugs from traditional and extreme habitats with new modes of action, antibiotics synthesised by symbiotic bacteria, metagenomic approach, combination therapy of antibiotics, *in situ* culture of microbial cells in the soil, repurposing of old antibiotics, antibiotic analogs with enhanced action, co-culture approach, genome mining approach, functional metagenomic approach, discovery of antibiotics from strange animals *e.g.* platypus milk, and synthesis of new derivatives of retinoid and polycarbonates.

Extreme Ecosystems

Rateb *et al.* [24] reported novel antibiotics from the hyper arid Atacama Desert such as chaxamycins. Atacama Desert, the driest place on earth, is an extreme ecosystem located in Northern Chile and is one of the oldest deserts in the world. It is also exposed to very high levels of UV radiation [24].

Interestingly, many novel *Streptomyces* species have been discovered from this extreme ecosystem which produces novel chemical structures with potent biological activities [25 - 27]. Among these newly reported compounds, there are novel antibiotics with antagonistic activity against superbugs.

Streptomyces leeuwenhoekii from Atacama Desert was found to produce **chaxamycins**, ansamycin like compounds with antibacterial activity against several drug-resistant pathogens including MRSA, VRE and PRSP, *etc* [24].

A list of novel antibiotics produced by various bioactive bacteria, their chemical composition and functions are shown in Table **1**.

Table 1. Lists of novel or new antibiotics obtained from different sources.

Antibiotic	Source	Chemical Composition	Function	References
Chaxamycins	*Streptomyces leeuwenhoekii*	Azamacrocyclic lactam	Anti-MRSA, anti-VRE	[24 - 27]
Kocurin	*Kocuria palustris*	Thiazolyl peptide	Anti-MRSA	[28]
Formicamycins	*Streptomyces formicae*	Pentacyclic polyketide	Anti-MRSA, anti-VRE	[29, 30]
Sceliphrolactam	*Streptomyces sp.*	Polyene macrocyclic lactam	anti- *C. albicans*	[31]
Macrotermycins	*Amycolatopsis sp.* M39	Glycosylated macrolactams	Antimicrobial activity	[32]
Natalamycin A	*Streptomyces sp.*	Geldanamycin analog	Antifungal activity	[33]
Gerumycins	*Pseudonocardia sp.*	Cyclic depsipeptide	Antifungal activity	[34]
Alchivemycin A	*Streptomyces endus* S-522	Polycyclic polyketide	Antimicrobial activity	[35]
Piperidamycins	*Streptomyces mauvecolor*	cyclohexadepsipeptide	Anti-bacterial	[36]
Phosphacetamycin	*Streptomyces aureus*	Phosphanate	Antimicrobial activity	[37]
TP-1161	*Nocardiopsis sp. TFS65-07*	thiopeptide	Anti-VRE	[38]
Armeniaspirols	*Streptomyces armeniacus DSM 19369*	Chlorinated spiro[4.4] non-8-ene-scaffold	Anti MRSA and anti-VRE	[39]
Cervimycins	*Streptomyces tendae*	Polyketide glycosides	Anti MRSA and anti-VRE	[40, 41]
Malacidins	Soil bacteria	Cyclic lipopeptides	Anti-MRSA	[42]
Pseudouridimycin (PUM)	Soil bacteria	Rifamycin analog	Anti-bacterial	[43, 44]
Zavicefta	Ceftazidme (an old drug) + avibactam (a new antibiotic)	Beta lactams	Anti-bacterial - KPCs	[45 - 49]
Octapeptins	Chemical synthesis	lipopeptides	Anti bacterial	[50]
Vancapticins	Vancomycins	lipoglycopeptides	Anti- *C.* difficile	[51]
Lugdunins	*Staphylococcus lugdunensis* (Human nasal bacteria)	Thiazolidine containing cyclic peptide	Anti MRSA and anti-VRE	[72]

(Table 1) cont.....

Antibiotic	Source	Chemical Composition	Function	References
Plazomycin	Sisomicin or ensamycin isolated from *Micromonospora* sp.	Aminoglycoside-s	Anti MRSA, anti-VRSA and anti-CRE	[75 - 78]

Symbiotic Bacteria

Bacteria and insects are ubiquitous in distribution and some species have naturally developed a symbiotic relationship through co-evolution in which the bacteria are located in specialized anatomical compartments of the insects. The attine ants live in a tripartite mutualism with the fungus *Leucoagaricus gongylophorus*, which provides food to the ants, along with antibiotic producing actinomycetes that protect the fungal gardens from other fungal invaders. Similar findings have been discovered from symbiotic relationship of wasp-*Streptomyces* and termite-*Streptomyces*.

Kocurin, an anti-MRSA antibiotic, has been reported from sponge-associated microorganisms. Kocurin is a new thiazolyl peptide derived from culture broths of a marine-derived *Kocuria palustris*. The structure was determined using a combination of spectroscopic and chemical methods such as HRMS, extensive 1D and 2D NMR analysis and mass spectrometry [28].

Formicamycins, a class of novel antibiotics, were isolated from a novel actinobacterial species, *Streptomyces formicae*, which is associated symbiotically with the African fungus growing plant–ant, *Tetraponera penzigi*. It is a novel pentacyclic polyketide that has a unique antagonistic activity against MRSA and VRE. Chemically, it is same as the fasamycins identified from the heterologous expression of clones isolated from environmental DNA, but has marked differences. Details of this interesting symbiosis have been reported by several workers [29, 30].

Sceliphrolactam, a 26-membered polyene macrocyclic lactam, is produced by a *Streptomyces* strain isolated from the exoskeleton of the mud dauber (wasp), *Sceliphron caementarium*. It was found to be antagonistic to amphotericin B-resistant *C. albicans*. The chemical structure of sceliphrolactam was deduced by 1D- and 2D-NMR, MS, UV and IR spectral analysis [31].

A termite-associated *Amycolatopsis* sp. M39 produces **macrotermycins** with broad-spectrum antimicrobial activity. Chemically, macrotermycins are glycosylated macrolactams and show selective inhibition of the termite fungal garden competitor *Pseudoxylaria* sp [32]. **Natalamycin A,** another termite-associated natural product, exhibits potent broad-range antifungal activity. It is a rare geldanamycin analog which is isolated from a *Streptomyces* sp. associated with a South African nest of *Macrotermes natalensis* termites. Moreover, its structure has been characterized by NMR spectroscopy and X-ray crystallography [33].

Pseudonocardia spp. isolated from exoskeletons of several genera of ants such as *Apterostigma dentigerum* was reported to produce **gerumycins**, piperazic acid containing cyclic depsipeptides with selective antagonistic activity against a fungal pathogen *Escovopsis* [34].

Co-Culture Approach

Co-culture approach, an effective method for inducing the cryptic metabolite production, has been reported by certain groups. **Alchivemycin A**, a novel polycyclic polyketide, was produced by *Streptomyces endus* S-522 when cultured with *Tsukamurella* sp. (a mycolic acid-containing bacterium) [35].

Genome Mining Approach

Unlocking the gene expression from cryptic biosynthetic pathways to identify novel natural products has been a challenge in the exploitation of the secondary metabolite diversity of bacteria especially actinomycetes. Various methods for cryptic gene cluster activation have been developed in the last decade to awaken silent or poorly expressed secondary metabolite pathways and increase production yields.

One of the approaches used has been that of ribosome engineering. Ochi *et al.* reported that drug-resistant mutants to act at the level of ribosomes *e.g.* rifampicin were able to activate antibiotic production in some of the mutants. A novel antibiotic class **piperidamycins** was produced by *Streptomyces mauvecolor* through this ribosome engineering approach [36].

Other approaches have been directed at targeting new compounds structurally related to known antibiotics on the basis of specific key biosynthetic genes involved in their synthesis and targeted genome mining for these genes present in cryptic pathways. **Phosphacetamycin** is a new phosphonate antibiotic discovered from *Streptomyces aureus* using this approach [37]. It inhibits the growth of both Gram positive and Gram negative bacteria and fungi. The structure, biological activity and biosynthetic gene clusters have been reported for phosphacetamycin.

Similar genome-based approaches based on existing information on thiopeptide gene clusters has facilitated the discovery of novel thiopeptides by bioinformatic analysis of genomic sequences from other bacteria, and several new clusters potentially encoding thiopeptides were identified from strains of *Salinispora, Streptomyces*, and *Nocardiopsis, etc.*

Marine sediment derived *Nocardiopsis* strain TFS65-07 was found to produce a novel antibiotic, **TP-1161**, by using genome based approach [38]. This antibiotic is a new thiopeptide containing a rare aminoacetone moiety. It has broad-spectrum antibacterial activity against Gram positive strains. It was also found to be antagonistic against vancomycin-resistant bacterial strains including vancomycin- resistant *enterococci* (VRE). The isolation and structural and biological characterization of TP-1161 have been reported.

OSMAC (One Strain- Many Compounds) Approach

Another new class of antibiotic **Armeniaspirols** with anti-MRSA and anti-VRE activities have been isolated from *Streptomyces armeniacus*, DSM 19369. These antibiotics characterized by a novel spiro[4.4]non-8-ene scaffold are only produced by *S. armeniacus* when cultivated in a malt-containing medium. 5-Chloro-Armeniaspirole, a derivative produced by a linear six steps, exhibits potent activity against a range of multidrug-resistant, Gram-positive bacteria pathogens [39].

Another example of use of OSMAC approach is discovery of a new thiopeptide antibiotic, **TP-1161**, from a *Nocardiopsis* derived from marine sediment with activity against gram-positive clinical isolates comparable to that of vancomycin [38].

Cave Bacteria

Cervimycins A-D, a class of novel polyketide glycosides, exhibit significant activities against MRSA and VRE. They are produced by *Streptomyces tendae* associated with an ancient cave. They have a rare acetyl and carbamoyl ring substituent along with terminal methylmalonyl and dimethylmalonyl residues. The chemical structures have been determined by NMR and chemical degradation studies [40, 41].

New Mode & Old Habitat

Sean Brady and his colleagues at Rockefeller University discovered a set of genes that produce a novel calcium dependent antibiotic, **malacidins**. They are commonly encoded in crowd sourced soil microbiomes of New York. The malacidins are active against multidrug-resistant pathogens, sterilize MRSA skin infections in rat and did not develop resistance under the laboratory conditions [42]. They attack the bacterial cell wall.

Rutgers University scientists discovered a new antibiotic, **pseudouridimycin** (PUM), which is effective against a broad spectrum of drug-sensitive and drug-resistant bacteria and cures bacterial infections in mice. It is derived from a microbe associated with Italian soil. It functions as rifamycin analogs with novel mechanism of action. PUM is the first nucleoside analog inhibitor that inhibits bacterial RNA polymerases but not human RNA polymerases [43, 44].

Combining the Old and the New

A new antibiotic has been developed from an old antibiotic in our arsenal to fight the superbugs. It has been introduced for clinical usage in the US.

The new drug, named **zavicefta**, is a combination of an old drug called **ceftazidme**, 3rd generation cephalosporin, with an entirely new antibiotic known as **avibactam**, a novel β-lactam β-lactamase inhibitor [45]. It is very effective in targeting superbugs. It is used in the treatment of infections of urinary tract and intra-abdomen infections caused by nasty multidrug resistant gram negative bacterial pathogens [46 - 48] including *Klebsiella pneumoniae* carbapenemases (KPCs). Superbugs develop resistance as the pathogens evolve enzymes such as β-lactamase that deactivate antibiotics such as ceftazidme. However, in combination with the new antibiotic avibactam, it becomes effective again. Since the new drug inhibits the enzyme that causes resistance and restores antibacterial activity to the old drug [49].

Scientists are now in an urgent race to develop new generation of drugs that can tackle even the nastiest of the superbugs. Such combinations of new with old drugs are one of the options in combating infections due to menacing drug-resistant super-pathogens.

Reuse Old Antibiotics

Octapeptins were discovered in the 1970s but were soon discarded as there were a plethora of antibiotics with commercial potential at that time. Now, due to development of resistance to polymixins or colistin by certain gram negative pathogens mainly *Pseudomonas aeruginosa, Acinetobacter baumannii* and *Klebsiella pneumoniae*, octapeptins are reused for the development of a novel class of antibiotics targeting polymyxin-resistant superbugs. Being structurally related non-ribosomal lipopeptide antibiotics, they show cross-resistance with polymyxins and have a broader spectrum of antibacterial activity [50].

Now, Australian scientists, Professor Matt Cooper from University of Queensland and his team, synthesized a new class of antibiotics named as **vancapticins.** These are lipoglycopeptide antibiotics developed by the Cooper Group against *C. diff-*

icile. This group aims to expand the usefulness of these compounds from a parenteral treatment to an oral treatment selectively targeting CDI targeting MRSA and MDR *S. pneumonia* [51].

Repurposing Old Drugs

Scientists of Hong Kong University found that **colloidal bi-subcitrate (CBS)**, a bismuth based peptic ulcer drug can potentially paralyse superbugs including carbapenem resistant *enterococci* (CRE) and carbapenem resistant *Klebsiella*. It works by inhibiting New Delhi metallo-β-lactamase 1 (NDM1), an enzyme that confers these bacteria with resistance against all beta-lactam antibiotics [52, 53].

Immunobiotics

There are reports of a new type of drugs called **immunobiotics**, which is a combination of power of antibiotics and human immune system. Immunobiotics are showing promising results against the resistant pathogens. Pires and his team tagged gram negative bacteria which have rigid cell walls such as drug resistant pathogens (*Pseudomona aeruginosa)* by combining colistin (a last resort antibiotic) with some epitopes stimulating the immune system without affecting human cells. The complex attracts the antibodies on the pathogens' surface, thereby directly killing the bacteria as well as boosting immune system at the same time. The new drug increases the effectiveness of the old antibiotic by resensitizing the drug resistant pathogens to the antibiotic [54].

Phage Therapy

Phage therapy is the use of bacteriophages in the treatment of bacterial infections by lysing the bacteria at the infection site of the host [55] has significant applications in human medicine, dentistry, veterinary science and agriculture [56]. Bacteriophages are bioengineered to specifically treat multidrug-resistant bacterial infections, thereby, preventing harm to the beneficial bacteria in the human body [57]. Some of them have the ability of digesting of the biofilms that bacteria make to protect themselves from antibiotics [58]. The use of bacteriophages against antibiotic resistant bacteria has started in Georgia (George Eliava Institute) and Wroclaw, Poland [59, 60]. In eastern countries, bacteriophage cocktails are common drugs sold in pharmacies [61, 62].

Antibiotics Plus Probiotics

Rockefeller University scientists of New York propose **lysibodies** as new types of molecules. Lysibodies, representing a broad class of anti-infectives, are hybrid antibodies produced by the combination of human, bacterial and viral components by fusing the carbohydrate-binding lysine molecule of viruses with human antibodies. This approach allows production of antibodies against poorly immunogenic carbohydrate epitopes of many Gram-positive pathogens. Lysibodies binds to the carbohydrates on the surface of bacterial cells, thereby enabling destruction by the human immune system. These hybrid antibodies may be helpful to tackle the problematic superbugs. Assaf Raz and his team reported the lysibodies responsible for phagocytosis by targeting the carbohydrates on the cell wall of *Staphylococcus aureus* [63].

Synthetic Antibiotics

Dr. Yi Yan Yang and his group has reported a new class of synthetic antimicrobial polymer, guanidium functionalized polycarbonates as effective antibiotics against superbugs. This polymer is biodegradable and produces no significant toxicity to human cells. It has a distinctive mechanism which allows targeting and eliminating five dangerous superbugs namely *Acinetobacter baumannii*, *E. coli*, *Klebsiella pneumoniae*, Methicillin-resistant *Staphylococcus aureus* (MRSA) and *Pseudomonas aeruginosa*. These synthetic polymers have the potential to target deadly infections caused by multi drug resistant pathogens [64].

James Hedrick of IBM Lab in collaboration with IBN developed synthetic polymers (ninja polymers). These polymers are negatively charged and bind with great affinity to the positively charged cell surface, thus killing the superbug. The cell's inner cytoplasm turns solid (gel like) thus making the bacterial cell dysfunctional [65].

The team of researchers of Brown University and Rhode Island Hospital, led by Prof. Eleftherios Mylonakis, reported two synthetic compounds belonging to the class called "retinoids" with antagonistic activity against the superbug MRSA which is resistant to the available antibiotics. The two synthetic retinoids, CD437 and CD1530, show high killing rates to both growing and persistor MRSA cells by disrupting lipid bilayer and a low probability of resistance selection. In addition, an analogue of CD437 exhibits anti-persister activity and improved cytotoxicity profile [66].

New Gel for Superbugs

A synthetic antimicrobial and synthetic peptide called "**SAAP-148**" was found to disrupt biofilm formation by potential superbugs such as MRSA and MDR *Acinetobacter baumanii*. In human skin samples and mice, the gel containing the peptide completely cleared wounds of MRSA resistant to methicillin and other antibiotics and antibiotic-resistant *A. baumanii*. Both these pathogens cause serious infections in hospital patients. The synthetic peptide prevents superbugs from forming biofilms (colonies of pathogens enveloped in a protective slime) that shields them from antibiotics and eliminate already formed biofilms and persister cells. Bacteria living in a biofilm can be 10 to 1,000 times as difficult to kill as their solitary counterparts. SAAP-148 could also wipe out microbes that survive in a dormant, drug-tolerant state [67].

Interestingly, unlike *S. aureus* and *A. baumanii* exposed to conventional antibiotics, the pathogens didn't develop strong resistance to SAAP-148 even after a couple of weeks' exposure to the compound. Scientists are planning to test the peptide against other pathogens too which give dangerous threat to humans. Studies of this promising gel in humans are slated to begin before the end of 2018 [67].

The researchers of Purdue University are developing a new synthetic antibiotic called **F6**, N-(1,3,4-oxadiazol-2-yl) benzamide analog, as bacteriostatic agent against MRSA and VRE. They developed this synthetic antibiotic after scanning a library of synthetic chemical compounds and homed in on the most promising compound called F6 [68, 69].

Even after over two weeks of exposure to this compound, the MIC of F6 against MRSA remained almost constant, proving that this antibiotic effectively inhibits the growth of methicillin-resistant *Staphylococcus aureus* superbug while the chances of the pathogen developing resistance seems quite low. F6 is reported to be nontoxic to humans and other mammals and effective against MRSA, VRSA, *Enterococcus faecalis* living in the human gut, vancomycin-resistant *Enterococcus* (VRE) and *Listeria monocytogenes* (thriving often in unpasteurized dairy products) [68].

The Purdue team's next plan is to make F6 derivatives with even greater potency and develop candidate antibiotic agents against MRSA [69].

Analogs of Natural Antibiotics

Teixobactin, an antimicrobial peptide (AMP), was discovered in 2015 through i-CHIP technology (a plastic chip of credit card size having tiny chambers, each containing a single soil bacterial cell, is buried into the soil allowing the cells to grow and produce novel antibiotics). Teixobactin is a “head to side chain” cyclodepsipeptide associated with a soil gram–negative proteobacterium [70]. It has four D-amino acids and a rare L-allo-enduracididine amino acid. Scientists at University of Lincoln, UK, have made analogs of teixobactin with simplified structure and substitutions of key amino acids such as leucine and isoleucine in the peptide antibiotic with other amino acid thus improving its effectiveness and commercial potential against deadly MRSA and VRE infections [71]. Soon, teixobactin derivatives may reach the market as effective antibiotics against drug-resistant pathogens such as MRSA and VRE.

Strange Habitats

To tackle superbugs, many scientists are searching for novel microorganisms in various kinds of strange environments and habitats that could have the potential to produce novel antibiotics.

Staphylococcus lugdunensis isolated from human nose produce novel antibiotics named **lugdunins**. This antibiotic associated with the nasal bacteria exhibit potent antagonistic effects against the nasty infections by resistant superbugs such as MRSA and VRE. In future, this bacterium might be a good probiotic to fight staph infections [72].

Similarly, new antibiotics have been discovered from men's beard which were found to kill certain forms of drug-resistant *E. coli* [1]. Beard bacteria may have the potential to combat the harmful effects of superbugs effectively. Dr Adam Roberts, a researcher of University College London recommends isolating bacteria from strange habitats to look for new drugs targeting superbugs [73].

Caspofungin is an antifungal drug used to treat the human pathogenic fungi by inhibiting fungal cell wall biosynthesis. The efficiency of caspofungin is enhanced when it is combined with **humidimycin (MDN - 0010)** which is a novel natural lassopeptide identified as a secondary metabolite produced by the strain *Streptomyces humidus* isolated from a soil collected in Almeria, Spain. It may be the presence of humidimycin which affects the important salvage pathways of cell wall biosynthesis of the pathogenic fungi. This finding demonstrates that the signaling pathways can be targeted to produce novel anti-infective agents [74].

Plazomycin (ZEMDRI) is a new antibiotic with FDA approval in 2018 for adults suffering from complicated urinary tract infections (cUTI), including pyelonephritis, caused by *Escherichia coli*, *Klebsiella pneumoniae*etc [75, 76]. This drug is also effective against MRSA and VRSA when it is given with dactomycin or ceftobiprole and against *Pseudomonas aeruginosa* when combined with cefepime, doripenem, imipenem or piperacillin/tazobactam [77]. It also exhibits potent antibacterial activity against carbapenem-resistant *Acinetobacter baumannii* (CRE) [78].

Dentigerumycins, **candicidins**, and **pseudonocardone** are novel antibiotics derived from symbiotic bacteria. Dentigerumycins and candicidins are suites of antifungals produced by *Streptomyces* spp. which inhibits fungal pathogens such as *Escovopsis* sp. without causing any harm to attine ant-fungal symbiont *L. gongylophorus* [79]. Pseudonocardones, angucycline family of antibiotics, are the natural products from *Pseudonocardia* sp. EC080529- 01 isolated from the cuticle of the fungus – growing ant *Apterostigma dentigerum* [80].

CONCLUDING REMARKS

Biodiversity hotspots are mostly located in under-developed and developing parts of the world. But the threats of superbugs will first be seen in the developed countries and will soon spread to poorer regions of the world. As most new antibiotics will be natural molecules derived from biodiversity (combinatorial chemistry hasn't held much promise so far), isolation of novel microbes from biodiversity rich areas in the poorer and scientifically backward parts of the world and discovery of novel antibiotics effective against superbugs are urgently warranted.

Networking, sharing, and collaboration between scientists in rich countries and those in poorer nations will hold great promise in our search for new drugs for superbugs.

Unless we take urgent initiatives, soon infections and deaths by drug resistant pathogens will be more menacing than those due to cancer, CVDs, and other lifestyle diseases.

CONSENT FOR PUBLICATION

Not applicable.

CONFLICT OF INTEREST

The authors confirm that this chapter contents have no conflict of interest.

ACKNOWLEDGEMENTS

D.S.N. would like to thank Department of Biotechnology (DBT), Govt. of India for sponsoring the host laboratory under the scheme “Establishment of State Biotech Hubs” sanction order no: BT/04/NE/2009. K. Shaheen received DST INSPIRE fellowship with sanction no. DST/INSPIRE Fellowship/2014/195 of Department of Science & Technology, Ministry of Science & Technology, Government of India, New Delhi – 110016.

REFERENCES

[1] https://www.dailymail.co.uk/health/article-5623417/Could-antibiotics-mens-beards-soil-w-apons-battle-against-superdrugs.html.

[2] https://www.drugwatch.com/ercp/superbug/.

[3] Nanotechnology solutions to combat superbugs. Nanowerk Spotlight 2013.

[4] Boucher HW, Talbot GH, Bradley JS, *et al.* Bad bugs, no drugs: no ESKAPE! An update from the Infectious Diseases Society of America. Clin Infect Dis 2009; 48(1): 1-12. [http://dx.doi.org/10.1086/595011] [PMID: 19035777]

[5] Rice LB. Federal funding for the study of antimicrobial resistance in nosocomial pathogens: no ESKAPE. J Infect Dis 2008; 197(8): 1079-81. [http://dx.doi.org/10.1086/533452] [PMID: 18419525]

[6] Tacconelli E, Carrara E, Savoldi A, *et al.* Discovery, research, and development of new antibiotics: the WHO priority list of antibiotic-resistant bacteria and tuberculosis. Lancet Infect Dis 2018; 18(3): 318-27. [http://dx.doi.org/10.1016/S1473-3099(17)30753-3] [PMID: 29276051]

[7] http://www.who.int2017 February 27;

[8] WHO: Global Priority List of Antibiotic-Resistant Bacteria To Guide Research, Discovery and Development of New Antibiotics 2017 February 25;

[9] Stat News: WHO Releases List of World's Most Dangerous Superbugs.

[10] Munoz-Price LS, Weinstein RA. Acinetobacter infection. N Engl J Med 2008; 358(12): 1271-81. [http://dx.doi.org/10.1056/NEJMra070741] [PMID: 18354105]

[11] Perez F, Hujer AM, Hujer KM, Decker BK, Rather PN, Bonomo RA. Global challenge of multidrug-resistant Acinetobacter baumannii. Antimicrob Agents Chemother 2007; 51(10): 3471-84. [http://dx.doi.org/10.1128/AAC.01464-06] [PMID: 17646423]

[12] Giske CG, Monnet DL, Cars O, Carmeli Y. Clinical and economic impact of common multidrug-resistant gram-negative bacilli. Antimicrob Agents Chemother 2008; 52(3): 813-21. [http://dx.doi.org/10.1128/AAC.01169-07] [PMID: 18070961]

[13] Talbot GH. What is in the pipeline for Gram-negative pathogens? Expert Rev Anti Infect Ther 2008; 6(1): 39-49. [http://dx.doi.org/10.1586/14787210.6.1.39] [PMID: 18251663]

[14] Jacoby GA, Munoz-Price LS. The new beta-lactamases. N Engl J Med 2005; 352(4): 380-91. [http://dx.doi.org/10.1056/NEJMra041359] [PMID: 15673804]

[15] Frontline PBS. Illinois "Nightmare Bacteria" Outbreak Raises Alarms.

[16] Lin YC, Chen TL, Ju HL, *et al.* Clinical characteristics and risk factors for attributable mortality in Enterobacter cloacae bacteremia. J Microbiol Immunol Infect 2006; 39(1): 67-72. [PMID: 16440126]

[17] Wisplinghoff H, Bischoff T, Tallent SM, Seifert H, Wenzel RP, Edmond MB. Nosocomial bloodstream infections in US hospitals: analysis of 24,179 cases from a prospective nationwide surveillance study. Clin Infect Dis 2004; 39(3): 309-17. [http://dx.doi.org/10.1086/421946] [PMID: 15306996]

[18] Bishop E, Melvani S, Howden BP, Charles PG, Grayson ML. Good clinical outcomes but high rates of adverse reactions during linezolid therapy for serious infections: a proposed protocol for monitoring therapy in complex patients. Antimicrob Agents Chemother 2006; 50(4): 1599-602. [http://dx.doi.org/10.1128/AAC.50.4.1599-1602.2006] [PMID: 16569895]

[19] Boucher HW, Sakoulas G. Perspectives on Daptomycin resistance, with emphasis on resistance in Staphylococcus aureus. Clin Infect Dis 2007; 45(5): 601-8. [http://dx.doi.org/10.1086/520655] [PMID: 17682996]

[20] Tsiodras S, Gold HS, Sakoulas G, *et al.* Linezolid resistance in a clinical isolate of Staphylococcus aureus. Lancet 2001; 358(9277): 207-8.

[http://dx.doi.org/10.1016/S0140-6736(01)05410-1] [PMID: 11476839]

[21] Pathobiology of Helicobacter pylori-induced Gastric Cancer.

[22] Medscape: Campylobacter Infections.

[23] Antimicrobial Susceptibilities of Multidrug-Resistant Campylobacter jejuni and E. coli Strains: *In Vitro* Activities of 20 Antimicrobial Agents.

[24] Castro JF, Razmilic V, Gomez-Escribano JP, Andrews B, Asenjo JA, Bibb MJ. Identification and Heterologous Expression of the Chaxamycin Biosynthesis Gene Cluster from Streptomyces leeuwenhoekii. Appl Environ Microbiol 2015; 81(17): 5820-31. [http://dx.doi.org/10.1128/AEM.01039-15] [PMID: 26092459]

[25] Rateb ME, Houssen WE, Arnold M, *et al.* Chaxamycins A-D, bioactive ansamycins from a hyper-arid desert Streptomyces sp. J Nat Prod 2011; 74(6): 1491-9. [http://dx.doi.org/10.1021/np200320u] [PMID: 21553813]

[26] Rateb ME, Houssen WE, Harrison WTA, *et al.* Diverse metabolic profiles of a Streptomyces strain isolated from a hyper-arid environment. J Nat Prod 2011; 74(9): 1965-71. [http://dx.doi.org/10.1021/np200470u] [PMID: 21879726]

[27] Nachtigall J, Kulik A, Helaly S, *et al.* Atacamycins A-C, 22-membered antitumor macrolactones produced by Streptomyces sp. C38. J Antibiot (Tokyo) 2011; 64(12): 775-80. [http://dx.doi.org/10.1038/ja.2011.96] [PMID: 22008702]

[28] Martín J, da S Sousa T, Crespo G, *et al.* Kocurin, the true structure of PM181104, an anti-methicillin-resistant Staphylococcus aureus (MRSA) thiazolyl peptide from the marine-derived bacterium Kocuria palustris. Mar Drugs 2013; 11(2): 387-98. [http://dx.doi.org/10.3390/md11020387] [PMID: 23380989]

[29] Qin Z, Munnoch JT, Devine R, *et al.* Formicamycins, antibacterial polyketides produced by *Streptomyces formicae* isolated from African *Tetraponera* plant-ants. Chem Sci (Camb) 2017; 8(4): 3218-27. [http://dx.doi.org/10.1039/C6SC04265A] [PMID: 28507698]

[30] Holmes NA, Devine R, Qin Z, Seipke RF, Wilkinson B, Hutchings MI. Complete genome sequence of Streptomyces formicae KY5, the formicamycin producer. J Biotechnol 2018; 265: 116-8. [http://dx.doi.org/10.1016/j.jbiotec.2017.11.011] [PMID: 29191667]

[31] Oh DC, Poulsen M, Currie CR, Clardy J. Sceliphrolactam, a polyene macrocyclic lactam from a wasp-associated Streptomyces sp. Org Lett 2011; 13(4): 752-5. [http://dx.doi.org/10.1021/ol102991d] [PMID: 21247188]

[32] Beemelmanns C, Ramadhar TR, Kim KH, *et al.* Macrotermycins A-D, Glycosylated Macrolactams from a Termite-Associated Amycolatopsis sp. M39. Org Lett 2017; 19(5): 1000-3. [http://dx.doi.org/10.1021/acs.orglett.6b03831] [PMID: 28207275]

[33] Kim Ramadhar TR, Beemelmanns C, *et al.* Natalamycin A An Ansamycin from a Termite-Associated Streptomyces sp. Chem Sci 2014; 5(11): 4333-8. [http://dx.doi.org/10.1039/C4SC01136H]

[34] Sit CS, Ruzzini AC, Van Arnam EB, Ramadhar TR, Currie CR, Clardy J. Variable genetic architectures produce virtually identical molecules in bacterial symbionts of fungus-growing ants. Proc Natl Acad Sci USA 2015; 112(43): 13150-4. [http://dx.doi.org/10.1073/pnas.1515348112] [PMID: 26438860]

[35] Onaka H, Mori Y, Igarashi Y, Furumai T. Mycolic acid-containing bacteria induce natural-product biosynthesis in Streptomyces species. Appl Environ Microbiol 2011; 77(2): 400-6. [http://dx.doi.org/10.1128/AEM.01337-10] [PMID: 21097597]

[36] Hosaka T, Ohnishi-Kameyama M, Muramatsu H, *et al.* Antibacterial discovery in actinomycetes strains with mutations in RNA polymerase or ribosomal protein S12. Nat Biotechnol 2009; 27(5): 462-

4.
[http://dx.doi.org/10.1038/nbt.1538] [PMID: 19396160]

[37] Evans BS, Zhao C, Gao J, *et al.* Discovery of the antibiotic phosacetamycin *via* a new mass spectrometry-based method for phosphonic acid detection. ACS Chem Biol 2013; 8(5): 908-13. [http://dx.doi.org/10.1021/cb400102t] [PMID: 23474169]

[38] Engelhardt K, Degnes KF, Kemmler M, *et al.* Production of a new thiopeptide antibiotic, TP-1161, by a marine Nocardiopsis species. Appl Environ Microbiol 2010; 76(15): 4969-76. [http://dx.doi.org/10.1128/AEM.00741-10] [PMID: 20562278]

[39] Couturier C, Bauer A, Rey A, Schroif-Dufour C, Broenstrup M. Armeniaspiroles, a new class of antibacterials: Antibacterial activities and total synthesis of 5-chloro-Armeniaspirole A. Bioorg Med Chem Lett 2012; 22(19): 6292-6. [http://dx.doi.org/10.1016/j.bmcl.2012.06.107] [PMID: 22921279]

[40] Herold K, Xu Z, Gollmick FA, Grafe U, Hertweck C. Biosynthesis of cervimycin C, an aromatic polyketide antibiotic bearing an unusual dimethylmalonyl moiety. Org Biomol Chem 2004; 2(17): 2411-4. [http://dx.doi.org/10.1039/B409221J] [PMID: 15326518]

[41] Harold Gollmick FA, Groth I, *et al.* Cervimycin A-D: A Polyketide Glycoside complex from a cave bacterium can defeat Vancomycin resistance. Chemistry 2006; 11(19): 5523-9.

[42] Hover BM, Kim SH, Katz M, *et al.* Culture-independent discovery of the malacidins as calcium-dependent antibiotics with activity against multidrug-resistant Gram-positive pathogens. Nat Microbiol 2018; 3(4): 415-22. [http://dx.doi.org/10.1038/s41564-018-0110-1] [PMID: 29434326]

[43] Maffioli SI, Zhang Y, Degen D, *et al.* Antibacterial Nucleoside-Analog Inhibitor of Bacterial RNA Polymerase. Cell 2017; 169(7): 1240-1248.e23. [http://dx.doi.org/10.1016/j.cell.2017.05.042] [PMID: 28622509]

[44] Rutgers University. New antibiotic effective against drug-resistant bacteria: First selective nucleoside-analog inhibitor of bacterial RNA polymerase. Science Daily 2017. www.sciencedaily.com/releases/2017/06/170615142842.htm.

[45] Briefing package: ceftazidime-avibactam. Anti-infective drugs advisory committee meeting (PDF) fdagov US Food and Drug Administration Retrieved 27 June 2015.

[46] Zhanel GG, Lawson CD, Adam H, *et al.* Ceftazidime-avibactam: a novel cephalosporin/β-lactamase inhibitor combination. Drugs 2013; 73(2): 159-77. [http://dx.doi.org/10.1007/s40265-013-0013-7] [PMID: 23371303]

[47] Actavis Announces FDA Acceptance of the NDA Filing for Ceftazidime-Avibactam, a Qualified Infectious Disease Product. Actavis-a global, integrated specialty pharmaceutical company- Actavis. Actavis plc Retrieved 1 June 2015.

[48] Ehmann DE, Jahic H, Ross PL, *et al.* Kinetics of avibactam inhibition against Class A, C, and D β-lactamases. J Biol Chem 2013; 288(39): 27960-71. [http://dx.doi.org/10.1074/jbc.M113.485979] [PMID: 23913691]

[49] Abboud MI, Damblon C, Brem J, *et al.* Interaction of Avibactam with Class B Metallo-β-Lactamases. Antimicrob Agents Chemother 2016; 60(10): 5655-62. [http://dx.doi.org/10.1128/AAC.00897-16] [PMID: 27401561]

[50] Velkov T, Roberts KD, Li J. Rediscovering the octapeptins. Nat Prod Rep 2017; 34(3): 295-309. [http://dx.doi.org/10.1039/C6NP00113K] [PMID: 28180225]

[51] Cooper group. Infectious diseases.. Institute of Molecular Bioscience, University of Queensland http://cooper.imb.uq.edu.au/research_infectious_disease.html.

[52] Wang R, Lai TP, Gao P, *et al.* Bismuth antimicrobial drugs serve as broad-spectrum metallo-β-

lactamase inhibitors. Nat Commun 2018; 9(1): 439.
[http://dx.doi.org/10.1038/s41467-018-02828-6] [PMID: 29382822]

[53] https://www.asianscientist.com/2018/05/in-the-lab/bismuth-ulcer-antimicrobial-resistance/.

[54] https://www.smithsonianmag.com/smart-news/new-immunobiotic-could-treat-antibiotic-resistant-superbugs-180969560.

[55] Killers Silent. Silent Killers: Fantastic Phages?. Archived from the original on 10 February 2013. Retrieved 14 November 2017.

[56] McAuliffe O, Ross RP, Fitzgerald GF, *et al.* The New Phage Biology: From Genomics to Applications (introduction).McGrath S, van Sinderen D Bacteriophage: Genet and Mol Biol.

[57] Lin DM, Koskella B, Lin HC. Phage therapy: An alternative to antibiotics in the age of multi-drug resistance. World Journal of Gastrointestinal Pharmacology and Therapeutics 2017; 8(3): 162-73. Archived from the original on 24 April 2018. Retrieved 23 April 2018.

[58] Salmond GP, Fineran PC. A century of the phage: past, present and future. Nat Rev Microbiol 2015; 13(12): 777-86.
[http://dx.doi.org/10.1038/nrmicro3564] [PMID: 26548913]

[59] Parfitt T. Georgia: an unlikely stronghold for bacteriophage therapy. Lancet 2005; 365(9478): 2166-7.
[http://dx.doi.org/10.1016/S0140-6736(05)66759-1] [PMID: 15986542]

[60] Golkar Z, Bagasra O, Pace DG. Bacteriophage therapy: a potential solution for the antibiotic resistance crisis. J Infect Dev Ctries 2014; 8(2): 129-36.
[http://dx.doi.org/10.3855/jidc.3573] [PMID: 24518621]

[61] McCallin S, Alam Sarker S, Barretto C, *et al.* Safety analysis of a Russian phage cocktail: from metagenomic analysis to oral application in healthy human subjects. Virology 2013; 443(2): 187-96.
[http://dx.doi.org/10.1016/j.virol.2013.05.022] [PMID: 23755967]

[62] Abedon ST, Kuhl SJ, Blasdel BG, Kutter EM. Phage treatment of human infections. Bacteriophage 2011; 1(2): 66-85.
[http://dx.doi.org/10.4161/bact.1.2.15845] [PMID: 22334863]

[63] Raz A, Serrano A, Lawson C, *et al.* Lysibodies are IgG Fc fusions with lysin binding domains targeting *Staphylococcus aureus* wall carbohydrates for effective phagocytosis. Proc Natl Acad Sci USA 2017; 114(18): 4781-6.
[http://dx.doi.org/10.1073/pnas.1619249114] [PMID: 28428342]

[64] Chin W, Zhong G, Pu Q, *et al.* A macromolecular approach to eradicate multidrug resistant bacterial infections while mitigating drug resistance onset. Nat Commun 2018; 9(1): 917.
[http://dx.doi.org/10.1038/s41467-018-03325-6] [PMID: 29500445]

[65] https://newatlas.com/synthetic-molecule-polymer-treat-resistant-bacteria/53676/.

[66] Kim W, Zhu W, Hendricks GL, *et al.* A new class of synthetic retinoid antibiotics effective against bacterial persisters. Nature 2018; 556(7699): 103-7.
[http://dx.doi.org/10.1038/nature26157] [PMID: 29590091]

[67] de Breij A, Riool M, Cordfunke RA, *et al.* The antimicrobial peptide SAAP-148 combats drug-resistant bacteria and biofilms. Sci Transl Med 2018; 10(423): 1-14.
[http://dx.doi.org/10.1126/scitranslmed.aan4044] [PMID: 29321257]

[68] Sintim H. New compound shown to be as effective as FDA-approved drugs against life-threatening infections. Medical Xpress 2018.https://medicalxpress.com/news/2018-06-compound-shown-effective-fda-approved-drugs.html.

[69] Opoku-Temeng C, Naclerio GA, Mohammad H, *et al.* N-(1,3,4-oxadiazol-2-yl)benzamide analogs, bacteriostatic agents against methicillin- and vancomycin-resistant bacteria. Eur J Med Chem 2018; 155: 797-805.
[http://dx.doi.org/10.1016/j.ejmech.2018.06.023] [PMID: 29957525]

[70] Abdel Monaim SAH, Jad YE, El-Faham A, de la Torre BG, Albericio F. Teixobactin as a scaffold for unlimited new antimicrobial peptides: SAR study. Bioorg Med Chem 2018; 26(10): 2788-96. [http://dx.doi.org/10.1016/j.bmc.2017.09.040] [PMID: 29029900]

[71] Parmar A, Iyer A, Prior SH, *et al.* Teixobactin analogues reveal enduracididine to be non-essential for highly potent antibacterial activity and lipid II binding. Chem Sci (Camb) 2017; 8(12): 8183-92. [http://dx.doi.org/10.1039/C7SC03241B] [PMID: 29568465]

[72] https://lactobacto.com/tag/staphylococcus-lugdunensis/.

[73] https://www.ehfblog.com/2016/02/growing-beard-bacteria-in-beards.html.

[74] Valiante V, Monteiro MC, Martín J, *et al.* Hitting the caspofungin salvage pathway of human-pathogenic fungi with the novel lasso peptide humidimycin (MDN-0010). Antimicrob Agents Chemother 2015; 59(9): 5145-53. [http://dx.doi.org/10.1128/AAC.00683-15] [PMID: 26055366]

[75] BioCentury - FDA approves plazomicin for cUTI, but not blood infections www.biocentury.com Retrieved 2018-06-28.

[76] Drugs@FDA: FDA Approved Drug Products www.accessdata.fda.gov Retrieved 2018-06-28.

[77] Zhanel GG, Lawson CD, Zelenitsky S, *et al.* Comparison of the next-generation aminoglycoside plazomicin to gentamicin, tobramycin and amikacin. Expert Rev Anti Infect Ther 2012; 10(4): 459-73. [http://dx.doi.org/10.1586/eri.12.25] [PMID: 22512755]

[78] García-Salguero C, Rodríguez-Avial I, Picazo JJ, Culebras E. Can Plazomicin Alone or in Combination Be a Therapeutic Option against Carbapenem-Resistant Acinetobacter baumannii? Antimicrob Agents Chemother 2015; 59(10): 5959-66. [http://dx.doi.org/10.1128/AAC.00873-15] [PMID: 26169398]

[79] Scott W, Behie SW, Bonet B, Zacharia VM, McClung DJ, Traxler MF. Molecules to Ecosystems: Actinomycete Natural Products. In Situ 2017; 7(2149): 1-11.

[80] Caldera EJ, Currie CR. The population structure of antibiotic-producing bacterial symbionts of Apterostigma dentigerum ants: impacts of coevolution and multipartite symbiosis. Am Nat 2012; 180(5): 604-17. [http://dx.doi.org/10.1086/667886] [PMID: 23070321]

CHAPTER 6

Antifungal Agents: Therapeutic Approaches and Future Perspectives

Rakhi Khunjamayum*, **Roshan Singh Asem**, **Laishram Jaya Devi**, **K. Tamreihao** and **Debananda S. Ningthoujam**

Advanced Level State Biotech Hub, Microbial Biotechnology Research Laboratory (MBRL), Department of Biochemistry, Manipur University, Imphal, India

Abstract: Fungi are versatile organisms that cause infectious diseases to millions of people. The disease caused by fungi are rapidly rising in immunocompromised patients. Commonly available antifungal drugs act on the cell wall and nucleic acid synthesis and, cell division. However, excessive use of the clinically available common antifungal drugs has led to the development of multidrug-resistant strains that no longer respond to treatment. The rapidly emerging multidrug-resistant *Candida auris* has caused severe infection and has become a serious burden on public health. Therefore, the search for new effective compounds especially from endophytes associated with medicinal plants that have a novel target and mechanism of action against the multidrug-resistant strains to combat the rapidly emerging infectious diseases caused by fungi, has become vital.

Keywords: Antifungal compounds, *Candida auris*, Fungal infections, Multidrug-resistant, Pathogenesis, Symptoms, Treatment.

INTRODUCTION

Emerging infectious diseases caused by pathogenic microorganisms like bacteria, fungi, virus or parasite are a significant burden to the public health and global economies. Variations in the existence of microorganisms have also led to the development of new threats to public health. Infectious diseases caused by fungi are thought to be driven mostly by socio-economic, environmental and ecological factors, but no comparative study has analysed these relations to understand the patterns of developing the diseases [1 - 3].

* **Corresponding author Rakhi Khunjamayum:** Advanced Level State Biotech Hub, Microbial Biotechnology Research Laboratory (MBRL), Department of Biochemistry, Manipur University, Imphal, India; Tel: +91 977 4101 970; E-mail: rakhikhunjamayum@gmail.com

K. Tamreihao, Saikat Mukherjee and Debananda S. Ningthoujam (Eds.)
All rights reserved-© 2019 Bentham Science Publishers

Fungi are a versatile group of microorganisms that are found in various habitats. They can cause mild superficial infections to severe invasive infections. They are believed to have emerged some 1.6 million years ago. There are about 1.5 million different fungal species (on Earth) occupying a broad diversity of habitats but, only about 300 are reported to be pathogenic to human. Majority of them can cause rare mycoses and very few are comparatively common pathogens. Fungal infections caused by *Candida*, *Cryptococcus* and *Aspergillus* are among the most frequent infections in human. The most common fungal infections in humans are those caused by dematophytes [4 - 7].

Fungal diseases were considered less important until recently. However, diseases caused by fungi are rising and this could lead to more outbreaks of diseases. Fungal infections in immunocompromised patients have become a worldwide health issue. Immunocompromised patients such as intensive-care, organ transplant, cancer, AIDS, tuberculosis and other bacterial infections are at more risk as their immune system is weak. They are increasing at an alarming rate causing enormous pressure and challenge to healthcare professionals for diagnosis and treatment. Invasive candidiasis and dermatomycoses have become the most common fungal diseases among the immunocompromised individuals. For example, disseminated nosocomial fungal infection is caused by *Candida albicans*, nosocomial fungal pneumonia by *Aspergillus fumigatus* and central nervous system mycosis in HIV-infected patients by *Cryptococcus neoformans*. During the few decades, some other fungal pathogens also emerged which includes azole-resistant *Candida albicans*, other *Candida* species and *Trichosporon*, *Fusarium* spp., Zygomycetes, dematiaceous moulds, *Penicillium marneffei*, *Coccidioides immitis* and *Histoplasma capsulatum*. These emerging fungal pathogens are developing at an alarming rate in immunocompromised hosts [8 - 10, 14].

Comparative studies on bacteria, resistance to antibiotics and fungi, resistance to antifungal agents has been reported. However, over the past 30-40 years, there is a huge rise in resistance to antifungal drugs. Since many of the currently available drugs have unwanted side effects, are ineffective against new or re-emerging fungi, the need of the hour is to discover new antifungal agents that exhibit potent activity against drug resistant fungal pathogens and display low toxicity to human cells [11, 12, 15, 16]. Further detailed search to identify the targets and mechanisms of action of the novel compound is urgently needed. Modern genomic approaches are being used to search for the molecular targets. Six new antifungal agents are approaching the clinic. These include three new triazoles *viz.,* voriconazole, ravuconazole and posaconazole. The other three include echinocandins, sordarins and morpholines [13].

The main objective of this chapter is to summarise the target and mechanism of action of some of the commonly available antifungal compounds. It will also deal with the common infectious diseases caused to human by pathogenic fungi and treatment of the diseases using clinically available antifungal drugs.

Antifungal Agents and Mechanism of Action

Earlier, from the beginning of the 20th century until the Second World War, potassium iodide was used as the standard compound for treating cutaneous infections caused by fungi. Potassium iodide was first derived from sea algae. It exhibited potent antifungal activity however, the mechanism of action remains unclear [17 - 19]. Griseofulvin, extracted from *Penicillium griseofulvum* have been widely used for the treatment of superficial fungal infections [13, 20, 21].

Six categories of antifungal agents are currently available. These include azoles, allylamines/thiocarbamates, polyenes, morpholines, pyrimidine analogs, and echinocandins. These antifungal agents exhibit antifungal activities by inhibiting the fungal cell wall and nucleic acid synthesis and interfering in cell division (Table **1**) [22, 23]. Some of the commonly used antifungal compounds and its mechanism of actions are discussed below:

Table 1. Mechanism of action and target of common antifungal agents.

Antifungal Agent(s)	Target	Mechanism of Action	Reference
Azoles	Cell membrane	Inhibits C-14 demethylation of lanosterol	[28, 29]
Echinocandins	Cell membrane	Inhibits 1,3-β-D-glucan synthase (GS)	[13]
Allylamines and thiocarbamates	Cell membrane	Inhibit oxidosqualene cyclase	[22, 29]
Morpholines	Cell membrane	Inhibit sterol Δ^{14} reductase and Δ^7-Δ^8 isomerase	[20]
Polyene	Cell membrane	Binds to cell wall and forms a hole	[20, 23, 24]
Pyrimidine analogues	Nucleic acid synthesis	Intracellular conversion of 5-FU to 5-fluorouridine monophosphate and 5-fluorodeoxyuridine monophosphate	[20, 23]
Griseofulvin	Cell division	Inhibits spindle formation	[68, 69]

Azoles

Azoles and echinocandins are the two main classes of drugs which are usually employed to combat invasive fungal infections. Azole-based antifungal agents include ketoconazole, itraconazole, fluconazole, voriconazole, posaconazole, isavuconazole, and ravuconazole. These drugs could inhibit fungal ergosterol biosynthesis pathway (Fig. **1**). They are proved to be important drugs for combating human fungal infections. Ketoconazole was introduced to the US market in 1981, however, due to the risk of hepatic injury, drug-drug interactions and reduced human steroid synthesis; it has been removed from the clinics [16, 24, 25].

The antifungal activity of azole was first described in 1944. Currently, azoles represent one of the important drug classes to control the infectious diseases caused to human, animals and plants by pathogenic fungi [26]. It blocks the ergosterol synthesis which is a major component of cytoplasmic membranes of fungi. Azoles inhibit cytochrome P450-dependant 14α-lanosterol demethylase (Cyp51) encoded by the ERG11 gene which converts lanosterol to ergosterol [13, 27]. Itraconazole inhibits NADPH-dependent 3-ketosteroid reductase (ERG 27), catalysing the reduction of 3-ketosteroid obtusifolione to obtusifoliol in *Cryptococcus neoformans* [28, 29]. However, increased use of azoles has led to a rise in drug resistant strains. A new azole agent has been discovered which includes isavuconazole, voriconazole and albaconazole. These new azole agents which are under clinical evaluations, showed potent antifungal activities against clinically resistant fungi [23, 30, 31].

Echinocandins

Echinocandins were discovered in 1974. Antifungal activity of the prototypes *viz*., echinocandin B and aculeacin A was studied through random screening in the 1970s and found that they exhibit limited spectrum of activity to candida infections. Due to severe adverse effects, echinocandin B has been removed from clinical use. However, it inspires the development of semi-synthetic agents, caspofungin, micafungin and anidulafungin. These three recently discovered echinocandins are currently approved as antifungal drugs [23, 24, 32].

Echinocandins are antifungal secondary metabolite, a semi-synthetic amphiphilic lipopeptides comprising a cyclic hexapeptide core with different lipid side chains. They exerted antifungal effects by inhibiting the catalytic subunit of 1,3-β-D-glucan synthase (GS), responsible for the synthesis of the fungal cell wall 1,3 β-D-glucan polysaccharides. Treatment of patients with echinocandins is inconvenient as it requires prolonged intravenous administration [13, 33 - 35].

Allylamines and Thiocarbamates

Allylamines and thiocarbamates are sterol synthesis inhibitors. Their antifungal effects are due to inhibition of ergosterol synthesis at the level of squalene epoxidase encoded by the *ERG1* gene which converts squalene to 2, 3-squalene epoxide (Fig. **1**). Examples of allylamines include naftifine and terbinafine. Allylamines and thiocarbamates have broad spectrum activity against fungal species. They are used for treating dermatophyte infections [22, 29].

Morpholines

Morpholines are also sterol inhibitors. A morpholine derivative amorolfine is used for treatment of tropical superficial mycoses. It inhibits subsequent step of the ergosterol pathway. It targets the Δ^{14} reductase enzyme, $Erg24_p$ and Δ^8 - Δ^7 isomerase enzyme late in the ergosterol pathway (Fig. **1**) [13 - 15, 20].

Polyene

Polyenes are actinomycetes-derived unsaturated macrolactones. Polyene antibiotics include nystatin, amphotericin B (AmB) and candicidin. Polyene macrolides such as nystatin A1 and amphotericin B belong to polyketide compound. Polyene disrupts selective permeability of ergosterol. They are used for the treatment of human mycotic infections especially vaginitis caused by *Candida albicans* [25, 36, 37]. Intravenous injection of polyenes continue to be the major treatment option for severe fungal infections, especially aspergillosis, cryptococcosis, candidiasis and numerous cases of histoplasmosis, blastomycosis, coccidioidomycosis, and other infections of Mucorales [38]. For more than 50 years, AmB has been used as the treatment for invasive fungal infections. It is regarded as the drug of choice for treating serious systemic and internal infections caused by *Candida*, *Cryptococcus*, *Aspergillus*, *Fusarium*, and *Scedosporium* [39 - 42]. AmB exhibits potent chemotherapeutic properties with broad spectrum antifungal activity. However, due to its extreme toxicity, medical application is limited. AmB is nephrotoxic and causes several other toxic side effects [43 - 46]. In order to reduce these negative effects, efforts have been made to develop less toxic AmB derivatives. New delivery formulations have been introduced using chemical methods. These new AmB derivatives include lipid-based amBisome, abelcet and amphocil. They are commercially available and have proved to be better alternatives to fungizone. In addition to antifungal activity, AmB also exhibits antiparasitic and antiviral activity [44, 47 - 52].

Nystatin was first discovered from *Streptomyces noursei* by the Division of Laboratories and Research of the New York State Department of Health in 1949 [53]. It is mostly used for the treatment of infections caused by *Candida* species. Nystatin also showed modest activity against *Aspergillus* species. For systemic use, nystatin is toxic and it can cause nausea [54]. Due to aggregate formation in the aqueous solutions, they are toxic to mammalian cells. But recently, a more soluble liposomal nystatin formulation nystran with less toxicity has been developed. This liposomal nystatin is active against a variety of *candida* species and some AmB resistant isolates [55 - 57].

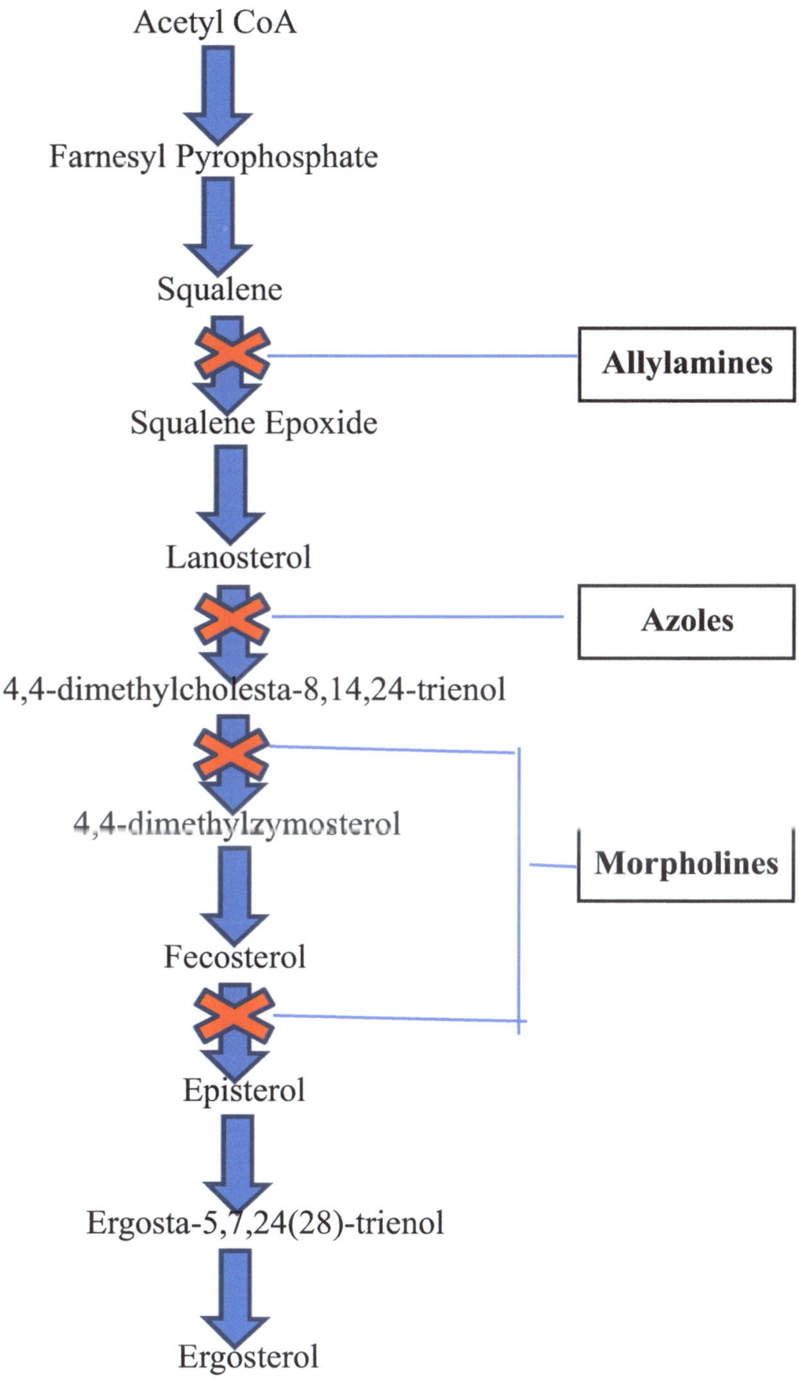

Fig. (1). Antifungal agents that inhibit the ergosterol biosynthesis pathway.

Polyene binds to the sterol component in the phospholipid-sterol membrane of the fungal cell wall and forms complexes, thus forming tiny holes or channels in the membrane [20, 23, 24]. These channels cause leakage of monovalent cellular components mainly potassium ions, sodium ions and chloride ions [58 - 61]. This leakage causes impairment of the membrane barrier function leading to proton influx, decline in intracellular pH, and dissipation of the proton gradient thereby inhibiting the growth [42, 62 - 64].

Pyrimidine Analogues

Pyrimidine analogues are antimetabolites which are used as antifungal agents. They interfere in nucleic acid synthesis. Pyrimidine analogues are used widely in the management of hematological and solid cancers. Examples of pyrimidine analogues include 5-fluorocytosine (5-FC) and 5-fluorouracil (5-FU). They exerted antifungal activity by inhibiting DNA and RNA synthesis. 5-FU is intracellularly converted to 5-fluorouridine monophosphate impairing RNA function and its polyadenylation thus inhibiting RNA synthesis. 5-FU is also converted to 5-fluorodeoxyuridine monophosphate. It inhibits the enzyme thymidylate synthase in thymine nucleotide formation thereby inhibiting DNA synthesis. 5-FC is used in combination with amphotericin B in order to avoid the recurrent occurrence of innate/acquired resistance of fungal pathogens [20, 23, 65 - 67].

Griseofulvin

Antifungal drug, Griseofulvin was isolated from *Penicillium griseofulvum* in 1939. It inhibits cell mitosis, nucleic acid and cell wall synthesis. It also acts by disrupting the spindle and cytoplasmic microtubule function by binding to alpha and beta tubulin [68, 69].

Common Fungal Diseases in Human – Causes, Symptoms, Pathogenesis and Treatment

Aspergillosis

***Causal Organism*:** Aspergillosis is caused by *Aspergillus* species. These species are ubiquitous in nature and mostly found in organic matter. More than 100 species of *Aspergillus* have been identified however, majority of the infections are caused by *Aspergillus fumigatus, Aspergillus niger* and rarely by *Aspergillus flavus* and *Aspergillus clavatus*. These species may cause a broad spectrum of diseases from hypersensitivity reactions to direct angioinvasion [70, 71].

Symptoms: Signs and symptoms of aspergillosis vary with the type of infections /illness developed.

- ***Allergic bronchopulmonary aspergillosis***: Asthma or cystic fibrosis patients have an allergic reaction to *Aspergillus*. Signs and symptoms include fever, cough with blood or mucus [72, 73].
- ***Aspergilloma***: Chronic lung (pulmonary) conditions such as emphysema, tuberculosis or advanced sarcoidosis can form cavities in the lungs. If such patients are infected by *Aspergillus* fungus fibre may enter the cavities, grow and form fungus balls. This fungus balls are known as aspergillomas. Aspergillomas may or may not produce any symptoms. However, if not treated on time it could worsen the underlying chronic lung condition and cause blood in cough (hemoptysis), wheezing, shortness of breath, weight loss, and fatigue [72, 74].
- ***Invasive aspergillosis***: It occurs when aspergillosis spreads from lungs to brain, heart, kidneys or skin. Invasive pulmonary aspergillosis occurs in immunocompromised individuals. It may be fatal if not treated. General signs and symptoms include fever, hemoptysis, shortness of breath, chest or joint pain, headaches, and skin lesions [75, 76].
- ***Chronic necrotizing pulmonary aspergillosis***: It infects the patients with underlying diseases such as steroid-dependent chronic obstructive pulmonary disease, alcoholism, *etc*. Signs and symptoms include fever, cough, weight loss, *etc* [70].

Pathogenesis

Disease development is through inhalation of *Aspergillus* species conidia. However, normal healthy host is not affected by the conidia even after inhalation. Host with weak immune system if inhaled, disease occurs with an overtly exuberant response resulting to allergic bronchoalveolar aspergillosis or allergic fungal rhinosinusitis [77 - 79].

Treatment

Treatment varies significantly with the types of disease. It may cause progressive destruction of lung tissue in patients who already has impaired pulmonary function. For allergic bronchopulmonary aspergillosis and aspergilloma, oral itraconazole (Fig. **2**) may be provided. It acts by blocking the ergosterol synthesis through cytochrome P450-dependant 14α-lanosterol demethylase which converts lanosterol to ergosterol [80]. For invasive aspergillosis and chronic necrotizing pulmonary aspergillosis, voriconazole is the drug of choice. The mechanism of action of voriconazole is similar to that of azoles [70, 81].

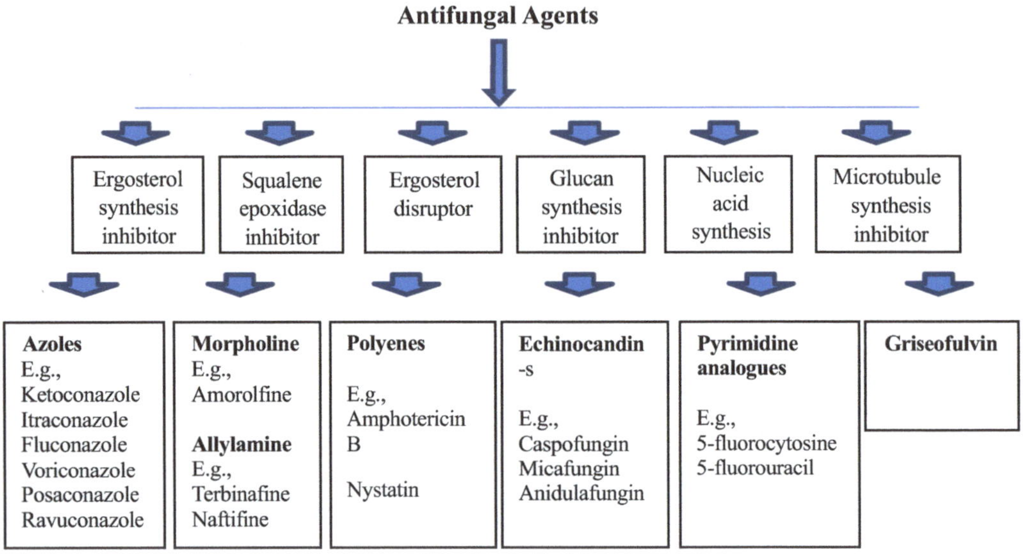

Fig. (2). Common agents/drugs used for treating fungal infection.

Candidiasis

Causal Organism: Candidiasis is caused by the yeast-like fungus *Candida*. There are number of *Candida* species that can cause diseases. However, the most common is *Candida albicans*. They normally live in the intestinal tract in latent state without causing infection but developed the symptoms when the strain become metabolically active and undergo multiplication. Candidiasis has three types *viz.,* candida infection of the mouth and throat, vaginal candidiasis and invasive candidiasis. Invasive candidiasis occurs when it enters the bloodstream and spread throughout the whole body [82].

Candida auris is a rapidly emerging fungal pathogen that can cause severe infections presenting a serious global health threat. It was first isolated from the ear discharge of a patient in 2009 in Japan [83, 84]. It is a multidrug-resistant, difficult to identify with standard laboratory methods and has caused outbreaks in healthcare settings. Recently, Centers for Disease Control and Prevention (CDC) has encouraged all the staff of the U.S laboratory to inform the state or local public health authorities and CDC if anyone identifies *Candida auris* [84].

Symptoms: Signs and symptoms of candidiasis infection includes patch of red, itchy skin, often leaking fluid, scabs, and pustules. They usually infect areas such as folds of buttocks, between the breasts, toes, fingers, *etc* [85]. It can also cause bloodstream, wound and ear infection [84].

***Pathogenesis*:** Candidiasis is usually transmitted during childbirth. It occurs when it enters the bloodstream and spread throughout the body. They are also transmitted through sexual contact [82, 84].

***Treatment*:** Azole-based antifungal agents are used for treatment of Candidiasis. Echinocandin (caspofungin, micafungin, or anidulafungin) or AmB are given to neutropenic patients. Fluconazole is injected through intra venom for candidemia patients [86, 87]. For treatment of *Candida auris* infections, echinocandin drugs (anidulafungin or caspfungin or micanfungin) are recommended (Fig. **2**) [84].

Blastomycosis

***Causal Organism*:** Blastomycosis is caused by *Blastomyces dermatitidis*. They are found in moist soil and in decomposing matters [88].

***Symptoms*:** Signs and symptoms of blastomycosis are similar to flu and other lung infections. It includes fever, cough, night sweats, muscle aches, weight loss, chest pain, and fatigue [88, 89].

Pathogenesis: It is caused by inhalation of *Blastomyces dermatitidis* spores. The spores further pass into the lower respiratory tract leading to pulmonary infection [90, 91].

Treatment: Itraconazole and AmB are the main drugs used for treating blastomycosis. Itraconazole is recommended to treat mild and moderate blastomycosis and AmB for severe blastomycosis in the lungs [92].

Coccidioidomycosis

***Causal Organism*:** Coccidioidomycosis is caused by pathogenic *Coccidioides*. It is also known as Valley Fever. They are commonly caused by *Coccidioides immitis* and *Coccidioides posadasii*. They are isolated from the soil of Southwestern United States and Central and South America [93].

***Symptoms*:** Signs and symptoms depend on the types of infection. Coccidioides have three forms *viz*., acute pulmonary coccidioidomycosis, chronic pulmonary coccidioidomycosis and disseminated coccidioidomycosis. Common symptoms include fever, cough with or without blood/mucus, fatigue, muscle aches, swelling of leg, joint pain, *etc* [94].

***Pathogenesis*:** Coccidioidomycosis infections are usually caused by inhalation of spores. The spores enter the terminal bronchioles, where they got enlarged forming spherules. The spherules get ruptured releasing the endospores and infect the tissues nearby and then spread throughout the body [95, 96].

***Treatment*:** Ketoconazole was the only drug approved by the US Food and Drug Administration for the treatment of coccidioidomycosis. However, for long-term treatment, it has been replaced with less-toxic triazoles such as fluconazole and itraconazole. Itraconazole is used for skeletal lesions treatment and fluconazole for pulmonary and soft tissue infection [97, 98].

Histoplasmosis

***Causal Organism*:** Histoplasmosis is caused by *Histoplasma capsulatum*. It can affect both immunocompromised and immunocompetent individuals. It is found in temperate climate throughout the world. However, it is endemic to Ohio and Mississippi river valleys, US. It lives in soil and material contaminated with large amount of birds or bats droppings [99].

***Symptoms*:** Fever, cough, extreme tiredness, chills, chest pain, *etc*. are some of the symptoms of histoplasmosis infection [100].

***Pathogenesis*:** Infections are acquired through inhalation of spores. The spores then enter the lungs, which is the site of infection. Further, spores are spread throughout the body infecting the organs with reticuloendothelial cells such as liver, spleen, lymph node, and bone marrow [101].

***Treatment*:** Treatment is not required for asymptomatic individuals. AmB is recommended for patients with severe infection. After 1-2 weeks once the patient is stable, AmB may be replaced by itraconazole [102].

Ringworm

***Causal Organism*:** Ringworm is also known as tinea or dermatophytosis. It is caused by *Trichophyton* and *Microsporum*. It usually infects the skin, hair and nails. When it infects the soles, it is called tinea pedis or athlete's foot. Infection on inner thighs and buttocks are referred to as tinea cruris or jock itch, on the beard area it's called tinea barbae, and if it's on the fingernails and toenails it is called tinea unguium or onychomycosis [103].

***Symptoms*:** Symptoms of ringworm depends on the sites of infection. It usually includes itchy skin, red-scaly or cracked skin, ring-shaped rash and, loss of hair in the infected area [103].

***Pathogenesis*:** Infection is acquired through deposition of viable spores or hyphae on the surface of susceptible individual. The fungal hyphae then grow in the stratum corneum which further continues to grow downward into the hair thereby invading keratin. The hyphae extend upwards at the rate of hair growth. Finally, the hair becomes brittle and broken. Infection at toenails and fingernails are called onychomycosis. The fungus spreads from plantar skin and invades the nail bed through hyponychium resulting in nail thickening, causing discoloured and brittle of nail. Dermatophytosis (fungal skin infection) spreads through direct contact with the fungus contaminated soil and also with infected animals or humans. This results in red, itchy, scaly and formation of circular rash. Hair loss in the affected area may occur [104, 105].

***Treatment*:** Drug of choice for the treatment of ringworm infection includes ketoconazole, griseofulvin and terbinafine (Fig. **2**) [106].

Sporotrichosis

***Causal Organism*:** The disease is also called as rose gardener's disease. It is a rare infection caused by *Sporothrix schenckii*. This fungus lives in soil and plant matters such as rose bushes, hay, *etc*. Sporotrichosis is of three type *viz*., cutaneous (skin) sporotrichosis, pulmonary (lung) sporotrichosis and disseminated sporotrichosis [107, 108].

***Symptoms*:** It depends on the area of infection. Signs and symptoms of cutaneous (skin) sporotrichosis are bump on finger, hand or arm. Cough, fever, chest pain and shortness of breath are the important symptoms of pulmonary (lung) sporotrichosis and symptoms of disseminated sporotrichosis includes joint pain, headache and seizures [109].

***Pathogenesis*:** Infection is acquired through exposure to contaminated plant materials. However, zoonotic transmission occurs through inhalation of infective fungal propagules. The mycosis can also be transmitted through animal bites or scratches. The infection spreads along lymphatic channel and then to the nearby tissues by direct extension, and finally to other parts of the body [119, 110, 111].

***Treatment*:** Itraconazole is used for the treatment of sporotrichosis.

CONCLUDING REMARKS

Since 1960s antifungal therapy has evolved. For decades, AmB was the only drug of choice for treating fungal infections until the introduction of the azoles family. Development and approval of azoles in 1980s was effective in treating the fungal infections. Further introduction of the six new antifungal agents *viz*., three triazoles, echinocandins, sordarins and other sterol synthesis inhibitors greatly improved in combating the diseases. Although much progress has been accomplished towards the identification of new antifungal compounds/drugs, excessive use of the same available drugs has led to the development of multi-drug resistant fungal strains. Therefore, infections/diseases caused by these multidrug resistant strains no longer respond to treatment. Further search for discovery of new antifungal compounds that have potent activity, novel mechanism of action against drug-resistant fungal strains and have less adverse effects to human health are urgently required to combat the diseases caused by drug-resistant fungal pathogens.

Most of the antifungal agents are derived from soil actinomycetes. It is of utmost important to explore antifungal agents from various habitats. A number of reports are now available on antifungal activity by bacterial/fungal endophytes isolated from various medicinal plants. Many of the compounds produced by these fungal endophytes exhibited broad spectrum antifungal activity and they could be promising source for development of novel antifungal bioactive agents.

CONSENT FOR PUBLICATION

Not applicable.

CONFLICT OF INTEREST

The authors confirm that this chapter contents have no conflict of interest.

ACKNOWLEDGEMENTS

Authors acknowledge the grant from the Department of Biotechnology (DBT), Government of India, given to the Advanced Level State Biotech Hub (BT/04/NE/2009) that facilitates the writing.

REFERENCES

[1] Ochiai A, Ogawa K, Fukuda M, *et al.* Rice Defensin OsAFP1 is a New Drug Candidate against Human Pathogenic Fungi. Sci Rep 2018; 8(1): 11434. [http://dx.doi.org/10.1038/s41598-018-29715-w] [PMID: 30061724]

[2] Ravikant KT. Gupte S, Kaur M. A review on emerging fungal infections and their significance. J Bacteriol Mycol 2015; 1(2): 39-41.

[3] Jones KE, Patel NG, Levy MA, *et al.* Global trends in emerging infectious diseases. Nature 2008; 451(7181): 990-3. [http://dx.doi.org/10.1038/nature06536] [PMID: 18288193]

[4] Garcia-Solache MA, Casadevall A. Global warming will bring new fungal diseases for mammals. MBio 2010; 1(1): 1. [http://dx.doi.org/10.1128/mBio.00061-10] [PMID: 20689745]

[5] Hawksworth DL. The magnitude of fungal diversity: the 1.5 million species estimate revisited. Mycol Res 2001; 105: 1422-32. [http://dx.doi.org/10.1017/S0953756201004725]

[6] Tedersoo L, Bahram M, Põlme S, *et al.* Fungal biogeography. Global diversity and geography of soil fungi. Science 2014; 346(6213)1256688 [http://dx.doi.org/10.1126/science.1256688] [PMID: 25430773]

[7] Ramanan P, Wengenack NL. Theel. Laboratory Diagnostics for Fungal Infections A Review of Current and Future Diagnostic Assays. Clin Chest Med 2017; 38: 535-54.

[8] Walsh TJ, Groll AH. Emerging fungal pathogens: evolving challenges to immunocompromised patients for the twenty-first century. Transpl Infect Dis 1999; 1(4): 247-61. [http://dx.doi.org/10.1034/j.1399-3062.1999.010404.x] [PMID: 11428996]

[9] Enoch DA, Ludlam HA, Brown NM. Invasive fungal infections: a review of epidemiology and management options. J Med Microbiol 2006; 55(Pt 7): 809-18. [http://dx.doi.org/10.1099/jmm.0.46548-0] [PMID: 16772406]

[10] Martinez-Rossi NM, Bitencourt TA, Peres NTA, *et al.* Resistance to antifungal drugs: mechanisms and prospectus. Front Microbiol 2018; 9: 1108. [http://dx.doi.org/10.3389/fmicb.2018.01108] [PMID: 29896175]

[11] Scorzoni L, de Paula E Silva AC, Marcos CM, *et al.* Antifungal therapy: new advances in the understanding and treatment of mycosis. Front Microbiol 2017; 8: 36. [http://dx.doi.org/10.3389/fmicb.2017.00036] [PMID: 28167935]

[12] Hope WW, McEntee L, Livermore J, *et al.* Pharmacodynamics of the orotomides against *Aspergillus fumigatus*: new opportunities for treatment of multidrug-resistant fungal disease. MBio 2017; 8(4): e01157-17. [http://dx.doi.org/10.1128/mBio.01157-17] [PMID: 28830945]

[13] Odds FC, Brown AJ, Gow NA. Antifungal agents: mechanisms of action. Trends Microbiol 2003; 11(6): 272-9. [http://dx.doi.org/10.1016/S0966-842X(03)00117-3] [PMID: 12823944]

[14] Sachin JA, Aanandhi MV. A brief review on current antifungal agents. Dit 2018; 10(1)

[15] White TC, Marr KA, Bowden RA. Clinical, cellular, and molecular factors that contribute to antifungal drug resistance. Clin Microbiol Rev 1998; 11(2): 382-402. [http://dx.doi.org/10.1128/CMR.11.2.382] [PMID: 9564569]

[16] Ghannoum MA, Rice LB. Antifungal agents: mode of action, mechanisms of resistance, and correlation of these mechanisms with bacterial resistance. Clin Microbiol Rev 1999; 12(4): 501-17. [http://dx.doi.org/10.1128/CMR.12.4.501] [PMID: 10515900]

[17] Richardson MD, Warnock DW. New directions in diagnosis.Fungal infection: diagnosis and management. 4. Manchester: Wiley-Blackwell Publishing 2012; 9.

[18] Harvey JC, Cantrell JR, Fisher AM. Actinomycosis: its recognition and treatment. Ann Intern Med 1957; 46(5): 868-85. [http://dx.doi.org/10.7326/0003-4819-46-5-868] [PMID: 13411897]

[19] Urabe H, Nagashima T. Mechanism of antifungal action of potassium iodide on sporotrichosis. Dermatol Int 1969; 8(1): 36-9. [http://dx.doi.org/10.1111/j.1365-4362.1969.tb05327.x] [PMID: 5343406]

[20] Malayeri FA, Rezaei AA, Raiesi O. Antifungal agents: polyene, azole, antimetabolite, other and future agents. J Bas Res Med Sci 2018; 5(2): 48-55. [http://dx.doi.org/10.29252/jbrms.5.2.48]

[21] Develoux M. [Griseofulvin]. Ann Dermatol Venereol 2001; 128(12): 1317-25. [PMID: 11908134]

[22] Campoy S, Adrio JL. Antifungals. Biochem Pharmacol 2017; 133: 86-96. [http://dx.doi.org/10.1016/j.bcp.2016.11.019] [PMID: 27884742]

[23] Su H, Han L, Huang X. Potential targets for the development of new antifungal drugs. J Antibiot (Tokyo) 2018; 71(12): 978-91. [http://dx.doi.org/10.1038/s41429-018-0100-9] [PMID: 30242283]

[24] Dudley RW. A brief review of antifungal drugs old and new. Mod Appl Pharm Pharmacol 2018; 2(1) 000530.
[http://dx.doi.org/10.31031/MAPP.2018.02.000530]

[25] Kathiravan MK, Salake AB, Chothe AS, *et al.* The biology and chemistry of antifungal agents: a review. Bioorg Med Chem 2012; 20(19): 5678-98.
[http://dx.doi.org/10.1016/j.bmc.2012.04.045] [PMID: 22902032]

[26] Geißel B, Loiko V, Klugherz I, *et al.* Azole-induced cell wall carbohydrate patches kill Aspergillus fumigatus. Nat Commun 2018; 9(1): 3098.
[http://dx.doi.org/10.1038/s41467-018-05497-7] [PMID: 30082817]

[27] Wiederhold NP. The antifungal arsenal: alternative drugs and future targets. Int J Antimicrob Agents 2018; 51(3): 333-9.
[http://dx.doi.org/10.1016/j.ijantimicag.2017.09.002] [PMID: 28890395]

[28] Gavarkar PS, Adnaik RS, Mohite SK. An overview of azole antifungals. Int J Pharm Sci Res 2013; 4: 4083-9.

[29] Prasad R, Shah AH, Rawal MK. Antifungals: mechanism of action and drug resistance.Yeast membrane transport. New York: Springer 2016; pp. 327-49.
[http://dx.doi.org/10.1007/978-3-319-25304-6_14]

[30] Del Poeta M. Special issue: novel antifungal drug discovery. J Fungi (Basel) 2016; 2(4): 33.
[http://dx.doi.org/10.3390/jof2040033] [PMID: 28058254]

[31] Liu N, Tu J, Dong G, Wang Y, Sheng C. Emerging new targets for the treatment of resistant fungal infections. J Med Chem 2018; 61(13): 5484-511.
[http://dx.doi.org/10.1021/acs.jmedchem.7b01413] [PMID: 29294275]

[32] Balkovec JM, Black RM, Hammond ML, *et al.* Synthesis, stability, and biological evaluation of water-soluble prodrugs of a new echinocandin lipopeptide. Discovery of a potential clinical agent for the treatment of systemic candidiasis and Pneumocystis carinii pneumonia (PCP). J Med Chem 1992; 35(1): 194-8.
[http://dx.doi.org/10.1021/jm00079a027] [PMID: 1732529]

[33] Rodrigues ME, Silva S, Azeredo J, Henriques M. Novel strategies to fight Candida species infection. Crit Rev Microbiol 2016; 42(4): 594-606.
[PMID: 25383647]

[34] Roemer T, Krysan DJ. Antifungal drug development: challenges, unmet clinical needs, and new approaches. Cold Spring Harb Perspect Med 2014; 4(5) a019703.
[http://dx.doi.org/10.1101/cshperspect.a019703] [PMID: 24789878]

[35] McCarthy MW, Kontoyiannis DP, Cornely OA, Perfect JR, Walsh TJ. Novel agents and drug targets to meet the challenges of resistant fungi. J Infect Dis 2017; 216 (suppl_3): S474-83.
[http://dx.doi.org/10.1093/infdis/jix130] [PMID: 28911042]

[36] Hammond SM, Lambert PA, Kliger BN. The mode of action of polyene antibiotics; induced potassium leakage in Candida albicans. J Gen Microbiol 1974; 81(2): 325-30.
[http://dx.doi.org/10.1099/00221287-81-2-325] [PMID: 4599408]

[37] Kim H-J, Han C-Y, Park J-S, *et al.* Nystatin-like Pseudonocardia polyene B1, a novel disaccharide-containing antifungal heptaene antibiotic. Sci Rep 2018; 8(1): 13584.
[http://dx.doi.org/10.1038/s41598-018-31801-y] [PMID: 30206268]

[38] d'Enfert C, Bougnoux ME. Polyenes.Human Fungal Infections. 3rd ed., Reference Module in Biomedical Research 2014.

[39] Kleinberg M. What is the current and future status of conventional amphotericin B? Int J Antimicrob Agents 2006; 27 (Suppl. 1): 12-6.
[http://dx.doi.org/10.1016/j.ijantimicag.2006.03.013] [PMID: 16707251]

[40] Ellis D. Amphotericin B: spectrum and resistance. J Antimicrob Chemother 2002; 49 (Suppl. 1): 7-10. [http://dx.doi.org/10.1093/jac/49.suppl_1.7] [PMID: 11801575]

[41] Enoch DA, Ludlam HA, Brown NM. Invasive fungal infections: a review of epidemiology and management options. J Med Microbiol 2006; 55(Pt 7): 809-18. [http://dx.doi.org/10.1099/jmm.0.46548-0] [PMID: 16772406]

[42] Baginski M, Czub J. Amphotericin B and its new derivatives - mode of action. Curr Drug Metab 2009; 10(5): 459-69. [http://dx.doi.org/10.2174/138920009788898019] [PMID: 19689243]

[43] Schaffner CP. Macrolide antibiotics. 1st ed. Orlando: Academic Press, Inc. 1984; pp. 457-507.

[44] Ostrosky-Zeichner L, Marr KA, Rex JH, Cohen SH, Amphotericin B. Amphotericin B: time for a new "gold standard". Clin Infect Dis 2003; 37(3): 415-25. [http://dx.doi.org/10.1086/376634] [PMID: 12884167]

[45] Cereghetti D, Carreira E. Amphotericin B: 50 years of chemistry and biochemistry. Synthesis 2006; 6: 914-42.

[46] Brown GD, Denning DW, Gow NAR, Levitz SM, Netea MG, White TC. Hidden killers: human fungal infections. Sci Transl Med 2012; 4(165)165rv13 [http://dx.doi.org/10.1126/scitranslmed.3004404] [PMID: 23253612]

[47] Barrett JP, Vardulaki KA, Conlon C, *et al.* A systematic review of the antifungal effectiveness and tolerability of amphotericin B formulations. Clin Ther 2003; 25(5): 1295-320. [http://dx.doi.org/10.1016/S0149-2918(03)80125-X] [PMID: 12867214]

[48] Kleinberg M. What is the current and future status of conventional amphotericin B? Int J Antimicrob Agents 2006; 27 (Suppl. 1): 12-6. [http://dx.doi.org/10.1016/j.ijantimicag.2006.03.013] [PMID: 16707251]

[49] Veerareddy PR, Vobalaboina V. Lipid-based formulations of amphotericin B. Drugs Today (Barc) 2004; 40(2): 133-45. [http://dx.doi.org/10.1358/dot.2004.40.2.799425] [PMID: 15045035]

[50] Dupont B. Overview of the lipid formulations of amphotericin B. J Antimicrob Chemother 2002; 49 (Suppl. 1): 31-6. [http://dx.doi.org/10.1093/jac/49.suppl_1.31] [PMID: 11801578]

[51] Antoniadou A, Dupont B. Lipid formulations of amphotericin B: where are we today? J Mycol Med 2005; 15: 230-8. [http://dx.doi.org/10.1016/j.mycmed.2005.06.005]

[52] Boswell GW, Buell D, Bekersky I. AmBisome (liposomal amphotericin B): a comparative review. J Clin Pharmacol 1998; 38(7): 583-92. [http://dx.doi.org/10.1002/j.1552-4604.1998.tb04464.x] [PMID: 9702842]

[53] Brown R, Hazen EL. Present knowledge of nystatin, an antifungal antibiotic. Trans N Y Acad Sci 1957; 19(5): 447-56. [PMID: 13422562]

[54] Waller DG, Sampson AP. Chemotherapy of infections.Medical Pharmacology and Therapeutics. 5th. UK 2018; pp. 581-629. [http://dx.doi.org/10.1016/B978-0-7020-7167-6.00051-8]

[55] Sloane MB. A new antifungal antibiotic, mycostatin (nystatin), for the treatment of moniliasis: a preliminary report. J Invest Dermatol 1955; 24(6): 569-71. [http://dx.doi.org/10.1038/jid.1955.77] [PMID: 13242889]

[56] Arikan S, Rex JH. Lipid-based antifungal agents: current status. Curr Pharm Des 2001; 7(5): 393-415. [http://dx.doi.org/10.2174/1381612013398031] [PMID: 11254895]

[57] Gupta AK, Sauder DN, Shear NH. Antifungal agents: an overview. Part II. J Am Acad Dermatol 1994; 30(6): 911-33.
[http://dx.doi.org/10.1016/S0190-9622(94)70112-1] [PMID: 7619094]

[58] de Kruijff B, Demel RA. Polyene antibiotic-sterol interactions in membranes of Acholeplasma laidlawii cells and lecithin liposomes. 3. Molecular structure of the polyene antibiotic-cholesterol complexes. Biochim Biophys Acta 1974; 339(1): 57-70.
[http://dx.doi.org/10.1016/0005-2736(74)90332-0] [PMID: 4546885]

[59] Gale EF. The release of potassium ions from *Candida albicans* in the presence of polyene antibiotics. J Gen Microbiol 1974; 80(2): 451-65.
[http://dx.doi.org/10.1099/00221287-80-2-451] [PMID: 4596987]

[60] Andreoli TE, Dennis VW, Weigl AM. The effect of amphotericin B on the water and nonelectrolyte permeability of thin lipid membranes. J Gen Physiol 1969; 53(2): 133-56.
[http://dx.doi.org/10.1085/jgp.53.2.133] [PMID: 5764743]

[61] Holz R, Finkelstein A. The water and nonelectrolyte permeability induced in thin lipid membranes by the polyene antibiotics nystatin and amphotericin B. J Gen Physiol 1970; 56(1): 125-45.
[http://dx.doi.org/10.1085/jgp.56.1.125] [PMID: 5514158]

[62] Chen WC, Chou DL, Feingold DS. Dissociation between ion permeability and the lethal action of polyene antibiotics on Candida albicans. Antimicrob Agents Chemother 1978; 13(6): 914-7.
[http://dx.doi.org/10.1128/AAC.13.6.914] [PMID: 354520]

[63] Palacios J, Serrano R. Proton permeability induced by polyene antibiotics. A plausible mechanism for their inhibition of maltose fermentation in yeast. FEBS Lett 1978; 91(2): 198-201.
[http://dx.doi.org/10.1016/0014-5793(78)81171-5] [PMID: 28247]

[64] Bracey D, Holyoak CD, Coote PJ. Comparison of the inhibitory effect of sorbic acid and amphotericin B on *Saccharomyces cerevisiae*: is growth inhibition dependent on reduced intracellular pH? J Appl Microbiol 1998; 85(6): 1056-66.
[http://dx.doi.org/10.1111/j.1365-2672.1998.tb05271.x] [PMID: 9871326]

[65] Haraguchi H, Taniguchi M, Motoba K, Shibata K, Oi S, Hashimoto K. Chrysodin, an antifungal antimetabolite. Agric Biol Chem 1990; 54(8): 2167-8.

[66] Arikan S, Rex J, Murray P, *et al.* Antifungal agents. Manual of clinical microbiology 2006; 2(9): 1949-60.

[67] Medoff G, Brajtburg J, Kobayashi GS, Bolard J. Antifungal agents useful in therapy of systemic fungal infections. Annu Rev Pharmacol Toxicol 1983; 23(1): 303-30.
[http://dx.doi.org/10.1146/annurev.pa.23.040183.001511] [PMID: 6307124]

[68] Elewski BE. Mechanisms of action of systemic antifungal agents. J Am Acad Dermatol 1993; 28(5 Pt 1): S28-34.
[http://dx.doi.org/10.1016/S0190-9622(09)80305-8] [PMID: 8496409]

[69] https://www.drugbank.ca/drugs/DB00400.

[70] Harman EM, Soo Hoo GW, Talavera F. Background of Aspergillosis Medscape medical news https://emedicine.medscape.com/article/296052-overview#a5.

[71] Ullmann AJ, Aguado JM, Arikan-Akdagli S, *et al.* Diagnosis and management of Aspergillus diseases: executive summary of the 2017 ESCMID-ECMM-ERS guideline. Clin Microbiol Infect 2018; 24 (Suppl. 1): e1-e38.
[http://dx.doi.org/10.1016/j.cmi.2018.01.002] [PMID: 29544767]

[72] Patterson TF, Thompson GR III, Denning DW, *et al.* Practice guidelines for the diagnosis and management of aspergillosis: update by the Infectious Diseases Society of America. Clin Infect Dis 2016; 63(4): e1-e60.
[http://dx.doi.org/10.1093/cid/ciw326] [PMID: 27365388]

[73] Allergic bronchopulmonary aspergillosis (ABPA). American Academy of Allergy, Asthma & Immunology. https://www.aaaai.org/conditions-and-treatments/related-conditions/allergic-bronchopulmonary-aspergillosis.

[74] Aspergillosis. Centers for Disease Control and Prevention. https://www.cdc.gov/fungal/diseases/aspergillosis/.

[75] Kauffman CA. Diagnosis of invasive aspergillosis https://www.uptodate.com/contents/search.

[76] Kauffman CA. Treatment and prevention of invasive aspergillosis https://www.uptodate.com/contents/search.

[77] Park SJ, Mehrad B. Innate immunity to Aspergillus species. Clin Microbiol Rev 2009; 22(4): 535-51. [http://dx.doi.org/10.1128/CMR.00014-09] [PMID: 19822887]

[78] Barnes PD, Marr KA. Aspergillosis: spectrum of disease, diagnosis, and treatment. Infect Dis Clin North Am 2006; 20(3): 545-561, vi. [http://dx.doi.org/10.1016/j.idc.2006.06.001] [PMID: 16984868]

[79] Challa S. Pathogenesis and Pathology of Invasive Aspergillosis. Curr Fungal Infect Rep 2018; 12(1): 23-32. [http://dx.doi.org/10.1007/s12281-018-0310-4]

[80] Giron JM, Poey CG, Fajadet PP, *et al.* Inoperable pulmonary aspergilloma: percutaneous CT-guided injection with glycerin and amphotericin B paste in 15 cases. Radiology 1993; 188(3): 825-7. [http://dx.doi.org/10.1148/radiology.188.3.8351356] [PMID: 8351356]

[81] Herbrecht R, Denning DW, Patterson TF, *et al.* Voriconazole *versus* amphotericin B for primary therapy of invasive aspergillosis. N Engl J Med 2002; 347(6): 408-15. [http://dx.doi.org/10.1056/NEJMoa020191] [PMID: 12167683]

[82] Centers for Disease Control and Prevention https://www.cdc.gov/fungal/diseases/candidiasis/index.html.

[83] Satoh K, Makimura K, Hasumi Y, Nishiyama Y, Uchida K, Yamaguchi H. *Candida auris* sp. nov., a novel ascomycetous yeast isolated from the external ear canal of an inpatient in a Japanese hospital. Microbiol Immunol 2009; 53(1): 41-4. [http://dx.doi.org/10.1111/j.1348-0421.2008.00083.x] [PMID: 19161556]

[84] Ku TSN, Walraven CJ, Lee SA. *Candida auris*: Disinfectants and Implications for Infection Control. Front Microbiol 2018; 9: 726. [http://dx.doi.org/10.3389/fmicb.2018.00726] [PMID: 29706945]

[85] https://medbroadcast.com/condition/getcondition/candidiasis.

[86] Nguyen MH, Peacock JE Jr, Tanner DC, *et al.* Therapeutic approaches in patients with candidemia. Evaluation in a multicenter, prospective, observational study. Arch Intern Med 1995; 155(22): 2429-35. [http://dx.doi.org/10.1001/archinte.1995.00430220087009] [PMID: 7503601]

[87] Pappas PG, Kauffman CA, Andes D, *et al.* Clinical practice guidelines for the management of candidiasis: 2009 update by the Infectious Diseases Society of America. Clin Infect Dis 2009; 48(5): 503-35. [http://dx.doi.org/10.1086/596757] [PMID: 19191635]

[88] Saccente M, Woods GL. Clinical and laboratory update on blastomycosis. Clin Microbiol Rev 2010; 23(2): 367-81. [http://dx.doi.org/10.1128/CMR.00056-09] [PMID: 20375357]

[89] Baumgardner DJ, Halsmer SE, Egan G. Symptoms of pulmonary blastomycosis: northern Wisconsin, United States. Wilderness Environ Med 2004; 15(4): 250-6. [http://dx.doi.org/10.1580/1080-6032(2004)015[0250:SOPBNW]2.0.CO;2] [PMID: 15636375]

[90] Chima-Melton C, Steele RW. Blastomycosis. Medscape. https://emedicine.medscape.com/article/296870-overview#a4

[91] Rooney PJ, Sullivan TD, Klein BS. Selective expression of the virulence factor BAD1 upon morphogenesis to the pathogenic yeast form of *Blastomyces dermatitidis*: evidence for transcriptional regulation by a conserved mechanism. Mol Microbiol 2001; 39(4): 875-89. [http://dx.doi.org/10.1046/j.1365-2958.2001.02300.x] [PMID: 11251809]

[92] Chapman SW, Dismukes WE, Proia LA, *et al.* Clinical practice guidelines for the management of blastomycosis: 2008 update by the Infectious Diseases Society of America. Clin Infect Dis 2008; 46(12): 1801-12. [http://dx.doi.org/10.1086/588300] [PMID: 18462107]

[93] Fungal Diseases Centers for Disease Control and Prevention https://www.cdc.gov/fungal/diseases/coccidioidomycosis/symptoms.html.

[94] Chung CR, Lee YC, Rhee YK, *et al.* Pulmonary coccidioidomycosis with peritoneal involvement mimicking lung cancer with peritoneal carcinomatosis. Am J Respir Crit Care Med 2011; 183(1): 135-6.https://www.thoracic.org/patients/patient-resources/resources/coccidioidomycosis.pdf. [http://dx.doi.org/10.1164/ajrccm.183.1.135] [PMID: 21193791]

[95] Li L, Dial SM, Schmelz M, Rennels MA, Ampel NM. Cellular immune suppressor activity resides in lymphocyte cell clusters adjacent to granulomata in human coccidioidomycosis. Infect Immun 2005; 73(7): 3923-8. [http://dx.doi.org/10.1128/IAI.73.7.3923-3928.2005] [PMID: 15972478]

[96] Ampel NM, Hoover SE. Pathogenesis of Coccidioidomycosis. Curr Fungal Infect Rep 2015; 9(4): 253-8. [http://dx.doi.org/10.1007/s12281-015-0242-1]

[97] Galgiani JN, Catanzaro A, Cloud GA, *et al.* Comparison of oral fluconazole and itraconazole for progressive, nonmeningeal coccidioidomycosis. A randomized, double-blind trial. Ann Intern Med 2000; 133(9): 676-86. [http://dx.doi.org/10.7326/0003-4819-133-9-200011070-00009] [PMID: 11074900]

[98] Hospenthal DR, Thompson GR, Oppenheimer AP, Arsura EL. Coccidioidomycosis and Valley Fever Treatment & Management Medscape 2018.https://emedicine.medscape.com/article/215978-treatment#d8.

[99] Fayyaz J, Vydyula R, Walczyszyn MP, Lessnau KD. Histoplasmosis Medscape 2018. https://emedicine.medscape.com/article/299054-overview#a4.

[100] Fungal Diseases Centers for Disease Control and Prevention https://www.cdc.gov/fungal/diseases/histoplasmosis/symptoms.html.

[101] Edwards JA, Rappleye CA. Histoplasma mechanisms of pathogenesis--one portfolio doesn't fit all. FEMS Microbiol Lett 2011; 324(1): 1-9. [http://dx.doi.org/10.1111/j.1574-6968.2011.02363.x] [PMID: 22092757]

[102] Fayyaz J, Vydyula R, Walczyszyn MP, Lessnau KD. Histoplasmosis. Medscape. 2018. https://emedicine.medscape.com/article/299054-treatment.

[103] Joseph BC. What Is Ringworm? Symptoms, Causes, and Treatment https://www.everydayhealth.com/ringworm/guide.

[104] Tainwala R, Sharma Y. Pathogenesis of dermatophytoses. Indian J Dermatol 2011; 56(3): 259-61. [http://dx.doi.org/10.4103/0019-5154.82476] [PMID: 21772583]

[105] Handler MZ, Stephany MP, Schwartz RA. Tinea Capitis Medscape 2018. https://emedicine.medscape.com/article/1091351-overview#a5.

[106] Dock E. Healthline Newsletter 2017.https://www.healthline.com/health/ringworm.

[107] Barros MB, de Almeida Paes R, Schubach AO. *Sporothrix schenckii* and Sporotrichosis. Clin Microbiol Rev 2011; 24(4): 633-54.
[http://dx.doi.org/10.1128/CMR.00007-11] [PMID: 21976602]

[108] Chakrabarti A, Bonifaz A, Gutierrez-Galhardo MC, Mochizuki T, Li S. Global epidemiology of sporotrichosis. Med Mycol 2015; 53(1): 3-14.
[http://dx.doi.org/10.1093/mmy/myu062] [PMID: 25526781]

[109] Fungal Diseases Centers for Disease Control and Prevention https://www.cdc.gov/fungal/diseases /sporotrichosis/index.html.

[110] Agudelo Higuita NI. Sporotrichosis Medscape 2018.https://emedicine.medscape.com/article/228723-overview#a5.

[111] Orofino-Costa R, Macedo PM, Rodrigues AM, Bernardes-Engemann AR. Sporotrichosis: an update on epidemiology, etiopathogenesis, laboratory and clinical therapeutics. An Bras Dermatol 2017; 92(5): 606-20.
[http://dx.doi.org/10.1590/abd1806-4841.2017279] [PMID: 29166494]

CHAPTER 7

Emerging Viral Diseases and Potential Therapeutic Agents for Their Control

Sumita Banerjee*

Department of Oral Pathology & Microbiology, Regional Institute of Medical Sciences, Dental College, Imphal, Manipur, 795004, India

Abstract: The emerging infectious human viral diseases have been a prime concern for public health since the last decade. Various new viruses or virulent strains of old viruses have emerged during this period. Appropriate knowledge of the viral pathogenesis is required to understand their emergence and possible therapies. Various factors are involved in the emergence of viruses and new human diseases. Some of these human diseases are zoonosis. Zoonosis can be defined as human diseases caused by animal pathogens, which that are transmitted to humans. The WHO has been continuously updating the prioritizing list for various infectious, and emerging viruses. In this chapter, we discussed some important emergent viral pathogens, such as Ebola virus, Crimean-Congo Haemorrhagic Fever virus, and Marburg virus, Hanta, Hendra, and SARS. Detailed understanding of the emergence, the modes of transmission and pathogenesis, and possible treatment plans are necessary to check the invasion and outbreak caused by these viruses.

Keywords: Emerging viral diseases, Crimean-Congo Haemorrhagic Fever virus, Ebola, Hanta, Hendra, SARS.

INTRODUCTION

Infectious diseases cause societal and economic problems causing nearly one in five human deaths worldwide. An emerging infectious pathogen is an infectious agent which has emerged in a population and its geographical ranges gets expanding rapidly, an old phenomena documented by Roman and Persian philosophers. They wrote about the devastating disease plague in the time of ancient Greece [1, 2]. There is historical evidence of the deadliest Pandemic Emerging infectious diseases (EIDs) such as 14th century Black Death (75 to 200 million deaths by the pneumonic plague); Spanish influenza pandemic in 1918-1919 (50 to 100 million deaths) [3]. HIV, the most potent killer of infectious origin had a

* **Corresponding author Sumita Banerjee:** Department of Oral Pathology & Microbiology, Regional Institute of Medical Sciences, Dental College, Imphal, Manipur, 795004, India; Tel: +91 813 2821 691;
E-mail: banerjeesumi10@gmail.com

K. Tamreihao, Saikat Mukherjee and Debananda S. Ningthoujam (Eds.)
All rights reserved-© 2019 Bentham Science Publishers

peak incidence in 1997, along with 3·3 million new infections.

After the development of antiretroviral drugs, the incidence number had declined in 2005, however, total number of HIV/AIDS infected people has reached 38·8 million in 2015 [4].

The first declared pandemic of the 21st century, in 2009, a swine-origin H1N1 influenza got spread rapidly to 213 countries [5]. In 2014, the WHO announced the Ebola outbreak in West Africa a "public health emergency of international concern" [6, 7]. Appearance of 335 infectious diseases in human population from 1940 to 2004 had been reported by Jones and co-workers of which nearly two-thirds originated in wildlife [8]. New patterns of deadly disease outbreaks caused by novel animal viruses are reported such as Nipah prevalence in Malaysia, hantavirus (United States), Hendra virus (Australia), SARS also known as severe acute respiratory syndrome virus and MERS also known as Middle East respiratory syndrome coronavirus. According to Jones and co-workers, EID origins are multifactorial and can be directly correlated ecological, environmental and socio-economic factors that can lead to identification of emerging disease 'hotspots' [9].

Possible Causes Behind the Emergence of New Viral Diseases

There is a plethora of determinants that can lead to the emergence of infectious diseases (Table **1**).

Table 1. Causes for Emergence or Re-emergence of Viral Diseases [1 - 9].

Factors Leading to Emergence	Determinants
Economic and social development	Population growth, density, distribution Environmental changes such as deforestation, dam building, global warming Increased global travel Increased international commerce Agribusiness, food processing, distribution Ecological changes and agricultural development
Poverty	Inadequate public health systems Open defecation Lack of safe water Breakdown of public Health measures and deficiencies in Public health infrastructure
Societal breakdown	Civil chaos War Changes in human demographics and behaviour

(Table 1) cont.....

Factors Leading to Emergence	Determinants
Human factors	Sexual activity Substance abuse
Biological factors	Natural mutation Antimicrobial resistance Immunosuppression
Climate change	It also plays important role in the emergence of an infectious disease

In some instances, the "emergence" of a viral disease represents the first identification of the cause of a well-recognized disease. Emergence of novel disease reflected a new found ability to identify the etiologic entity [10].

***Disease Caused by an Existing Virus*:** Many times, a virus which is already existing can cause epidemic or endemic because of increased ratio of cases to infections. an already wide spreading virus in a population can emerge as a cause of epidemic or endemic disease, due to an increase in the ratio of cases to infections. This can be caused by enhancement of virus virulence or increased host susceptibility such as Poliomyelitis which caused summer outbreaks of acute infantile paralysis in United States and Sweden in nineteenth century. Through extensive vaccination efforts, eradicating polio is perhaps the largest worldwide public health initiative in history [6]. Unfortunately, poliovirus has begun to re-emerge in once polio-free countries and infections now occurred in susceptible children, resulting in outbreaks of infantile paralysis [11 - 13].

Increase in Viral Virulence: An emergence of the dramatic outbreak of viral infections can be attributed to sudden increases in virulence factor. In early 1983, a lethal outbreak of avian influenza was reported in Pennsylvania. Initially, the infections were mild but the 2nd attack in the same region was severely wide spreading making it pandemic. However, the viral strains from both the isolates had exactly similar genomes. The virulent strain had a point mutation in hemagglutinin enabling hemagglutinin cleavage and made it capable for replication outside respiratory tract, thereby increased virulence [7]. The most challenging viral adaptation mechanism is gene mutation and RNA viruses very commonly acquire this mutation. RNA viruses have a mutation rate of 10^{-4} to 10^{-6} /bp/generation [14]. Mutations facilitate the viral population to adapt to a new host or changing environment. Reassortment, and recombination are the two other adaptation mechanisms. Reassortment is very common for Influenza virus. When two viral strains of *e.g.*, avian and human influenza viruses) infects the host simultaneously, a new virus progeny with recombined genome could appear and the host further gets susceptible to the new strain of viruses due to the lack of available immunity to the specific strain. The pandemic attack by emerging

Influenza strains, in 1957, 1968 and 2009, was caused by a process known as gene shuffling [15]. Enteroviruses which infect the gastrointestinal tract for a long period of time shows most recombination [16]. Similarly, in Polio vaccine which has three polio virus strains, recombinations are observed. These strains undergo mutations as well as recombinations, thereby increasing neuropathogenicity [17, 18].

***Accumulation of Susceptible Hosts*:** Emergence of viral infection depends on the number of susceptible hosts. If the number is below the critical level for perpetuation, the disease may "fade out" and disappear. In an isolated population, the virus may remain absent for many years. In this time interval, accumulation of further population susceptible for the disease will contribute for the re-emergence of the disease and may cause a disease outbreak. For example, from 1900 to 1950, Iceland had a population of two hundred thousand people only. So the number of susceptible host for measles virus was dramatically reduced. With the increase in tourist and travelers the measles virus was reintroduced to the population even giving it an epidemic proportion [6].

Appearance of a New Virus to a Specific Population: Sometimes, a virus enters and spreads in a place where it had never been found. It can be contributed due to human migration and business. West Nile virus (WNV) in emerged in such a way in the United States in 1999. WNV are confined to the Middle East area due to localization of its specific mosquito vectors. However, increased flight travel introduced the mosquitoes in New York resulting in emergence of a new infectious and significant disease. Few American mosquitoes served as WNV vectors for and American crows were very much susceptible contributing to the pandemic nature of the disease.

Similar kind of outbreak occurred on the island of Reunion in the Indian Ocean during 2005-2006 by the Chikungunya virus (CHIKV). Though this mosquito-borne arbovirus caused febrile illness along with arthralgia and arthritis, they made a new colonization in India and Asia, which was then followed in America. So far, transmission of CHIKV is reported in around 40 countries/territories in Central, South, North America and the Caribbean [9].

Zoonotic Host: Emerging viral diseases can also be caused by zoonotic infections in animals which gets transferred to humans. The transmission happens due to virus-laden droplets, direct contact, or aerosols, or through insect vectors. The epidemiological dynamics are shown (Table **2**).

In case of most of the zoonotic viruses, humans act as dead end host where the infection cannot be spread directly from one human to another like rabies [6]. Humans get infected by exposure to aerosol where when a rodent bite (in caves dwelled by roosting bats). Inhalation of contaminated aerosol also plays an important role in disease transmission, such as in Junin (Argentine hemorrhagic fever), Machupo (Bolivian hemorrhagic fever), and Lassa. Human to human transmission of viruses are also observed (Table **2**). Many viruses in this emerging group cause a high mortality in humans. Mostly, these infections spread to the persons who are with intimate contact with the person like family members and care givers [3].

Our chapter focuses on examples of recent emerging and re-emerging viral diseases, possible therapeutic approaches and any knowledge gaps.

Table 2. Zoonotic Virus Infections of Humans and the Extent of Human-to-Human Transmission [10 - 14].

Family	Viruses	Zoonosis	Etiology
Arenaviridae	Chapare virus Guanarito virus Junin virus Lassa virus Lujo virus Machupo virus Sabia virus	- - - - - Mouse Rodents	- Venezuelan hemorrhagic fever Argentine hemorrhagic fever Lassa fever - Bolivian Hemorrhagic fever Brazilian hemorrhagic fever
Bunyaviridae	Andes virus Crimean-Congo haemorrhagic fever virus (CCHFV) Severe fever with Thrombocytopenia syndrome virus (SFTSV)	Rodents Ticks Arthropod	Hantavirus cardiopulmonary syndrome Crimean Congo hemorrhagic fever Severe fever with thrombocytopenia
Coronaviridae	MERS-Cov SARS-Cov	- Bats	Severe acute respiratory syndrome Seasonal/Swine/Bird Flu Severe acute respiratory syndrome
Filoviridae	Ebola virus Marburg virus	- -	Ebola hemorrhagic fever Marburg hemorrhagic Fever
Flavirideae	Zinka virus Dengue virus West Nile Virus	Mosquitoes Mosquitoes Mosquitoes	Fever, congenital microcephaly Dengue fever West Nile fever and encephalitis
Hepeviridae	Hepatitis E virus (HRV)	Swine, Boar	Chronic hepatitis E Neuropathy
Lyssaviruses	Australian Bat lyssavirus (ABLV) European Bat lyssavirus(EBLV) Irkut virus (IRKV)	Bat Bat Bat	Fatal encephalitic disease Fatal encephalitic disease Fatal encephalitic disease
Orthomyxoviridae	Influenza virus	Swine, Bird	Swine flu, Bird flu

(Table 2) cont.....

Family	Viruses	Zoonosis	Etiology
Paramyxoviridae	Hendra virus Nipah virus	Bat Bat	Hendra disease Nipah disease
Retroviridae	HIV		AIDS
Togaviridae	Chikungunya virus	Mosquito	Chikungunya fever

Major Emerging Viruses

Crimean-Congo Hemorrhagic Fever (CCHF)

According to WHO prioritization list published in 2015, Crimean-Congo haemorrhagic fever (CCHF) is a potent viral emerging disease of public health concern. It is a tick-borne virus (*Nairovirus*) of *Bunyaviridae* family. It causes viral haemorrhagic fever outbreaks and a fatality rate of 10-40%. It is endemic in Middle East, Africa, Balkans, and Asia.

Pathogenicity

Crimean-Congo haemorrhagic fever virus has a host in Hyalommatick larvae which is frequently found on blackbirds [19, 20]. Exposure to Hyalomma ticks results in contracting the disease. CCHFV is circulated in an enzootic tick–vertebrate–tick cycle. Sero-epidemiological studies detected CCHFV antibodies in domestic cattle, donkeys, sheep horses, pigs, and goats, from Europe, Africa, Asia [21]. Human-to-human transmission of CCHFV also happens in healthcare. High mortality among health care workers occurs while providing medical care due to contact with the infected blood or body secretions. The nosocomial transmission occurs in health care personnel due to splash and needle-stick injuries [12]. The pathogenesis of CCHF is mainly due to interaction of the viral cells with host immune cell and endothelial cells. The pathogenesis depends on activation of endothelial cells. The endothelial cell activation is related to the up-regulation of activated soluble molecules like cytokines. It creates toxicity, thereby increased vasodilatation, vascular permeability, hypotension, multiple organ failure, shock, and death. The clearance of CHEF becomes difficult due to delayed adaptive immune response. The virus replicates uncontrolled and systematically spread throughout the body. Delayed interferon induction, activation of dendritic cells and macrophages, lymphocyte apoptosis, weak antibody response, and hemophagocytosis are caused due to infective immune suppression [22, 23]. The acute phage of infection is preceded by the prodromal symptoms such as sudden onset of severe headache, dizziness, fever, chills, photophobia, and back and abdominal pains. It is associated with neuropsychiatric changes such as mood changes, feelings of confusion and aggression, and violent behavior [24]. In addition, enlarged spleen and liver is observed in 30% of patients. The average mortality rate can be very high as 70% [24] The pathogenesis of CCHF is not very clearly understood for various reasons such as: (i) sporadic infections (ii) requirement of biosafety level 4 (BSL-4) containment laboratories, and (iii) a lack of animal disease models. CCHF pathogenesis details are mostly derived from liver biopsies and blood analyses of patients [25]. The major causes attributed to the fatal nature of the disease are cerebral severe dehydration, severe anemia, hemorrhage, and shock associated with, lung edema, prolonged diarrhea, and pleural effusion. Multiple organ failure is the most important cause of mortality [24]

Diagnosis

For testing animals or humans for viremia, detection of viral nucleic acid in plasma or serum is observed using conventional [26] or real-time reverse transcriptase (RTPCR) [27 - 29], or by viral antigen demonstration [30]. Blood and liver samples are generally sent as specimens for viral identification. Appropriate safety measures should be taken to prevent risk of laboratory infections. CCHFV research should be done in appropriate biosafety facilities. For viral isolation and cell culture, Vero cells are commonly used. Infectivity CCHFV is demonstrated by immunofluorescence in infected cells [30]. SW-13 cell lines are also choice for viral isolation and they produce plaques in 4 days. Identification of viral isolates are confirmed by fluorescence focus assay and plaque assay in CER cells [31]. For detection of viral nucleic acid, molecular diagnostic assays, such as RT-PCR is used [32]. Compared to virus culture, molecular diagnostic assays are preferred because of their rapidity [26]. The RT-PCR is sensitive technique, but because of CCHFV genetic diversity, primer designing is difficult. However, real-time RT-PCR is very sensitive in detecting strains from different geographic locations is [29]. A low-density microarray detects as few as 6.3 genome copies per reaction is developed and validated in clinical specimens collected from of CCHF over 20 years by a WHO reference laboratory [33].

Treatment

Supportive or palliative treatment is the main treatment modality by the management of symptoms. The viral disease is characterized by severe fluid loss and management is done with intravenous fluids. Considering the hemorrhagic nature of the disease, fresh frozen plasma, blood products platelets, are suggested depending on the amount of blood loss [34]. No approved antiviral treatment for CCHF exists. Ribavirin, approved by WHO, is used for CCHFV treatment as it inhibits CCHFV viral replication in vitro and in vivo. However, lack of large placebo-controlled, prospective randomized controlled trials exist [35 - 37]. Recently Favipiravir (T-705), a drug showed better survival benefit in mouse model compared to ribavirin [38]. Recent advance studies have proved that Monoclonal antibody therapy may be used as antivirals for CCHF treatment of [39].

Ebola Viral Disease and Marburg Viral Disease

Ebola (EBOV) and Marburg (MARV) viruses have gained 2nd position in prioritization list published by WHO in 2018 and is one of the concerning emerging viral disease due to its high mortality rate (90%) [39]. Ebola hemorrhagic fever (EHF), named after the Ebola River, was first discovered in 1979 during an outbreak in Democratic Republic of the Congo. 21 additional outbreaks of Ebola disease have been reported till date and the most sever was the outbreak in Gulu, Uganda in 2000-2001 which claimed around 53% mortality rate [40]. After the outbreak of Ebola in Guinea, considering the severity of the disease in March 2014, WHO declared the disease as "public health emergency of international concern" [41]. The Ebola virus infection is life threatening and can involve isolated cases those have been imported from endemic areas and may contribute to a devastating outbreak [42]. VHF can be life-threatening. In Ebola virus, the viral protein 35 (VP35), is a multifunctional dsRNA binding protein which modulates viral replication, evasion of innate immune, and pathogenesis. The viral RNA polymerase (encoded by L gene), partially uncoat nucleocapsid and transcribes viral genes into positive-strand mRNAs, which get translated into structural and non-structural proteins [43]. All known MARV strains are deviated from one specie that is *Lake Victoria Marburg* virus, while EBOV strains deviated from four different species: *Sudan ebolavirus* (SEBOV), *Zaire ebolavirus* (ZEBOV), *Reston ebolavirus* (REBOV) and *Côte d'Ivoire ebolavirus* (CIEBOV). The fifth species is the newly discovered *Bundibugyo ebolavirus* (BEBOV). The pathogenicity in human species varies species wise; ZEBOV is most pathogenic with 90% fatality rate. CIEBOV and REBOV cause lethal infections in non-human primates and are non-pathogenic to human [44, 45].

Pathogenicity

Ebola virus (EBOV) and Marburg virus infections are hemorrhagic. Replications of EBOV and MARV release high levels of inflammatory cytokines which in turn cause coagulation abnormalities and fluid distribution problems. The final disease process is manifested as hemorrhage and vascular leakage; leading to multiple organ failure and shock [46, 47]. During entry, macrophages along with other cells of the phagocytic system are the main targets of the viruses. The infective macrophages deliver the virus to liver, spleen, lymph nodes. endothelium, kidney pancreas, and adrenal gland [48, 49]. Marked leukopenia with a left shift and typical lymphocytes are other key findings in blood smears. Viral GP is the main cause of neutropenia supposed to be a result of apoptosis. The deaths of lymphocytes are also contributed by the impaired production of pro-inflammatory cytokines. Impaired stimulation of T cells also plays an important role [49].

Diagnosis

The symptom of the disease process is not specific and does not have any defined symptoms. Therefore, it's difficult to identify the epidemics. Diagnostic processes are based upon virus identification for outbreak all suspected cases and consideration of them as at high risk of exposure. For better managements of the epidemic, exposure risks and case definitions must be considered [50, 51]. Case definition of EVD mostly includes index case: very first case (probable or confirmed) reported as the origin of the epidemic [51]. The alert case is considered when a person reports of bloody diarrhea, sudden high fever or sudden death or bleeding, or bleeding in urine [51]. Most important points considered as a suspect case with person reporting, dead or alive, who has (or had): fever (>38.5 ^{0}C or 101.5 ^{0}F) and most importantly with additional signs of muscle pain, vomiting, abdominal pain, severe headache, diarrhea, or unexplained hemorrhage. It can be caused due to handling of bush animals in disease-endemic areas [51]. The probable cases are also considered if a person evaluated by a clinician, has symptoms similar to EVD, it might be a dead person who has an epidemiological link to a confirmed case [51]. Positive signal with Ebola virus antigen or Ebola IgG antibody is critical marker of the potent risk assessment marker [51]. There are different methods for Laboratory diagnosis for Ebola like measuring particle components in infected individuals or measuring the host-specific immune responses to infection and detection of viral particles. For acute infections, RT-PCR and antigen detection, ELISA are the main diagnostic assays. Viral antigen and nucleic acid is found in blood from Day 3 to Day 7-16 after the prodromal period [46, 52]. The most commonly used assays detecting antibodies are direct IgG, IgM ELISA, as well as IgM capture ELISA. An IgG-specific antibody starts developing within 6 and 18 days after onset of the illness and they persist for a longtime. An IgM or rising IgG titer (four-fold) signifies presumptive diagnosis [52].

Prevention and Treatment

Scientists working in high containment facilities such as health care workers in Africa and people residing in the affected areas in Africa run a risk of potential exposures. In 2014, CDC began recommending use of medical personal protective equipment (PPE); also, a designated person, who has appropriate training in biosafety, should monitor the procedures to ensure they are performed as per guidelines [53]. Several concurrent strategies and strict infection control measures should be followed to prevent transmission to healthcare workers. Individuals with Ebola exposure should be monitored and signs and symptoms of the disease should be quickly identified. Individual house based treatment kit for Ebola virus was developed in after 2010 outbreak which helped the family members of Ebola patients to treat the patient without compromising their own health. These kits included protective clothing as well as chlorine powder and other cleaning supplies. Proper knowledge and suitable disinfection methods can significantly reduce the chance of the spread of the disease. Ebola virus gets eliminated by heat (normally heating is required for 30 to 60 minutes at 60 ^{0}C or boiling for 5 minutes). To disinfect surfaces, some lipid solvents such as some detergents, bleaching powder, alcohol-based products [54 - 56].

Isolation and Quarantine

Isolation refers to separating sick people from non-sick people. In case of severely infective viral diseases isolation is the best methods to prevent the spread of the disease. Quarantine refers to separating individuals with disease exposure until they either show signs of the disease or are no longer at risk. During the 2014 Ebola disease outbreak. Liberia closed schools following the United States quarantine protocol to prevent the spread of the disease [57, 58].

Environmental Infection Control

It is the best method to prevent the chance of spread of the disease in the hospital environment. Monitoring should continue for 21 days after the last known exposure; manifestation supporting Ebola infections should be reported immediately [54].

Breastfeeding and Infant Care

Ebola virus shows vertical transmission. So according to the CDC guideline, the infant should not be in contact with the mother if the infant can receive adequate care and nutrition in other ways [59, 60]. Though the virus is no longer detectable in the blood during the convalescent period, but it can be present in mother's body fluid such as in urine, breast-milk, therefore, precautions should be taken during this period. To prevent sexual transmission through semen, WHO recommends that men should abstain from sex (including oral sex) for three months' symptoms as well as the use of condoms are mandatory. However, no recommendations yet exist if infected women can resume sexual activity and/or breast feeding [61].

Pregnancy

According to CDC and American College of Obstetrics and Gynecology guidelines, strict infection control precautions have to be taken while handling all pregnant patients with Ebola virus disease. The most severe complication associated with delivery in case of Ebola infection is high risk of fatal death and pregnancy associated hemorrhage. However, no data is available suggesting preference of cesarean or vaginal delivery or when the baby should be delivered [62].

Vaccines

Due to pathogenicity of the virus, no conventional vaccines such as consisting of inactivated/killed virus, or prepared from the attenuated virus, could be developed for Ebola because of the risk of incomplete inactivation of the virus or of reversion to a fully active form. New molecular biology and recombinant genetic technology based approaches are expected to develop in near future [63, 64]. Two vaccines are reported to be used in human; cAd3-ZEBOV, which has been developed by GlaxoSmithKline (tested US National Institute of Allergy and Infectious Diseases (NIAID) and rVSV, tested by New Link Genetics Corporation after being licensed from the Public Health Agency of Canada. These vaccines showed promising rates of efficacy in non-human primates, however, testing on human is yet to be done [64, 65].

Challenges to Therapy

No approved specific treatment modality is available for EVD. The preliminary approach for treatment of Ebola virus is to prevent hypovolemic or hemorrhagic shock due to fluid or blood loss. Supportive care of complications, such as electrolyte abnormalities, hematologic abnormalities, refractory shock, septic shock hemorrhage, hypoxia hypovolemia, multi-organ failure should be given. Maintaining the adequate cardiovascular function is one of the prime challenges [66, 67].

Antiviral Therapy

There are no approved medications for treatment of Ebola virus exists. Ebola virus treatments are under development and have not been fully tested for safety and effectiveness. Currently, Non-clinical and clinical data are made available for:

- Three nucleoside polymerase inhibitors: BCX4430, Brincidofovir, and Favipiravir;
- Two oligonucleotide based products: TKM-100802 and AVI-7537;

• A cocktail of monoclonal antibodies: ZMapp

Hantavirus

Hantaviruses (family Bunyaviridae, genus Hantavirus) are a large family of over 300 viruses that are serologically and phylogenetically related and infect animals, plants, humans, and arthropods [68 - 70]. They are enveloped RNA viruses of rodents that have been detected in Europe, Asia and America. Hanta virus existed for a long time, but American hanta viruses have been reported as major emerging zoonotic pathogens threatening humans only in the last decade [71 - 73]. As reported with other Bunyaviruses, the genomes of hanta viruses consist of 3 different single-stranded RNA segments that are mostly negative stranded. The viral RNA polymerase acts as a precursor glycoprotein that is processed into 2 separate envelope glycoproteins (termed G1 and G2) which encode the viral RNA polymerase(transcriptase), and a nucleocapsid protein, respectively [73]. Electron microscopic studies with hanta virus infected cells shows hantavirus have morphologies typical of the other members of the Bunyaviridae family. The viral components are spherical or ovoid, having 80–120 nm in diameter and can also form elongated particles (170 nm) which are common for Bunya viruses. When the virus stained negatively and viewed under electron microscope, a prominent chessboard-like (ordered mosaic) pattern composed of square surface approximately measuring approximately 838 nm morphologic subunits are pictured as negatively stained hantaviruses are observed through electron microscopy [71 - 74]. The list of various species of hanta viruses is growing and the taxonomy of hantaviruses is complex. The Committee on Taxonomy of Viruses (ICTV) has set one criterion for hantavirus species recognition with a 7% cut off level for protein diversity. As the vectors for Bunyaviruses varies considerably, distinguishment is made between arthropod-borne (arboviruses) and rodent-borne (roboviruses). Transmission of hanta viruses to humans is not contact dependent. The contamination happens through the respiratory route involving inhalation of aerosols which are virus-contaminated of rodent excreta [75 - 77]. Infection by Hanta virus in human most commonly involves two systems like renal and pulmonary causing distinguishing syndromes like hemorrhagic fever with renal syndrome (HFRS) and hanta virus pulmonary syndrome (HPS), each with varying degrees of severity [72 - 80].

Clinical Features

The viruses currently recognized as agents of HFRS are Dobrava-Belgrade, Hantaan, Puumala, and Seoul viruses. HFRS manifests as mild, moderate, or severe disease. Severe form of HFRS is usually attributed to Dobrava and Hantaan viruses. Moderate HFRS is caused by Seoul virus and mild form is attributed to Puumala virus. Like most other viral infections HFRS is characterized by the development prodromal symptoms of an acute influenza-like febrile illness which finally leads to hemorrhagic manifestations and renal failure. The incubation period for severe HFRS caused by Dobrava and Hanta viruses is 2 to 3 weeks, with a subsequent febrile phase (prodrome) that shows characterization of influenza-like symptoms lasting for 3 to 5 days. Hemorrhage can occur during the febrile phase and is manifested as a flushing of the face or injection in the conjunctiva and mucous membranes. On day 4 of the febrile phase sudden and extreme albuminuria is a characteristic feature of severe HFRS. There is formation of a hypotensive phase lasting from several hours to few days as evidenced by thrombocytopenia and most often associated with petechial rash. Shock occurs in about 15% of the patients. The most common cause of death is renal failure characterized by oliguric phase [81].

Clinical Features of Hantavirus Pulmonary Syndrome (HPS)

Hantavirus pulmonary syndrome is found in America. In 1993, it was first recognized as a hantavirus disease. Sin Nombre virus (SNV) has caused most HPS cases in North America. HPS is a more severe disease having mortality rate of 40%. HPS like other viral diseases is characterized by a distinctive febrile phase as prodromal period followed by hematologic manifestations, cardiac depression, and pulmonary infection [75, 76]. In case of American hanta virus infections extra thoracic findings are often seen. Usually, in HPS while caused by SNV, fourteen to seventeen-day incubation period is observed after having the exposure [82]. Renal involvement during SNV though presents, but is not a major consideration [83]. The febrile phase usually lasts for 3-5 days. There is headache, myalgia, malaise, and fever. Following the febrile phase of disease there can also be thrombocytopenia associated with anorexia, abdominal pain, nausea, and vomiting [74 - 76]. SNV-induced HPS is manifested by involvement of cardiopulmonary, which coincides with patient's hospitalization timing. The clinical presentation is dominated by gastrointestinal manifestations but can be associated with cough. Tachycardia, Tachypnea and postural hypotension are typical; however, chest information is not contributory. Abnormal laboratory findings become common starting with a decrease or low platelet count [74, 76, 84, 85]. Other laboratory findings include elevated hematocrit and circulating immunoblasts, which can be considered as typical lymphocytes [86]. Pulmonary functions are distinctly abnormal with low PAO_2 level. There are low pulse oximetry findings and often low $PACO_2$ is observed. The disease is associated with severe interstitial edema after onset of cardiopulmonary involvement by 48 hours [74 - 76].

Pathogenesis

The early events occurring with human hanta virus infection are not yet fully understood. Hantaviruses target endothelial cells. After infection, the viremia develops and proceeds to kidney and lungs infection. The virus infects the microvasculature of endothelial cells, especially in lungs and accounts for the severe edema associated with HPS [74, 76, 80, 81]. Generally, we don't see cytopathic effects in hantavirus-infected human cells and the pattern of infection for both HFRS and HPS are immunopathologic [87, 88]. Though the exact cause of kidney failure in HERS is not clear but Acute Tubulointerstitial Nephritis are seen in biopsies of HFRS patients [74, 76]. Interstitial pneumonitis, hyaline membrane formation and mononuclear cell infiltrates are the main pulmonary histopathologic findings of SNV infection [82, 83]. Though the Hanta virus infections of rodents are asymptomatic and persistent, but the new generation viral strains are capable of causing pathology in their reservoir hosts. Edema of alveolar septa and Immune infiltrates are observed in liver and lungs in Peromyscus leucopus infected with New York strain of the virus [89]. Similar findings were observed in Peromyscus maniculatus infected with SNV [90]. Unfortunately, neither situation mimics HPS, ruling these hosts out as models for the study of HPS. Fortunately, there are Andes group of virus that induces a disease with pathology almost similar like that of typical HPS in hamsters [91] providing the first animal model for the study of HPS.

Serological and Molecular Tests

Serological analysis is the key tool for the detection of antibodies formed against Old World hantaviruses in infected individuals. Standard immunofluorescence assays are used by using serum drawn from a patient. Other than that fluorescein-labelled goat anti-human antibodies, and slides containing hantavirus-infected cells is also being used. Immunoglobulin (Ig) M and IgG enzyme linked immunosorbent assays are also available and often used [92]. It is quite difficult to recognize the causative virus species because of cross-neutralizing primary antibody against several Old World hantavirus genotypes that is formed during HFRS. Therefore, there is a need of additional, testing by other methods [92]. Reverse Transcriptase–Polymerase Chain Reaction (RT-PCR) technique has been widely used for detection of Old World hanta viruses [92 - 94].

For RNA analysis, the sample is serum or blood acquired from the autopsy tissue or acute phase of infection. Various laboratory tests are done for final diagnosis of HPS, for SNV induced HPS as well.

For American patients, the widely used screening is the IgM capture enzyme-linked immunosorbent assay since the hanta virus antibodies in United States general population are very scanty IgG level is at its peak in first week of illness. It remains detectable for long period of time. These specific IgG levels can also be measured by enzyme-linked immunosorbent assay [95]. For HPS infection, RT-PCR is performed on acute-phase serum specimens within first 10 days of illness [96]. The success of this technique depends on primer choice and if nested reaction has been used for improved detection efficiency. Considering the pathogenic nature of the virus, virus isolation as well as the molecular biology techniques is performed in BSL-3 or BSL-4 facilities [96]. Primary isolation of hanta viruses is done on an African green monkey kidney cell line, also known as VERO E6. VERO E6 cell line is preferred for the viral isolation because the virus does not produce any cytopathic effects. The viral isolation from infected cell is performed by RNA isolation after about 2 weeks of incubation and detection of hanta virus RNA is done by RT PCR.

Treatment

There is no U.S. Food and Drug Administration (FDA) approved drugs available for the treatment of hemorrhagic fever viruses. Drugs are also not available for HFRS and NE. Experimentally it has been proved that that Ribavirin has antiviral activity against *Bunyaviridae* and the *Arenaviridae*. The drug reduces mortality and was proven effective for the treatment of lethal encephalitic suckling mice infected with HTNV [97]. Ribavirin has been proved to improve disease diagnosis if given early during disease course. When given during the first stage of the disease, it causes significant reduction to the mortality rate [98, 99]. But there are significant side effects for the use of Ribavirin like anemia which might even lead to blood transfusion. It has been found to cause renal insufficiency. Although no human trial reports are available, however passively transferring neutralizing monoclonal antibodies (MAbs) or polyclonal sera to HTNV in hamster and rats can passively protect animals while challenged with hanta viruses [100].

While doing passive immunization with neutralizing MAbs to PUUV in primates, it protects them from subsequent PUUV challenge [101]. Passive transfer of sera from rhesus macaques while vaccinated with M segment of ANDV will protect against lethal challenge with ANDV in hamsters [102]. A post hanta virus prophylaxis treatment regimen is effective, as it is found in viral diseases such as hepatitis A and B, varicella, and rabies.

Systemic administration of Ig will not lead to achievement of these criteria for pathogen challenge in the lung in HPS cases. The abrupt onset of respiratory failure, acute nature of disease, and high chances of shock development in HPS, the disease calls rapid and targeted treatments to the site of infection. There are no FDA approved vaccines, antivirals, or immune therapeutics available for HPS disease. There are high chances of development of cardiogenic shock.

Prevention

The prime target for the prevention of diseases caused by hanta viruses is based on rodent control. Identification and reduction of rodent shelter and food sources in and around the home is the main concern. Elimination of rodents inside the home and preventing them from entering the home are found to be effective to control Hanta virus spread [103]. Significant precautionary measures should be taken for persons who are exposed to wild rodents in their occupation [104], as well as precautions for hikers and campers [105, 106]. Vaccination protocol is advisable for the high risk population like military personal. The basic target for the development of vaccine is the viral glycoproteins, which elicit a protective neutralization response [107]. Four Hantavirus vaccines are developed using inactivated SEO and HTN viruses. They are found to be safe and effective in China [108]. In 1991, an effective vaccine Hantavax, was derived from suckling mouse brain and found to be quite effective [109]. An inactivated vaccine based on cell culture against Hanata virus was developed in Korea. It was more protective than Hantavax [110]. Other group of vaccine includes DNA vaccine. A DNA vaccine developed with SEOV M segment produced neutralizing antibodies which protected SEOV infection in Hamsters [111]. DNA vaccination with HTNV M segment elicits neutralizing antibodies against several HFRS-causing hantaviruses [112]. Other DNA vaccines targeting ADNV and SNV are also effective in mice models [113, 114]. A novel bivalent HTN/AND viral DNA vaccine has recently shown to elicit memory response as well as produce antibodies neutralizing viruses causing HPS and HFRS [115]. Nucleocapsid proteins of HTNV, PUUV, and DOBV of *Saccharomyces cerevisiae* is a useful tool for vaccine development against hantavirus [116]. The recombinant proteins of Hanta Virus which were obtained from transgenic plants elicited specific immune responses [117]. Besides, with use of reverse genetics for negative-stranded RNA viruses [118], generation of vaccines from attenuated hantavirus is possible in future.

Hendra Virus

Hendra virus (HeV), a zoonotic paramyxovirus, reported in 1994 in Hendra, Australia [119]. It was the first species that was identified as a new viral genus *Henipavirus* in order Mononegavirales and family *Paramyxoviridae.* It is distinct from Nipah virus and Cedar virus [120, 121]. HeV virus was isolated from equine lung tissue from an outbreak of severe febrile respiratory disease in horses. Two people who had close contact with infected horses developed influenza-like illness (ILI). The infection has caused death of one of these patients due to severe interstitial pneumonia. HeV was isolated from the kidney of the fatal human case. On inoculation into experimental horses, the virus produced the similar symptoms in as the wild form. The virus could be re-isolated from tissues including lung, kidney, and lymph nodes. It confirmed HeV as the etiologic agent.

In between 1994 to 2010 around 14 sporadic events of outbreaks have been reported and all of them mostly involve coastal Queensland or the north-eastern corner of New South Wales (NSW). The first case of west of the Great Dividing Range was reported in 2011 and 2012 where 26 HeV incidents was reported. These events confirmed HeV as an emerging zoonotic disease and other animals like dogs were also reported to be infected [122] Human involvement was strongly associated with direct contamination and was mostly reported in the field workers in the horse farm. The treating veterinarians and nurses get contaminated easily during performing other routine procedures [123]. HeV attack rate for persons exposed to infected equine body fluids has been estimated at 10% (6). The HeV infection has been proved to be very fatal and has the mortality rate up to 57%. Most of the deaths are reported to be due to multiorgan failure with interstitial pneumonia and encephalitis [124]. Association with HeV was confirmed by serological test having positivity for neutralizing antibodies to HeV and the viral genome. The HeV antigen was found in brain during necropsy. The viral species is not maintained in the horses only. There is no evidence of neutralizing antibody in the Queensland horses supporting the statement and therefore other sources of virus were investigated [125]. In survey, sera from 46 species in 34 species of fauna were sampled. None of the samples were found to be positive for antibody against HeV, however while extending the work to fruit bats (flying foxes) revealed a seroprevalence of over 25% in these animals [126]. Serological evidences have proved that all the four species of flying fox such as the black flying-fox (*Pt. alecto*), grey-headed flying-fox (*Pteropuspolio cephalus*), little red flying-fox (*Pt. scapulatus*) and the spectacled flying-fox (*Pt. conspicillatus*) harvest HeV. HeV was first isolated in free-living bats from a fetus (*Pt. alecto)* as well as from a fetus and uterine fluid (*Pt. poliocephalus*) [127] and from urine collected from flying fox roosts [128].

Pathogenesis

The viral genetic material is usually recovered on nasal swab from experimental Horses after two to three days of exposure [129]. Viremia generally increases during incubation period and in clinical phase of infection and the number is consistent with local replication in the upper respiratory tract or nasopharynx. The rapid onset of fever is signs of typical viremia and viral genome can also be recovered from oral secretions and urine. The viral involvement of the tissues and organs more widely establishes the typical symptoms. Post mortem reports from acutely affected animal organ have revealed presence of pulmonary edema, congestion, and consolidation. There is presence of typical blood-tinged foam in the airways and dilation of subpleural lymphatic [130]. It is common to find congestion of intra-abdominal lymph nodes, subpleural hemorrhage, and enlarged, submandibular, sternal, edematous and bronchial lymph nodes [129]. Vasculitis is the most prominent light microscopic features in both natural and experimental HeV infection of horses that affects predominantly smaller blood vessels in a wide range of tissues including kidney(glomeruli), brain (and meninges), lymphoid tissues, lung, and female reproductive tract and also the nasal mucosa, adrenal gland, liver, heart and gastrointestinal tract. During the infection, necrotizing lymphadenitis is a common feature associated with extensive necrotizing alveolitis along with marked fibrinous alveolar exudates. In renal involvement, syncytial cells are found within renal glomeruli. Similar kinds of cells are evident to lymphoid tissues, vascular endothelium, lymphatic endothelium, and in alveolar walls. Immunohistochemical techniques are quite useful for the demonstration of HeV antigen in affected tissues using appropriate techniques. Virus is also isolated from fresh carcass, especially from lung, kidney, and lymphoid tissues and also from brain and spinal cord, meninges, cerebrospinal fluid, heart upper respiratory tract, and adrenal gland. Virus isolation attempts can have error in post-mortem delay examination. CNS involvement is associated with focal, nonsuppurative meningoencephalitis along with gliosis and perivascular cuffing. Generally low levels of HeV genome are found in brain [131].

Laboratory Diagnosis

As the clinical signs associated with HeV infection are not pathognomonic, confirmation can only be done by laboratory analysis. Sample collection procedure is critical and the zoonotic potentiality of the disease should be considered. Guided protocol has to be followed for collection of samples and submission of specimen to diagnostic laboratories. The subclinical nature of the disease makes it very difficult to control the human transmission. For live horse, samples involve blood in EDTA and oral, nasal, and rectal swabs for PCR testing. If positive results have been found in PCR, the virus isolation attempts must be done in a BSL4 laboratory. Whole blood must be collected for serological testing and analyzed by ELISA or neutralization test in BSL4 laboratory [132]. The viral load is highest in a dead horse. Therefore, the post mortem examination becomes very hazardous and not indicated in confirmed cases. Necropsy is conducted by equipped operators with appropriate infrastructure.

Therapy

There is no existing therapy for HeV infected horses. If diagnostically confirmed, euthanasia has to be carried out.

Post Exposure Therapeutics for People

Exposure of humans to HeV through affected horses may occur. All horses can't be vaccinated against HeV and outbreaks often occur in temperate as well as tropical climates. In 2008, Zhu and co-authors identified and characterized a human monoclonal antibody, m102.4, that neutralized Nipah virus and HeV virus *in vitro* [133]. While post exposure to animals in laboratory, m102.4 was found to prevent Nipah and Hendra-associated morbidity and mortality in ferrets [134] (Middleton unpublished data) and in African Green monkeys [135]. These studies paved the pathway for preclinical safety testing of m102.4. In 2014, a Phase 1 human clinical trial commenced.

SARS

Severe acute respiratory syndrome (SARS) is a recently encountered human infection associated with pneumonia and was first reported in Guangdong Province, China, in November 2002 [136] in a Hong Kong hotel. The single hotel floor became the solely responsible cause for the international spread of SARS [137]. Around 14 hotel guests was a carrier to the virus to Toronto, Vietnam, Hong Kong, and Singapore and contributed for the severe outbreaks. Almost no information was available regarding this disease and as a result all the hospital staff responding to the earliest cases. As a result, the disease spread within the hospitals by infecting staff, patients, and visitors. Gradually it covered the larger community [138]. By the mid-February 2003, the disease had spread to Hong Kong and showed its widespread nature by subsequently involving more than 8000 patients in over 30 countries across five continents. With the help of the war foot action strategies by World Health Organization (WHO), the SARS was successfully contained in less than four months [137].

Etiology

Key information regarding this life threatening disease process was gathered by March 2003 including the information about the causative organism, which was identified as a new coronavirus (SARS CoV) The virus was found to follow Koch's postulates and was recognized as vector born disease. SARS virus is capable of producing cytopathic activity in Vero E6 tissue culture cells and samples collected from Oropharyngeal specimens from patients shows similar findings. Ultrastructural features studied by Electron microscope had revealed characteristic features of coronaviruses. Immunohistochemical and immunofluorescence staining also supported the fact by showing reactivity using polyclonal antibodies from group I coronavirus. Consensus primers from corona virus were designed for amplifying a coronavirus identifying gene by reverse transcriptase-polymerase chain reaction (RT-PCR). Uniformity of coron virus was confirmed from clinical samples of affected patients. Serological evidence proved antibodies specific to the new coronavirus were present in the serum SARS patients [139 - 144]. A completely new group of virus under Coronavirus family, named as cynomolgus macaques (*Macaca fascicularis*) causing pneumonia and necropsy in experimental animals proved the similar pattern of pulmonary damage as seen in human beings with SARS. This newly identified coronavirus is known as SARS CoV and it is the cause of SARS. Coronaviruses are the largest of any of the RNA viruses having large envelop with a positive stranded RNA genome ranging in size from 27 to 30 kb. In humans, coronaviruses associate with common cold. In other animals, these viruses affect multisystem leading to highly virulent enteric, respiratory, and neurological diseases as well as hepatitis. Analysis of the complete genome sequence of SARS CoV published in May 2003 and it was found that this virus is a unique corona virus. They are not even originated from a chance in genetic recombination between known coronaviruses [145] has unique sequence of genes has proved its origin from animal host [146, 147].

Clinical Features

SARS has an incubation period generally ranging between 2–10 day. The onset of clinical symptoms to hospital admission is within 3 to 5 days [148]. The major clinical features for SARS include flu like symptoms such as myalgia, malaise, dry cough, chills/rigor, headache fever, and dyspnea. Less common symptoms include productive cough, sore throat, rhinorrhea, nausea, vomiting, and diarrhea. 73% of patients of Amoy Gardens outbreak of SARS was clinically related to watery diarrhea, together with recurrence of fever and the gastrointestinal symptoms were reported in one week in the clinical course [149]. The diarrhea is usually watery without containing blood or mucus. SARS was reported to develop severe acute neurological symptoms like status epilepticus and the virus had been detected in the CSF of the affected people [150, 151].

The clinical course of SARS has a typical pattern: the phase 1 is designated as viral replication and is characterized by an increased viral load and clinically symptoms involving fever, myalgia and systemic symptoms which improves few days [149]. In case of phase 2, there is distinct immunopathological involvement which is characterized by recurrence of fever, decreased oxygen saturation along with radiological evidence of pneumonia with decrease in viral load. This severe condition in majority of the cases improves with the medication specifically using steroid therapy. However, in severe cases intensive care unit admission may be required. Even in case of progressive lesion, it may lead to acute respiratory distress that requires invasive ventilatory support [149, 152, 153]. The infective stage of the disease process is associated with the acute phase of the disease along with viral shedding from stool, nasopharynx, and urine within day 10 till day 21 after the symptoms have appeared.

Laboratory Findings

Serological studies have revealed immunological involvement in the disease process as characterized by Lymphopenia associated with destruction of both CD4 and CD8 lymphocytes. The disease process is also associated with coagulopathy and symptoms are similar to low grade disseminated intravascular coagulation (DIC). The serum enzymatic profile is also altered and manifested as raised lactate dehydrogenase, alanine transaminases, and creatine kinase [154, 155]. Other biochemical markers like lactate dehydrogenase and creatine kinase levels can be correlated with affected cardiovascular function. It results in decreased left ventricular ejection fraction which is considered of having significant prognostic values [156]. Other cardiological manifestation includes reversible subclinical diastolic impairment occurring in acute SARS [156]. Hepatic involvement can also be associated with altered liver function test and mostly reported in 29.6% and 75.9% of patients [157]. The principal organ affected by SARS is the lungs. The radiographic appearance of the lungs correlates with disease progression although 20% to 25% patients show normal chest radiograph [158]. In the early stage of the disease, parenchymal opacity can be detected by high resolution computed tomography of the thorax [159]. The distinctive features revealed in the chest radiography are the predominant involvement of lung periphery and the lower zone, in addition to the absence of cavitation, hilar lymphadenopathy, or pleural effusion [158, 159]. The radiographic features have significant prognostic values and can also be correlated with the treatment outcome. The prognostic radiographic feature mostly includes radiographic progression from unilateral focal air-space opacity. Other usual radiological findings of SARS involving lungs include ground glass opacification which may or may not be associated with consolidation, intralobular interstitial and thickened interlobular septal, with predominantly a peripheral and lower lobe involvement [159]. In case of SARS, the characteristic peripheral alveolar opacities have similarities as in bronchiolitis obliterans organizing pneumonia [159]. As the clinical, radiographic, biochemical parameters of SARS are not exclusively pathognomonic, WHO and the Centers for Disease Control and Prevention issued updated case definitions for SARS during the outbreak. A suspected case of SARS defined by WHO (revised; 1 May 2003) [160] is as a person observed after 1st November 2002 with distinctive features (Tables **3**, **4**).

Table 3. WHO case definitions of SARS in the post outbreak period [154 - 159].

Clinical Case Definition of SARS	Laboratory Case Definition of SARS
A person with a history of Fever>38 °C,	A person with symptoms and signs that clinically suggest SARS along with positive laboratory findings for SARS CoV based on one or more of diagnostic criteria
One or more symptoms of lower respiratory tract illness (shortness of breath, cough)	PCR positive for SARS CoV validated by At least two different clinical specimens or – The same clinical specimen collected on two or more occasions during the illness (sequential nasopharyngeal aspirates), or – Two different repeat PCR using a RNA extract from the original clinical sample
Radiographic evidences of lung infiltrates suggesting pneumonia or respiratory distress syndrome or necropsy findings confirming pathology of pneumonia or respiratory distress syndrome without identifying the cause	Seroconversion by ELISA or immunofluorescence
In case where no alternative diagnosis fails to explain the illness.	Virus isolation: Isolation of SARS CoV from cell culture of any any specimen; PCR confirmation

Treatment

The basic management steps for SARS depend on rapid diagnostic procedures, disease severity assessment, and usage of broad spectrum antimicrobials until the infective agent is identified (Table **5**). Infection control measures play a pivotal role in disease management. Symptomatic management is to be considered while patients are in hospital. Procedures and practices that promote aerosolization like nebulizers, continuous positive airway pressure, high-flow oxygen, non-invasive ventilation, bronchoscopy, tracheal intubation, chest physiotherapy, suctioning and humidification should be avoided to reduce the risk of infection to healthcare workers. Patients with impending respiratory failure should be managed under critical care unit and early incubation should be considered. Considering the biphasic nature of the illness and evidence from pathological studies steroids is considered valuable to manage the disease process. Basic mechanism behind the steroid therapy is modulation of cytokine dysregulation and found to be more effective in later stages of the disease [162]. The steroids are more effective in controlling the fever and reduce the oxygen supplementation [163]. Pulse therapies for steroids have some advantages over daily treatment [164]. In the early stages of SARS epidemic Ribavarin was considered one of the preferred drug. But Ribavarin is losing its priority as it has been proved that this drug has no *in vitro* activity against SARS CoV. On the other hand, this drug is having its own significant toxicity of bone marrow depression including hemolysis (in about 76% of patients) and decrease in hemoglobin of 2 g/dl (in about 49%) [165]. There are various experimental treatments for severe ill patients. The therapeutic molecules include intravenous immunoglobulins, tumor necrosis factor, alpha-blockers, convalescent serum, proteinase inhibitors, interferons traditional Chinese medicines *etc.*, but the outcome is yet awaited [166].

Table 4. Centres for Disease Control and Prevention: Updated interim case definition for SARS [161].

Clinical Criteria	Early illness – Presence of two or more of the features: fever (might be subjective), chills, rigors, myalgia, headache, diarrhoea, sore throat, rhinorrhoea
	Mild to moderate respiratory illness Temperature 100.4 °F or 38 °C) and lower respiratory illness (for example, cough, dyspnoea, difficulty breathing)
	Severe respiratory illness mild to moderate respiratory illness, radiographic evidence of pneumonia, or acute respiratory distress syndrome, necropsy findings consistent with pneumonia, or acute respiratory distress syndrome without an identifiable cause
Epidemiological Criteria	Possible exposure to SARS: Travel to a foreign or domestic location with documented or suspected SARS transmission –
	Close contact with a person with mild-to-moderate or severe respiratory illness and with history of travel in the 10 days before onset of symptoms to a foreign or domestic location with documented or suspected SARS transmission
Laboratory Criteria	Detection of serum antibody to SARS CoV as validated by the Centres for Disease Control and Prevention (CDC) enzyme immunoassay) Isolation of SARS CoV in cell culture from a clinical specimen,
	Detection SARS CoV RNA by RT-PCR as validated CDC and with subsequent confirmation in a designated laboratory
Exclusion Criteria	A person may be excluded if: An alternative diagnosis can fully explain the illness
	Absence of antibody to SARS CoV in a serum specimen

(Table 4) cont.....

<table>
<tr><td>Clinical Criteria</td><td>Early illness
– Presence of two or more of the features:
fever (might be subjective), chills, rigors, myalgia, headache, diarrhoea, sore throat, rhinorrhoea</td></tr>
<tr><td rowspan="2">SARS Disease Classification</td><td>Probable case of SARS CoV disease: person who shows clinical criteria for severe respiratory illness and the epidemiological criteria for likely exposure to SARS CoV</td></tr>
<tr><td>Confirmed case of SARS CoV disease: person who has a clinically compatible illness (that is, early, mild to-moderate, or severe) that is laboratory confirmed</td></tr>
</table>

Table 5. Management of severe acute respiratory syndrome (SARS) (adapted from the BTS/BIS SARS guidelines50) [162 - 166].

<table>
<tr><td></td><td colspan="2">Suspected SARS</td><td colspan="2">Probable SARS</td></tr>
<tr><td>Case Definition</td><td>Non-severe</td><td>Severe</td><td>Non-severe</td><td>Severe</td></tr>
<tr><td></td><td colspan="2">A person with clinical presentation after 1 Feb 2003 with all 3:
High fever >38 °C
Cough or breathing difficulty
H/o travel, to an area with local transmission 2
and/or
Close contact with a person with probable SARS</td><td colspan="2">A suspect case with:
1 CXR pneumonia and no response to usual Rx
and/or
RDS</td></tr>
<tr><td>Infection Control Issues</td><td colspan="2">1 N95 mask for patient to wear 1
1 Consult in identified area away from others 1
1 HCW to adhere to local infection control measures 1
(gown, gloves, mask, hand washing)
1 Inform hospital infection control and CCDC</td><td colspan="2">Admit to negative pressure isolation room
Transfer to regional centre
Inform regional designated SARS ID unit</td></tr>
<tr><td>Clinical Issues</td><td colspan="4">1 Confirm travel/contact history + obtain history of close contact/household contacts
1 Consider other causes of community acquired pneumonia
1 Note comorbidity (severity risk)
1 Assess severity (BTS guidelines</td></tr>
<tr><td>Investigative Issues</td><td colspan="4">1 Laboratory testing for SARS (PHLS website): sputum, urine, stool, EDTA blood, acute serology
1 CXR
1 Pulse oximetry and blood gases if SpO_2 <92% on air
1 FBC, U&E, LFT, LDH, CK, CRP
1 Other microbiological samples (e.g. blood cultures)</td></tr>
</table>

(Table 5) cont.....

<table>
<tr><th></th><th>Suspected SARS</th><th>Probable SARS</th></tr>
<tr><td>Management</td><td colspan="2">Consider home management for non-severe cases
Hospitalization for severe cases
Patient to record temperature bd in non- severe cases where as antibiotics as for severe CAP (b-lactam +macrolide)
In case of non-severe Paracetamol for fever but severe cases should be closely monitored
Fluids and bed rest, severe cases Avoid CT scan</td></tr>
<tr><td>Discharge</td><td colspan="2">Afebrile for 48 hours + resolving cough + lab tests returning to normal + CXR improved
Record temperature bd; if >37.9 °C ´ 2 report to healthcare facility
Stay at home with minimum contacts for 7 days
Follow-up at minimum of one week (? at home)
Convalescent serology at 3 weeks</td></tr>
</table>

CONSENT FOR PUBLICATION

Not applicable.

CONFLICT OF INTEREST

The authors confirm that this chapter contents have no conflict of interest.

ACKNOWLEDGEMENTS

Declare none.

REFERENCES

[1] Krause RM. The origin of plagues: old and new. Science 1992; 257(5073): 1073-8. [http://dx.doi.org/10.1126/science.257.5073.1073] [PMID: 1509258]

[2] Morens DM, Folkers GK, Fauci AS. Emerging infections: A perpetual challenge. Lancet Infect Dis 2008; 8(11): 710-9. [http://dx.doi.org/10.1016/S1473-3099(08)70256-1] [PMID: 18992407]

[3] Jaiyan DK, Liu J, Hai R, Zhu H. Emerging and Reemerging Human Viral Diseases. Ann Microbiol Res 2018; 2(1): 31-44.

[4] Estimates of global, regional, and national incidence, prevalence, and mortality of HIV, 1980-2015: the Global Burden of Disease Study 2015. Lancet HIV 2016; 3(8): e361-87. [http://dx.doi.org/10.1016/S2352-3018(16)30087-X] [PMID: 27470028]

[5] Moses IM. Swine-origin Influenza A (H1N1) Virus: An Update. Chapter 9.

[6] Tripp RA. Addressing the Re-emergence of Poliovirus. J Antivir Antiretrovir 2014; 6: 1. [http://dx.doi.org/10.4172/jaa.1000e116]

[7] World Health Organisation. Statement on the 1st meeting of the IHR Emergency Committee on the 2014 Ebola outbreak in West Africa 2014. The United Nations, https://www. who.int/mediacentre/news/statements/2014/ebola-20140808/en/.

[8] Jones KE, Patel NG, Levy MA, *et al.* Global trends in emerging infectious diseases. Nature 2008; 451(7181): 990-3.

[http://dx.doi.org/10.1038/nature06536] [PMID: 18288193]

[9] Josseran L, Paquet C, Zehgnoun A, *et al.* Chikungunya disease outbreak, Reunion Island. Emerg Infect Dis 2006; 12(12): 1994-5.
[http://dx.doi.org/10.3201/eid1212.060710] [PMID: 17354339]

[10] James W. Le Duc, Nathanson N. Emerging Viral Diseases. Chapter 16. 216-231.

[11] Pliaka V, Kyriakopoulou Z, Markoulatos P. Risks associated with the use of live-attenuated vaccine poliovirus strains and the strategies for control and eradication of paralytic poliomyelitis. Expert Rev Vaccines 2012; 11(5): 609-28.
[http://dx.doi.org/10.1586/erv.12.28] [PMID: 22827246]

[12] Kew OM, Sutter RW, de Gourville EM, Dowdle WR, Pallansch MA. Vaccine-derived polioviruses and the endgame strategy for global polio eradication. Annu Rev Microbiol 2005; 59: 587-635.
[http://dx.doi.org/10.1146/annurev.micro.58.030603.123625] [PMID: 16153180]

[13] Fine PE, Carneiro IA. Transmissibility and persistence of oral polio vaccine viruses: implications for the global poliomyelitis eradication initiative. Am J Epidemiol 1999; 150(10): 1001-21.
[http://dx.doi.org/10.1093/oxfordjournals.aje.a009924] [PMID: 10568615]

[14] Lauring AS, Frydman J, Andino R. The role of mutational robustness in RNA virus evolution. Nat Rev Microbiol 2013; 11(5): 327-36.
[http://dx.doi.org/10.1038/nrmicro3003] [PMID: 23524517]

[15] Holmes EC, Ghedin E, Miller N, *et al.* Whole-genome analysis of human influenza A virus reveals multiple persistent lineages and reassortment among recent H3N2 viruses. PLoS Biol 2005; 3(9)e300
[http://dx.doi.org/10.1371/journal.pbio.0030300] [PMID: 16026181]

[16] Lukashev AN, Shumilina EY, Belalov IS, *et al.* Recombination strategies and evolutionary dynamics of the Human enterovirus A global gene pool. J Gen Virol 2014; 95(Pt 4): 868-73.
[http://dx.doi.org/10.1099/vir.0.060004-0] [PMID: 24425417]

[17] Kirkegaard K, Baltimore D. The mechanism of RNA recombination in poliovirus. Cell 1986; 47(3): 433-43.
[http://dx.doi.org/10.1016/0092-8674(86)90600-8] [PMID: 3021340]

[18] Jarvis TC, Kirkegaard K. Poliovirus RNA recombination: mechanistic studies in the absence of selection. EMBO J 1992; 11(8): 3135-45.
[http://dx.doi.org/10.1002/j.1460-2075.1992.tb05386.x] [PMID: 1379178]

[19] Athar MN, Baqai HZ, Ahmad M, *et al.* Short report: Crimean-Congo hemorrhagic fever outbreak in Rawalpindi, Pakistan, February 2002. Am J Trop Med Hyg 2003; 69(3): 284-7.
[http://dx.doi.org/10.4269/ajtmh.2003.69.284] [PMID: 14628945]

[20] Akinci E, Yilmaz M, Bodur H, *et al.* Analysis of lymphocyte subgroups in Crimean-Congo hemorrhagic fever. Int J Infect Dis 2009; 13(5): 560-3.
[http://dx.doi.org/10.1016/j.ijid.2008.08.027] [PMID: 19112036]

[21] Paragas J, Whitehouse CA, Endy TP, Bray M. A simple assay for determining antiviral activity against Crimean-Congo hemorrhagic fever virus. Antiviral Res 2004; 62(1): 21-5.
[http://dx.doi.org/10.1016/j.antiviral.2003.11.006] [PMID: 15026198]

[22] Tang Q, Saijo M, Zhang Y, *et al.* A patient with Crimean-Congo hemorrhagic fever serologically diagnosed by recombinant nucleoprotein-based antibody detection systems. Clin Diagn Lab Immunol 2003; 10(3): 489-91.
[PMID: 12738657]

[23] Akıncı E, Bodur H, Leblebicioglu H. Pathogenesis of Crimean-Congo hemorrhagic fever. Vector Borne Zoonotic Dis 2013; 13(7): 429-37.
[http://dx.doi.org/10.1089/vbz.2012.1061] [PMID: 23663164]

[24] Swanepoel R, Gill DE, Shepherd AJ, Leman PA, Mynhardt JH, Harvey S. The clinical pathology of

Crimean-Congo hemorrhagic fever. Rev Infect Dis 1989; 11 (Suppl. 4): S794-800. [http://dx.doi.org/10.1093/clinids/11.Supplement_4.S794] [PMID: 2749111]

[25] Akinci E, Yilmaz M, Bodur H, *et al.* Analysis of lymphocyte subgroups in Crimean-Congo hemorrhagic fever. Int J Infect Dis 2009; 13(5): 560-3. [http://dx.doi.org/10.1016/j.ijid.2008.08.027] [PMID: 19112036]

[26] Burt FJ, Leman PA, Smith JF, Swanepoel R. The use of a reverse transcription-polymerase chain reaction for the detection of viral nucleic acid in the diagnosis of Crimean-Congo haemorrhagic fever. J Virol Methods 1998; 70(2): 129-37. [http://dx.doi.org/10.1016/S0166-0934(97)00182-1] [PMID: 9562407]

[27] Drosten C, Göttig S, Schilling S, *et al.* Rapid detection and quantification of RNA of Ebola and Marburg viruses, Lassa virus, Crimean-Congo hemorrhagic fever virus, Rift Valley fever virus, dengue virus, and yellow fever virus by real-time reverse transcription-PCR. J Clin Microbiol 2002; 40(7): 2323-30. [http://dx.doi.org/10.1128/JCM.40.7.2323-2330.2002] [PMID: 12089242]

[28] Duh D, Saksida A, Petrovec M, Dedushaj I, Avsic-Zupanc T. Novel one-step real-time RT-PCR assay for rapid and specific diagnosis of Crimean-Congo hemorrhagic fever encountered in the Balkans. J Virol Methods 2006; 133(2): 175-9. [http://dx.doi.org/10.1016/j.jviromet.2005.11.006] [PMID: 16343650]

[29] Wölfel R, Paweska JT, Petersen N, *et al.* Virus detection and monitoring of viral load in Crimean-Congo hemorrhagic fever virus patients. Emerg Infect Dis 2007; 13(7): 1097-100. [http://dx.doi.org/10.3201/eid1307.070068] [PMID: 18214191]

[30] Shepherd AJ, Swanepoel R, Gill DE. Evaluation of enzyme-linked immunosorbent assay and reversed passive hemagglutination for detection of Crimean-Congo hemorrhagic fever virus antigen. J Clin Microbiol 1988; 26(2): 347-53. [PMID: 3125221]

[31] Shepherd AJ, Swanepoel R, Leman PA, Shepherd SP. Comparison of methods for isolation and titration of Crimean-Congo hemorrhagic fever virus. J Clin Microbiol 1986; 24(4): 654-6. [PMID: 3095367]

[32] Drosten C, Kümmerer BM, Schmitz H, Günther S. Molecular diagnostics of viral hemorrhagic fevers. Antiviral Res 2003; 57(1-2): 61-87. [http://dx.doi.org/10.1016/S0166-3542(02)00201-2] [PMID: 12615304]

[33] Wölfel R, Paweska JT, Petersen N, *et al.* Low-density macroarray for rapid detection and identification of Crimean-Congo hemorrhagic fever virus. J Clin Microbiol 2009; 47(4): 1025-30. [http://dx.doi.org/10.1128/JCM.01920-08] [PMID: 19225100]

[34] Song JW, Baek LJ, Nagle JW, Schlitter D, Yanagihara R. Genetic and phylogenetic analyses of hantaviral sequences amplified from archival tissues of deer mice (Peromyscus maniculatus nubiterrae) captured in the eastern United States. Arch Virol 1996; 141(5): 959-67. [http://dx.doi.org/10.1007/BF01718170] [PMID: 8678841]

[35] Sung JJ, Wu A, Joynt GM, *et al.* Severe acute respiratory syndrome: report of treatment and outcome after a major outbreak. Thorax 2004; 59(5): 414-20. [http://dx.doi.org/10.1136/thx.2003.014076] [PMID: 15115870]

[36] Zhong NS, Zeng GQ. Our strategies for fighting severe acute respiratory syndrome (SARS). Am J Respir Crit Care Med 2003; 168(1): 7-9. [http://dx.doi.org/10.1164/rccm.200305-707OE] [PMID: 12773318]

[37] Ho JC, Ooi GC, Mok TY, *et al.* High-dose pulse versus nonpulse corticosteroid regimens in severe acute respiratory syndrome. Am J Respir Crit Care Med 2003; 168(12): 1449-56. [http://dx.doi.org/10.1164/rccm.200306-766OC] [PMID: 12947028]

[38] Oestereich L, Rieger T, Neumann M, Bernreuther C, *et al.* Evaluation of antiviral efficacy of ribavirin,

arbidol, and T-705 (favipiravir) in a mouse model for Crimean-Congo hemorrhagic fever PLoSNegl Trop Dis 2014; 8: e2804 73..

[39] Mehedi M, Falzarano D, Seebach J, *et al.* A new Ebola virus nonstructural glycoprotein expressed through RNA editing. J Virol 2011; 85(11): 5406-14. [http://dx.doi.org/10.1128/JVI.02190-10] [PMID: 21411529]

[40] McElroy AK, Erickson BR, Flietstra TD, *et al.* Ebola hemorrhagic Fever: novel biomarker correlates of clinical outcome. J Infect Dis 2014; 210(4): 558-66. [http://dx.doi.org/10.1093/infdis/jiu088] [PMID: 24526742]

[41] Fauci AS. Ebola--underscoring the global disparities in health care resources. N Engl J Med 2014; 371(12): 1084-6. [http://dx.doi.org/10.1056/NEJMp1409494] [PMID: 25119491]

[42] Bannister B, Puro V, Fusco FM, Heptonstall J, Ippolito G. Framework for the design and operation of high-level isolation units: consensus of the European Network of Infectious Diseases. Lancet Infect Dis 2009; 9(1): 45-56. [http://dx.doi.org/10.1016/S1473-3099(08)70304-9] [PMID: 19095195]

[43] Bagherani N, Smoller BR, Kannangara AP, *et al.* An Overview on Ebola 2015; 2: 64-73.

[44] Kugelman JR, Sanchez-Lockhart M, Andersen KG, *et al.* Evaluation of the potential impact of Ebola virus genomic drift on the efficacy of sequence-based candidate therapeutics. MBio 2015; 6(1)e02227-14 Marzi A, Feldmann H, Geisbert TW, Falzarano D. Vesicular stomatitis virus-based vaccines for prophylaxis and treatment of filovirus infections. J Bioterror Biodef. 2011, 45. [http://dx.doi.org/10.1128/mBio.02227-14] [PMID: 25604787]

[46] Feldmann H, Geisbert TW. Ebola haemorrhagic fever. Lancet 2011; 377(9768): 849-62. [http://dx.doi.org/10.1016/S0140-6736(10)60667-8] [PMID: 21084112]

[47] Mehedi M, Falzarano D, Seebach J, *et al.* A new Ebola virus nonstructural glycoprotein expressed through RNA editing. J Virol 2011; 85(11): 5406-14. [http://dx.doi.org/10.1128/JVI.02190-10] [PMID: 21411529]

[48] Ansari AA. Clinical features and pathobiology of Ebolavirus infection. J Autoimmun 2014; 55: 1-9. [http://dx.doi.org/10.1016/j.jaut.2014.09.001] [PMID: 25260583]

[49] Ströher U, Feldmann H. Progress towards the treatment of Ebola haemorrhagic fever. Expert Opin Investig Drugs 2006; 15(12): 1523-35. [http://dx.doi.org/10.1517/13543784.15.12.1523] [PMID: 17107278]

[50] Chippaux JP. Outbreaks of Ebola virus disease in Africa: the beginnings of a tragic saga. J Venom Anim Toxins Incl Trop Dis 2014; 20(1): 44. [http://dx.doi.org/10.1186/1678-9199-20-44] [PMID: 25320574]

[51] Koenig KL, Majestic C, Burns MJ. Ebola Virus Disease: essential public health principles for clinicians. West J Emerg Med 2014; 15(7): 728-31. [http://dx.doi.org/10.5811/westjem.2014.9.24011] [PMID: 25493109]

[52] Olupot-Olupot P. Ebola in children: epidemiology, clinical features, diagnosis and outcomes. Pediatr Infect Dis J 2015; 34(3): 314-6. [http://dx.doi.org/10.1097/INF.0000000000000638] [PMID: 25522340]

[53] Thippeswamy NB. Ebola Virus Disease: New Horizons in Biotechnology. India. 2015; 007-14.

[54] Ethiopian Public Health Institute. Ebola viral disease interim Guideline. Addis Ababa, Ethiopia 2014; pp. 1-83.

[55] Peters CJ. Hemorrhagic Fevers in the African Health Care Setting. Centers for Disease Control and Prevention. J Infect Dis 1998.

[56] Baron RC, McCormick JB, Zubeir OA. Ebola virus disease in southern Sudan: hospital dissemination and intrafamilial spread. Bull World Health Organ 1983; 61(6): 997-1003. [PMID: 6370486]

[57] Centers for Disease Control. gov.About Quarantine andIsolation. 2014.

[58] Lewis D. Liberia shuts schools, considers quarantine to curbEbola. Reuters 2014.

[59] Kortepeter MG, Bausch DG, Bray M. Basic clinical and laboratory features of filoviral hemorrhagic fever. J Infect Dis 2011; 204 (Suppl. 3): S810-6. [http://dx.doi.org/10.1093/infdis/jir299] [PMID: 21987756]

[60] Centers for Disease Control Ebola Hemorrhagic FeverPrevention. 2014.

[61] Kilmarx PH, Clarke KR, Dietz PM, *et al.* Ebola virus disease in health care workers--Sierra Leone, 2014. MMWR Morb Mortal Wkly Rep 2014; 63(49): 1168-71. [PMID: 25503921]

[62] Jamieson DJ, Uyeki TM, Callaghan WM, Meaney-Delman D. RasmussenSA . What obstetrician-gynecologists should know about Ebola: a perspective from the Centers for Disease Control and Prevention ObstetGynecol 124: 1005-10.2014;

[63] Jocelyn Y. Antiviral InteliStrat in the 2014 Ebola Virus Outbreak in West Africa: Current Perspectives for Prevention and Treatment. Journal of Human Virology & Retrovirology 2014; 1: 4.

[64] Hampton T. Largest-ever outbreak of Ebola virus disease thrusts experimental therapies, vaccines into spotlight. JAMA 2014; 312(10): 987-9. [http://dx.doi.org/10.1001/jama.2014.11170] [PMID: 25162140]

[65] Cheepsattayakorn A, Cheepsattayakorn R. Ebola Virus Disease: Updated Path physiology and Clinical Aspects. Ann Clin Pathol 2015; 3: 1048.

[66] Woldu AM, Lenjisa LJ, Tegegne TG, Satessa GD. Emerging Therapeutic Approaches to Combat the Pandemicity of the Deadly Ebola Virus. American Journal of Phytomedicine and Clinical Therapeutics 2014.

[67] Kalra S, Kelkar D, Galwankar SC, *et al.* The emergence of ebola as a global health security threat: from 'lessons learned' to coordinated multilateral containment efforts. J Glob Infect Dis 2014; 6(4): 164-77. [http://dx.doi.org/10.4103/0974-777X.145247] [PMID: 25538455]

[68] Bishop DH, Calisher CH, Casals J, *et al.* Bunyaviridae. Intervirology 1980; 14(3-4): 125-43. [http://dx.doi.org/10.1159/000149174] [PMID: 6165702]

[69] Fenner F. The classification and nomenclature of viruses.Summary of results of meetings of the International Committee on Taxonomy of Viruses Intervirology. 1975; 6: 1-12. [http://dx.doi.org/10.1159/000149448]

[70] Knipe DM, Howley PM, Griffin DE, Eds. Fieldsvirology. 4th ed.

[71] Elliot RM, Schmaljohn CS, Collett MS. Bunyaviridae genome structure and gene expression.Current Topics in Microbiology and Immunology. New York, NY: Springer-Verlag 1991; pp. 91-141.

[72] Nichol ST. Bunyaviruses.Field's Virology. 4th ed. Philadelphia, Pa: LippincottWilliams&Wilkins 2001; Vol. 2: pp. 1603-33.

[73] Schmaljohn CS, Hooper JW. Bunyaviridae: the viruses and their replication.Field's Virology. 4th ed. Philadelphia, Pa: Lippincott Williams & Wilkins 2001; Vol. 2: pp. 1581-602.

[74] Martin ML, Lindsey-Regnery H, Sasso DR, McCormick JB, Palmer E. Distinction between Bunyaviridae genera by surface structure and comparison with Hantaan virus using negative stain electron microscopy. Arch Virol 1985; 86(1-2): 17-28. [http://dx.doi.org/10.1007/BF01314110] [PMID: 2412528]

[75] Xu ZY, Guo CS, Wu YL, Zhang XW, Liu K. Epidemiological studies of hemorrhagic fever with renal syndrome: analysis of risk factors and mode of transmission. J Infect Dis 1985; 152(1): 137-44. [http://dx.doi.org/10.1093/infdis/152.1.137] [PMID: 2861242]

[76] Tsai TF. Hemorrhagic fever with renal syndrome: mode of transmission to humans. Lab Anim Sci 1987; 37(4): 428-30.
[PMID: 2889846]

[77] Lee HW, van der Groen G. Hemorrhagic fever with renal syndrome. Prog Med Virol 1989; 36: 62-102.
[PMID: 2573914]

[78] Monroe MC, Morzunov SP, Johnson AM, *et al.* Genetic diversity and distribution of Peromyscus-borne hantaviruses in North America. Emerg Infect Dis 1999; 5(1): 75-86.
[http://dx.doi.org/10.3201/eid0501.990109] [PMID: 10081674]

[79] Peters CJ, Khan AS. Hantavirus pulmonary syndrome: the new American hemorrhagic fever. Clin Infect Dis 2002; 34(9): 1224-31.
[http://dx.doi.org/10.1086/339864] [PMID: 11941549]

[80] Schmaljohn C, Hjelle B. Hantaviruses: a global disease problem. Emerg Infect Dis 1997; 3(2): 95-104.
[http://dx.doi.org/10.3201/eid0302.970202] [PMID: 9204290]

[81] Lednicky JA. Hantaviruses. a short review. Arch Pathol Lab Med 2003; 127(1): 30-5.
[PMID: 12521363]

[82] Young JC, Hansen GR, Graves TK, *et al.* The incubation period of hantavirus pulmonary syndrome. Am J Trop Med Hyg 2000; 62(6): 714-7.
[http://dx.doi.org/10.4269/ajtmh.2000.62.714] [PMID: 11304061]

[83] Peters CJ, Simpson GL, Levy H. Spectrum of hantavirus infection: hemorrhagic fever with renal syndrome and hantavirus pulmonary syndrome. Annu Rev Med 1999; 50: 531-45.
[http://dx.doi.org/10.1146/annurev.med.50.1.531] [PMID: 10073292]

[84] Nolte KB, Feddersen RM, Foucar K, *et al.* Hantavirus pulmonary syndrome in the United States: a pathological description of a disease caused by a new agent. Hum Pathol 1995; 26(1): 110-20.
[http://dx.doi.org/10.1016/0046-8177(95)90123-X] [PMID: 7821907]

[85] Zaki SR, Greer PW, Coffield LM, *et al.* Hantavirus pulmonary syndrome. Pathogenesis of an emerging infectious disease. Am J Pathol 1995; 146(3): 552-79.
[PMID: 7887439]

[86] Chapman LE, Ellis BA, Koster FT, *et al.* Discriminators between hantavirus-infected and -uninfected persons enrolled in a trial of intravenous ribavirin for presumptive hantavirus pulmonary syndrome. Clin Infect Dis 2002; 34(3): 293-304.
[http://dx.doi.org/10.1086/324619] [PMID: 11774075]

[87] Peters CJ, Mills JN, Spiropoulou C, Zaki SR, Rollin PE. Hantaviruses. InGuerrant RL, Walker DH, Weller PF, eds. Tropical Infectious Diseases: Principles,Pathogens, and Practice. New York, NY: WB Saunders. 1998.

[88] Peters CJ. Hantavirus pulmonary syndrome in the Americas.Emerging Infections 2. Washington, DC: AmericanSociety for Microbiology Press 1998; pp. 17-64.
[http://dx.doi.org/10.1128/9781555816957.ch2]

[89] Lyubsky S, Gavrilovskaya I, Luft B, Mackow E. Histopathology of Peromyscus leucopus naturally infected with pathogenic NY-1 hantaviruses: pathologic markers of HPS viral infection in mice. Lab Invest 1996; 74(3): 627-33.
[PMID: 8600313]

[90] Netski D, Thran BH, St Jeor SC. Sin Nombre virus pathogenesis in Peromyscus maniculatus. J Virol 1999; 73(1): 585-91.
[PMID: 9847363]

[91] Hooper JW, Larsen T, Custer DM, Schmaljohn CS. A lethal dose model forhantavirus pulmonary syndrome. Virology 2001; 289: 6-14.

[http://dx.doi.org/10.1006/viro.2001.1133]

[92] Lundkvist A, Hukic M, Hörling J, Gilljam M, Nichol S, Niklasson B. Puumala and Dobrava viruses cause hemorrhagic fever with renal syndrome in Bosnia-Herzegovina: evidence of highly cross-neutralizing antibody responses in early patient sera. J Med Virol 1997; 53(1): 51-9. [http://dx.doi.org/10.1002/(SICI)1096-9071(199709)53:1<51::AID-JMV9>3.0.CO;2-P] [PMID: 9298732]

[93] Plyusnin A, Vapalahti O, Lankinen H, *et al.* Tula virus: a newly detected hantavirus carried by European common voles. J Virol 1994; 68(12): 7833-9. [PMID: 7966573]

[94] Plyusnin A, Hörling J, Kanerva M, *et al.* Puumala hantavirus genome in patients with nephropathia epidemica: correlation of PCR positivity with HLA haplotype and link to viral sequences in local rodents. J Clin Microbiol 1997; 35(5): 1090-6. [PMID: 9114386]

[95] Padula PJ, Colavecchia SB, Martínez VP, *et al.* Genetic diversity, distribution, and serological features of hantavirus infection in five countries in South America. J Clin Microbiol 2000; 38(8): 3029-35. [PMID: 10921972]

[96] Terajima M, Hendershot JD III, Kariwa H, *et al.* High levels of viremia in patients with the Hantavirus pulmonary syndrome. J Infect Dis 1999; 180(6): 2030-4. [http://dx.doi.org/10.1086/315153] [PMID: 10558964]

[97] Hujakka H, Koistinen V, Kuronen I, *et al.* Diagnostic rapid tests for acute hantavirus infections: specific tests for Hantaan, Dobrava and Puumala viruses versus a hantavirus combination test. J Virol Methods 2003; 108(1): 117-22. [http://dx.doi.org/10.1016/S0166-0934(02)00282-3] [PMID: 12565162]

[98] Martinez VP, Bellomo C, San Juan J, *et al.* Person-to-person transmission of Andes virus. Emerg Infect Dis 2005; 11(12): 1848-53. [http://dx.doi.org/10.3201/eid1112.050501] [PMID: 16485469]

[99] Padula PJ, Edelstein A, Miguel SD, López NM, Rossi CM, Rabinovich RD. Hantavirus pulmonary syndrome outbreak in Argentina: molecular evidence for person-to-person transmission of Andes virus. Virology 1998; 241(2): 323-30. [http://dx.doi.org/10.1006/viro.1997.8976] [PMID: 9499807]

[100] Severson WE, Schmaljohn CS, Javadian A, Jonsson CB. Ribavirin causes error catastrophe during Hantaan virus replication. J Virol 2003; 77(1): 481-8. [http://dx.doi.org/10.1128/JVI.77.1.481-488.2003] [PMID: 12477853]

[101] Choi Y, Ahn CJ, Seong KM, Jung MY, Ahn BY. Inactivated Hantaan virus vaccine derived from suspension culture of Vero cells. Vaccine 2003; 21(17-18): 1867-73. [http://dx.doi.org/10.1016/S0264-410X(03)00005-7] [PMID: 12706671]

[102] Laakkonen J, Kallio-Kokko H, Oktem MA, *et al.* Serological survey for viral pathogens in Turkish rodents. J Wildl Dis 2006; 42(3): 672-6. [http://dx.doi.org/10.7589/0090-3558-42.3.672] [PMID: 17092901]

[103] Cosgriff TM. Mechanisms of disease in Hantavirus infection: pathophysiology of hemorrhagic fever with renal syndrome. Rev Infect Dis 1991; 13(1): 97-107. [http://dx.doi.org/10.1093/clinids/13.1.97] [PMID: 1673261]

[104] Lednicky JA. Hantaviruses. a short review. Arch Pathol Lab Med 2003; 127(1): 30-5. [PMID: 12521363]

[105] Schmaljohn CS, Dalrymple JM. Analysis of Hantaan virus RNA: evidence for a new genus of bunyaviridae. Virology 1983; 131(2): 482-91. [http://dx.doi.org/10.1016/0042-6822(83)90514-7] [PMID: 6419460]

[106] Papa A, Nemirov K, Henttonen H, *et al.* Isolation of Dobrava virus from Apodemus flavicollis in

Greece. J Clin Microbiol 2001; 39(6): 2291-3. [http://dx.doi.org/10.1128/JCM.39.6.2291-2293.2001] [PMID: 11376073]

[107] Laakkonen J, Kallio-Kokko H, Oktem MA, *et al.* Serological survey for viral pathogens in Turkish rodents. J Wildl Dis 2006; 42(3): 672-6. [http://dx.doi.org/10.7589/0090-3558-42.3.672] [PMID: 17092901]

[108] Schountz T, Prescott J, Cogswell AC, *et al.* Regulatory T cell-like responses in deer mice persistently infected with Sin Nombre virus. Proc Natl Acad Sci USA 2007; 104(39): 15496-501. [http://dx.doi.org/10.1073/pnas.0707454104] [PMID: 17875986]

[109] Cho HW, Howard CR, Lee HW. Review of an inactivated vaccine against hantaviruses. Intervirology 2002; 45(4-6): 328-33. [http://dx.doi.org/10.1159/000067925] [PMID: 12602351]

[110] Choi Y, Ahn CJ, Seong KM, Jung MY, Ahn BY. Inactivated Hantaan virus vaccine derived from suspension culture of Vero cells. Vaccine 2003; 21(17-18): 1867-73. [http://dx.doi.org/10.1016/S0264-410X(03)00005-7] [PMID: 12706671]

[111] Hooper JW, Kamrud KI, Elgh F, Custer D, Schmaljohn CS. DNA vaccination with hantavirus M segment elicits neutralizing antibodies and protects against seoul virus infection. Virology 1999; 255(2): 269-78. [http://dx.doi.org/10.1006/viro.1998.9586] [PMID: 10069952]

[112] Hooper JW, Custer DM, Thompson E, Schmaljohn CS. DNA vaccination with the Hantaan virus M gene protects Hamsters against three of four HFRS hantaviruses and elicits a high-titer neutralizing antibody response in Rhesus monkeys. J Virol 2001; 75(18): 8469-77. [http://dx.doi.org/10.1128/JVI.75.18.8469-8477.2001] [PMID: 11507192]

[113] Custer DM, Thompson E, Schmaljohn CS, Ksiazek TG, Hooper JW. Active and passive vaccination against hantavirus pulmonary syndrome with Andes virus M genome segment-based DNA vaccine. J Virol 2003; 77(18): 9894-905. [http://dx.doi.org/10.1128/JVI.77.18.9894-9905.2003] [PMID: 12941899]

[114] Hooper JW, Custer DM, Smith J, Wahl-Jensen V. Hantaan/Andes virus DNA vaccine elicits a broadly cross-reactive neutralizing antibody response in nonhuman primates. Virology 2006; 347(1): 208-16. [http://dx.doi.org/10.1016/j.virol.2005.11.035] [PMID: 16378630]

[115] Bharadwaj M, Mirowsky K, Ye C, *et al.* Genetic vaccines protect against Sin Nombre hantavirus challenge in the deer mouse (Peromyscus maniculatus). J Gen Virol 2002; 83(Pt 7): 1745-51. [http://dx.doi.org/10.1099/0022-1317-83-7-1745] [PMID: 12075094]

[116] Razanskiene A, Schmidt J, Geldmacher A, *et al.* High yields of stable and highly pure nucleocapsid proteins of different hantaviruses can be generated in the yeast Saccharomyces cerevisiae. J Biotechnol 2004; 111(3): 319-33. [http://dx.doi.org/10.1016/j.jbiotec.2004.04.010] [PMID: 15246668]

[117] Khattak S, Darai G, Süle S, Rösen-Wolff A. Characterization of expression of Puumala virus nucleocapsid protein in transgenic plants. Intervirology 2002; 45(4-6): 334-9. [http://dx.doi.org/10.1159/000067926] [PMID: 12602352]

[118] Palese P, Zheng H, Engelhardt OG, Pleschka S, García-Sastre A. Negative-strand RNA viruses: genetic engineering and applications. Proc Natl Acad Sci USA 1996; 93(21): 11354-8. [http://dx.doi.org/10.1073/pnas.93.21.11354] [PMID: 8876139]

[119] Murray K, Selleck P, Hooper P, *et al.* A morbillivirus that caused fatal disease in horses and humans. Science 1995; 268(5207): 94-7. [http://dx.doi.org/10.1126/science.7701348] [PMID: 7701348]

[120] Chua KB, Goh KJ, Wong KT, *et al.* Fatal encephalitis due to Nipah virus among pig-farmers in Malaysia. Lancet 1999; 354(9186): 1257-9. [http://dx.doi.org/10.1016/S0140-6736(99)04299-3] [PMID: 10520635]

[121] Marsh GA, de Jong C, Barr JA, *et al.* Cedar virus: a novel Henipavirus isolated from Australian bats. PLoS Pathog 2012; 8(8)e1002836
[http://dx.doi.org/10.1371/journal.ppat.1002836] [PMID: 22879820]

[122] Symons R. Re: Canine case of Hendra virus and Hendra virus vaccine. Aust Vet J 2011; 89(10): N24.

[123] Playford EG, McCall B, Smith G, *et al.* Human Hendra virus encephalitis associated with equine outbreak, Australia Emerg Infect Dis 2008; 16(2): 219-3. 2010.

[124] O'Sullivan JD, Allworth AM, Paterson DL, *et al.* Fatal encephalitis due to novel paramyxovirus transmitted from horses. Lancet 1997; 349(9045): 93-5.
[http://dx.doi.org/10.1016/S0140-6736(96)06162-4] [PMID: 8996421]

[125] Young PL, Halpin K, Selleck PW, *et al.* Serologic evidence for the presence in Pteropus bats of a paramyxovirus related to equine morbillivirus. Emerg Infect Dis 1996; 2(3): 239-40.
[http://dx.doi.org/10.3201/eid0203.960315] [PMID: 8903239]

[126] Field H, Young P, Yob JM, Mills J, Hall L, Mackenzie J. The natural history of Hendra and Nipah viruses. Microbes Infect 2001; 3(4): 307-14.
[http://dx.doi.org/10.1016/S1286-4579(01)01384-3] [PMID: 11334748]

[127] Halpin K, Young PL, Field HE, Mackenzie JS. Isolation of Hendra virus from pteropid bats: a natural reservoir of Hendra virus. J Gen Virol 2000; 81(Pt 8): 1927-32.
[http://dx.doi.org/10.1099/0022-1317-81-8-1927] [PMID: 10900029]

[128] Smith I, Broos A, de Jong C, *et al.* Identifying Hendra virus diversity in pteropid bats. PLoS One 2011; 6(9)e25275.
[http://dx.doi.org/10.1371/journal.pone.0025275] [PMID: 21980413]

[129] Marsh GA, Haining J, Hancock TJ, *et al.* Experimental infection of horses with Hendra virus/Australia/horse/2008/Redlands. Emerg Infect Dis 2011; 17(12): 2232-8.
[http://dx.doi.org/10.3201/eid1712.111162] [PMID: 22172152]

[130] Hooper PT, Ketterer PJ, Hyatt AD, Russell GM. Lesions of experimental equine morbillivirus pneumonia in horses. Vet Pathol 1997; 34(4): 312-22.
[http://dx.doi.org/10.1177/030098589703400407] [PMID: 9240840]

[131] Tan CT, Goh KJ, Wong KT, *et al.* Relapsed and late-onset Nipah encephalitis. Ann Neurol 2002; 51(6): 703-8.
[http://dx.doi.org/10.1002/ana.10212] [PMID: 12112075]

[132] Accessed March 14, 2014] Guidelines for veterinarians handling potential Hendra virus infection in horses Version 5.0. 2013. Available at:. http://www.daff.qld.gov.au/__data/assets/pdf_file/0009/97713/2355-guidelines-for-veterinarians-sept-2013.pdf132

[133] Zhu Z, Bossart KN, Bishop KA, *et al.* Exceptionally potent cross-reactive neutralization of Nipah and Hendra viruses by a human monoclonal antibody. J Infect Dis 2008; 197(6): 846-53.
[http://dx.doi.org/10.1086/528801] [PMID: 18271743]

[134] Bossart KN, Zhu Z, Middleton D, *et al.* A neutralizing human monoclonal antibody protects against lethal disease in a new ferret model of acute nipah virus infection. PLoS Pathog 2009; 5(10)e1000642.
[http://dx.doi.org/10.1371/journal.ppat.1000642] [PMID: 19888339]

[135] Bossart KN, Geisbert TW, Feldmann H, *et al.* A neutralizing human monoclonal antibody protects african green monkeys from hendra virus challenge. Sci Transl Med 2011; 3(105)105ra103.
[http://dx.doi.org/10.1126/scitranslmed.3002901] [PMID: 22013123]

[136] Murray K, Selleck P, Hooper P, *et al.* A morbillivirus that caused fatal disease in horses and humans. Science 1995; 268(5207): 94-7.
[http://dx.doi.org/10.1126/science.7701348] [PMID: 7701348]

[137] Peiris JS, Lai ST, Poon LL, *et al.* SARS study group. Coronavirus as a possible cause of severe acute

respiratory syndrome. Lancet 2003; 361(9366): 1319-25. [http://dx.doi.org/10.1016/S0140-6736(03)13077-2] [PMID: 12711465]

[138] Lee N, Hui D, Wu A, *et al.* A major outbreak of severe acute respiratory syndrome in Hong Kong. N Engl J Med 2003; 348(20): 1986-94. [http://dx.doi.org/10.1056/NEJMoa030685] [PMID: 12682352]

[139] Fouchicr RA, Kuiken T, Schutten M, *et al.* Aetiology: Koch's postulates fulfilled for SARS virus. Nature 2003; 423(6937): 240. [http://dx.doi.org/10.1038/423240a] [PMID: 12748632]

[140] Peiris JS, Lai ST, Poon LL, *et al.* SARS study group. Coronavirus as a possible cause of severe acute respiratory syndrome. Lancet 2003; 361(9366): 1319-25. [http://dx.doi.org/10.1016/S0140-6736(03)13077-2] [PMID: 12711465]

[141] Ksiazek TG, Erdman D, Goldsmith CS, *et al.* SARS Working Group. A novel coronavirus associated with severe acute respiratory syndrome. N Engl J Med 2003; 348(20): 1953-66. [http://dx.doi.org/10.1056/NEJMoa030781] [PMID: 12690092]

[142] Drosten C, Günther S, Preiser W, *et al.* Identification of a novel coronavirus in patients with severe acute respiratory syndrome. N Engl J Med 2003; 348(20): 1967-76. [http://dx.doi.org/10.1056/NEJMoa030747] [PMID: 12690091]

[143] Martina BE, Haagmans BL, Kuiken T, *et al.* Virology: SARS virus infection of cats and ferrets. Nature 2003; 425(6961): 915. [http://dx.doi.org/10.1038/425915a] [PMID: 14586458]

[144] Rota PA, Oberste MS, Monroe SS, *et al.* Characterization of a novel coronavirus associated with severe acute respiratory syndrome. Science 2003; 300(5624): 1394-9. [http://dx.doi.org/10.1126/science.1085952] [PMID: 12730500]

[145] Marra MA, Jones SJ, Astell CR, *et al.* The Genome sequence of the SARS-associated coronavirus. Science 2003; 300(5624): 1399-404. [http://dx.doi.org/10.1126/science.1085953] [PMID: 12730501]

[146] Ruan YJ, Wei CL, Ee AL, Vega VB, *et al.* Comparative full-length genomesequence analysis of 14 SARS coronavirus isolates and common mutationsassociated with putative origins of infection. Lancet 2003;361: 1779-85. Erratum: Lancet 2003; 361: 1832.

[147] Brown EG, Tetro JA. Comparative analysis of the SARS coronavirus genome: a good start to a long journey. Lancet 2003; 361(9371): 1756-7. [http://dx.doi.org/10.1016/S0140-6736(03)13444-7] [PMID: 12781529]

[148] Poutanen SM, Low DE, Henry B, *et al.* Identification of severe acute respiratory syndrome in Canada. N Engl J Med 2003; 348(20): 1995-2005. [http://dx.doi.org/10.1056/NEJMoa030634] [PMID: 12671061]

[149] Lee N, Hui D, Wu A, *et al.* A major outbreak of severe acute respiratory syndrome in Hong Kong. N Engl J Med 2003; 348(20): 1986-94. [http://dx.doi.org/10.1056/NEJMoa030685] [PMID: 12682352]

[150] Fowler RA, Lapinsky SE, Hallett D, *et al.* Toronto SARS Critical Care Group. Critically ill patients with severe acute respiratory syndrome. JAMA 2003; 290(3): 367-73. [http://dx.doi.org/10.1001/jama.290.3.367] [PMID: 12865378]

[151] Leung WK, To KF, Chan PK, *et al.* Enteric involvement of severe acute respiratory syndrome-associated coronavirus infection. Gastroenterology 2003; 125(4): 1011-7. [http://dx.doi.org/10.1016/j.gastro.2003.08.001] [PMID: 14517783]

[152] Tanaka N, Matsumoto T, Kuramitsu T, *et al.* High resolution CT findings in community-acquired pneumonia. J Comput Assist Tomogr 1996; 20(4): 600-8. [http://dx.doi.org/10.1097/00004728-199607000-00019] [PMID: 8708064]

[153] Tsui PT, Kwok ML, Yuen H, Lai ST. Severe acute respiratory syndrome: clinical outcome and prognostic correlates. Emerg Infect Dis 2003; 9(9): 1064-9. [http://dx.doi.org/10.3201/eid0909.030362] [PMID: 14519241]

[154] Tsang KW, Ho PL, Ooi GC, *et al.* A cluster of cases of severe acute respiratory syndrome in Hong Kong. N Engl J Med 2003; 348(20): 1977-85. [http://dx.doi.org/10.1056/NEJMoa030666] [PMID: 12671062]

[155] Peiris JS, Chu CM, Cheng VC, *et al.* HKU/UCH SARS Study Group. Clinical progression and viral load in a community outbreak of coronavirus-associated SARS pneumonia: a prospective study. Lancet 2003; 361(9371): 1767-72. [http://dx.doi.org/10.1016/S0140-6736(03)13412-5] [PMID: 12781535]

[156] Li SS, Cheng CW, Fu CL, *et al.* Left ventricular performance in patients with severe acute respiratory syndrome: a 30-day echocardiographic follow-up study. Circulation 2003; 108(15): 1798-803. [http://dx.doi.org/10.1161/01.CIR.0000094737.21775.32] [PMID: 14504188]

[157] Wong WM, Ho JC, Ooi GC, *et al.* Temporal patterns of hepatic dysfunction and disease severity in patients with SARS. JAMA 2003; 290(20): 2663-5. [http://dx.doi.org/10.1001/jama.290.20.2663] [PMID: 14645306]

[158] Wong KT, Antonio GE, Hui DS, *et al.* Severe acute respiratory syndrome: radiographic appearances and pattern of progression in 138 patients. Radiology 2003; 228(2): 401-6. [http://dx.doi.org/10.1148/radiol.2282030593] [PMID: 12759474]

[159] Wong KT, Antonio GE, Hui DS, *et al.* Thin-section CT of severe acute respiratory syndrome: evaluation of 73 patients exposed to or with the disease. Radiology 2003; 228(2): 395-400. [http://dx.doi.org/10.1148/radiol.2283030541] [PMID: 12738877]

[160] World Health Organisation. Case definitions for surveillance of severe acuterespiratory syndrome (SARS). Available at:. http://www.who.int/csr/sars/csedefinition/en/print.html (accessed 10 July 2003).

[161] Centers for Disease Control and Prevention. Public health guidance for community-level preparedness and response to severe acute respiratorysyndrome (SARS) version 2. Supplement B: SARS surveillance. Appendix B1:revised CSTE SARS surveillance case definition. Available at:. http://www.cdc.gov/ncidod/sars/guidance/B/pdf/b.pdf.

[162] Vijayanand P, Wilkins E, Woodhead M. Severe acute respiratory syndrome (SARS): a review. Clin Med (Lond) 2004; 4(2): 152-60. [http://dx.doi.org/10.7861/clinmedicine.4-2-152] [PMID: 15139736]

[163] So LK, Lau AC, Yam LY, *et al.* Development of a standard treatment protocol for severe acute respiratory syndrome. Lancet 2003; 361(9369): 1615-7. [http://dx.doi.org/10.1016/S0140-6736(03)13265-5] [PMID: 12747883]

[164] Ho JC, Ooi GC, Mok TY, *et al.* High-dose pulse versus nonpulse corticosteroid regimens in severe acute respiratory syndrome. Am J Respir Crit Care Med 2003; 168(12): 1449-56. [http://dx.doi.org/10.1164/rccm.200306-766OC] [PMID: 12947028]

[165] Knowles SR, Phillips EJ, Dresser L, Matukas L. Common adverse events associated with the use of ribavirin for severe acute respiratory syndrome in Canada. Clin Infect Dis 2003; 37(8): 1139-42. [http://dx.doi.org/10.1086/378304] [PMID: 14523782]

[166] Cinatl J, Morgenstern B, Bauer G, Chandra P, *et al.* Treatment of SARS with human interferons. Lancet 2003;362:293-4. Erratum: Lancet 2003; 362: 748.

CHAPTER 8

Leprosy: Clinical / Diagnostic Features and Current Status of Anti-leprosy Drugs

Khullakpam Shaheen*, **Ibemhal D. Asem** and **Debananda Singh Ningthoujam**

Advanced Level State Biotech Hub, Microbial Biotechnology Research Laboratory (MBRL), Department of Biochemistry, Manipur University, Canchipur, Imphal, Manipur 795003, India

Abstract: Leprosy, also called Hansen's disease, is known since ancient times. It is a curable, slow, progressive lifelong contagious disease, caused by an intracellular, rod shaped, aerobic, slow growing bacterium, *Mycobacterium leprae*. Leprosy affects the skin, peripheral nerves, and mucosal portion of upper respiratory tract and may also affect other organs. Leprosy is not critically contagious. Early diagnosis and treatments prevent nerve involvement, which is considered to be the hallmark of leprosy. Its diagnosis is carried out from a number of distinct clinical presentations which should be complemented by skin bacilloscopy and histopathology. Highly effective MDT (multidrug therapy) is used as a medication which aims to eliminate the causal organism in the shortest possible time. It involves three major drugs: dapsone, rifampicin (Rifadin), and clofazimine (Lamprene). The WHO has been providing free treatment for all people suffering from leprosy since 1995. This chapter focuses on the clinical and diagnostic features of leprosy as well as the current drugs used in the treatment along with their pharmacokinetics.

Keywords: Clofazimine, Dapsone, Hansen's disease, Leprosy, *Mycobacterium leprae*, MDT, Pharmacokinetics, Rifampicin.

INTRODUCTION

Leprosy or Hansen's disease, is a lifelong infectious disease. It mainly affects superficial tissue; especially the skin and peripheral nerves, the mucosal portion of the upper tract of respiration, and the eyes. The disease affects all individuals irrespective of age and sex. Children are more prone to leprosy than adults [1]. For more than hundred years, it is endured to be a poorly known disease characterised by suffering of humans and isolation from the society as it was considered to be associated with social stigma (punishment of God).

* **Corresponding author Khullakpam Shaheen:** Advanced Level State Biotech Hub, Microbial Biotechnology Research Laboratory (MBRL), Department of Biochemistry, Manipur University, Canchipur, Imphal, Manipur 795003, India; Tel: +91 977 4594 596; E-mail: khshaheen@manipuruniv.ac.in

K. Tamreihao, Saikat Mukherjee and Debananda S. Ningthoujam (Eds.)
All rights reserved-© 2019 Bentham Science Publishers

History

Leprosy has often been accompanied by refusing stigmas since ancient times. Leprosy outbreaks have always caused panic. Leprosy was feared as an untreatable, disfiguring, infectious and contagious disease in the Chinese, Egyptian, and Indian civilizations [1] although in reality, it is not proven to be contagious. The first human suffering from leprosy was identified by DNA of the wrapped remains of a man discovered in a tomb close to Jerusalem [2]. The disease was perhaps originated in Egypt and some other Middle Eastern countries since 2400 BC and could spread all over the world due to the probable lack of knowledge (Fig. **1**). The implementation of Multi Drug Therapy (MDT) by the World Health Organization (WHO) since past 20 years has provided this disease a less widespread infection with less than one case per 10,000 populations. However, it remains to be a persistent health problem in Brazil, Congo, Madagascar, Mozambique, Nepal, and Tanzania [3]. In present, according to the WHO, about 180,000 people all over the world, mainly in Africa and Asia, are infected with leprosy while around 100 people are diagnosed with leprosy every year in the United States, mostly in South California, Hawaii, and some U.S. territories [1].

Causes

The first causal organism of leprosy in humans, *Mycobacterium leprae,* was identified by G. A. Hansen (Fig. **2**) in Norway in 1873 [4]. The discovery revoked leprosy as a hereditary disease or association with social stigma or a punishment from the gods.

M. leprae (Fig. **3**) is an intracellular, aerobic, acid-fast rod shaped slow growing bacterium [6]. In addition to humans, leprosy could be detected in nine-banded armadillo, three species of primates (African chimpanzee, Sooty mangabey, and Cynomolgus macaque), and red squirrels [7]. In November 2016, a threatened species of red squirrels, *Sciurus vulgaris* was reported in England to have leprosy [8]. *M. leprae* can also be cultured in the laboratory by injecting into the mice footpads [9]. With a doubling time of 14 days, this bacterium is famous for its notoriously slow growth. Therefore, *M. leprae* has not yet been successfully cultured *in vitro* [10, 11]. The genome of *M. leprae* has been sequenced which shows the presence of genes with less than 50% coding capacity and a large number of pseudogenes while the remaining genes define the minimal set of genes necessary for bacterial *in vivo* survival and genes possibly required for infection and pathogenesis in leprosy [12].

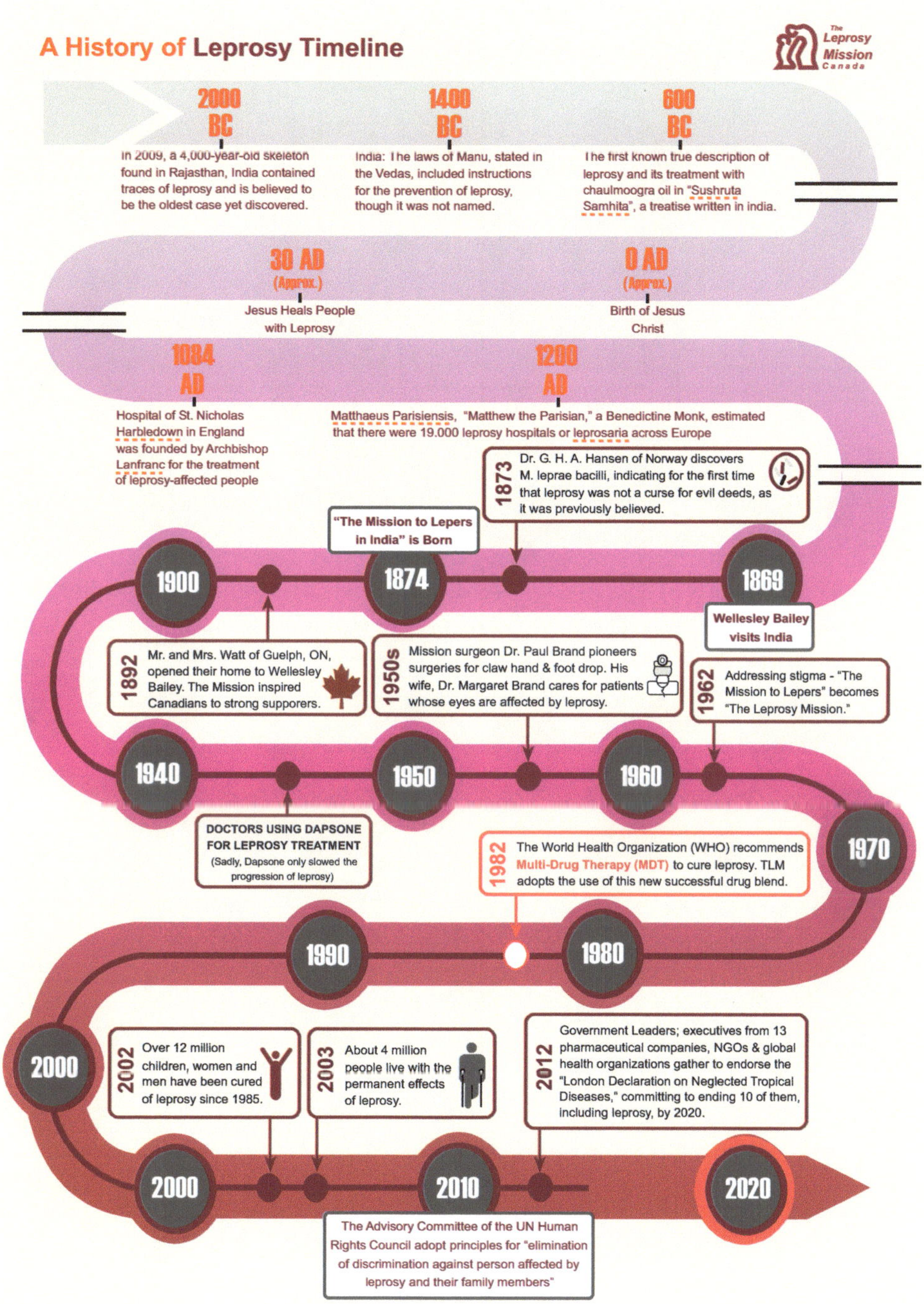

Fig. (1). History of leprosy; Source: Effect: hope (the leprosy mission Canada) (Courtesy: Leprosy Mission Canada).

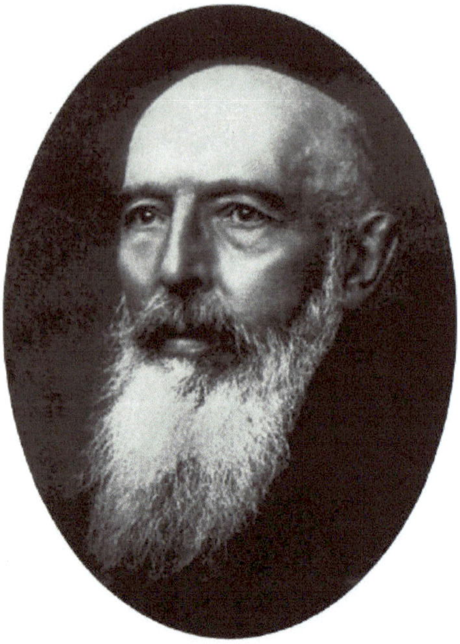

Fig. (2). Gerhard Armaner Hansen, the man who discovered *Mycobacterium leprae*. Photograph by J.F. Lehman, Munich, 1912. Public domain (Courtesy the U.S. National Library of Medicine).

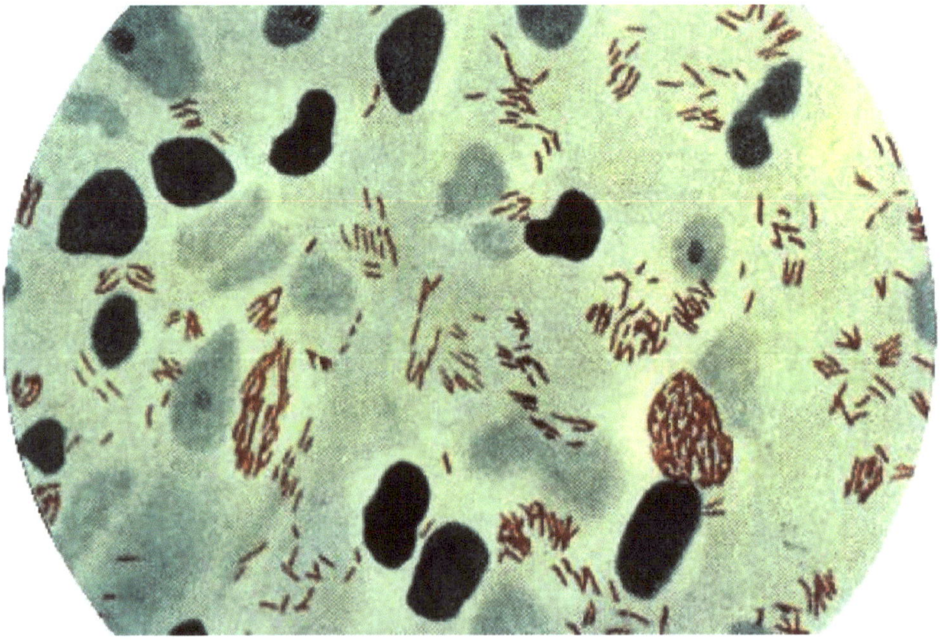

Fig. (3). Micrograph of *Mycobacterium leprae* (red) taken from a leprosy skin lesion. Photograph: CDC/Public domain.

Mycobacterium lepromatosis is a recently identified mycobacterium isolated from diffuse lepromatous leprosy affected fatal case in 2008 whose significance is still not clearly understood [13, 14]. Diffuse lepromatous leprosy (DLL) is a unique and severe form of leprosy, which is endemic in Mexico, and characterized clinically by diffuse, non-nodular cutaneous infiltration, manifesting recurrent crops of large sharply demarcated skin lesions.

Signs and Symptoms

Leprosy is not highly infectious or very contagious [5]. Leprosy primarily affects the skin and the peripheral nerves, later affecting the eyes and the thin nasal tissue lining. Leprosy may affect other organs. Symptoms of leprosy are pale colored deforming skin sores, lumps or bumps that exist for several weeks or months [1].

Depending on the immune response of an individual to *M. Leprae,* the indications of leprosy may vary. To differentiate between various forms of leprosy, the classification system of the WHO uses clinical manifestations such as the skin lesions number and nerve involvement as well as skin smears into two major types as paucibacillary (PB) leprosy and multibacillary (MB) leprosy in which there can be a vast range of clinical presentations [15].

In general, reddish or copper colored, flat or raised skin lesions or nodules, often with less pigmentation than the surrounding skin, can be found. There are single or multiple skin lesions often found on the face, buttocks, and extremities. It may lead to thickening of the skin and peripheral nerves, ulcerations of the skin, and hoarseness. There may be peripheral nerve involvement leading to loss of sensation, muscle weakness, as well as testicular involvement leading to sexual dysfunction or sterility. Moreover, eye involvement including eye pain, eye redness, inability to close the eyelids, corneal ulcers, blindness and loss of eyebrows & eyelashes can be seen during the course of infection, which may finally lead to the destruction of the nasal cartilage.

Classification of Leprosy

Various types of approaches are there for classification of leprosy.

According to WHO, leprosy can be classified into two major groups based on the bacterial proliferation [16].

1. Paucibacillary (PB) leprosy- two to five lesions with negative smear that result at all sites
2. Multibacillary (MB) leprosy- more than five skin lesions with or without positive skin smear that may result at any site.

Another classification system that is used universally in evaluating patients in clinical studies is the Ridley-Jopling classification which has five different classifications of leprosy namely tuberculoid leprosy (TT), borderline tuberculoid leprosy (BT) mid-borderline leprosy (BB), borderline lepromatous leprosy (BL), and lepromatous leprosy (LL) [17, 18].

For leprosy treatment purposes, the patients could be classified into two groups as paucibacillary (TT, BT) and multibacillary (BB, BL, LL) [19].

The common clinical features of leprosy are given in Table **1**.

Table 1. Clinical features of Leprosy.

Features	TT	BT	BB	BL	LL	Reference
No. of lesions	1 to 3	1 to 10	10 to 30	Numerous, asymmetrical (>30)	Innumerab-le, symmetric-al	[20]
Size	Variable, usually large	Variable, some are large	Variable	Small, some can be large	Small	[20]
Surface changes	Hypopigmente-d	Dry, scaly, look bright and infiltrated	Dull or slightly shiny	Shiny	Shiny	[20]
Sensatio-ns	Nil	Greatly reduced	Fairly reduced	Lightly reduced	Nominally reduced	[20]
Hair growth	Nil	Greatly diminished	Fairly reduced	Lightly reduced	Initially not affected	[20]
Skin smear	Negative	Negative or 1+	1-3+	3-5+	Plenty, including globi (6+)	[20]
Lepromi-n test	Strongly positive	Weakly positive	Negative	Negative	Negative	[20]

Some other forms of leprosy include indeterminate leprosy, polyneuritic leprosy and histoid leprosy.

Indeterminate leprosy, a curtain raiser to the determinate forms of leprosy [21, 22], is characterized by an ill-defined, bizarre hypopigmented macule(s) with a smooth or scaly surface.

In polyneuritic leprosy, neural signs without any evidence of skin lesions are found in which the affected nerves are thickened, tender, or both [23].

Histoid leprosy is comparatively not common and confers histopathologic expression of multibacillary leprosy. It is clinically distinct and bacteriologic in nature [24]. It may come as a primary manifestation of the disease or in result to secondary drug resistance to irregular and inadequate monotherapy of dapsone. It is distinctly seen as numerous cutaneous nodules and plaques primarily over the back, buttocks, face, and bony prominences.

Leprosy Reactions

Leprosy reactions include severe events of inflammations clinically occurring during the chronic course of disease leading to problems even after completion of treatment. The morbidity is increased due to nerve damage. They are classified as follows:

1. ***Type I Reaction or Reversal Reactions (RR)***: This reaction occurs in borderline patients (BT, BB and BL) and is distinguished by edema and erythema of existing skin lesions, new skin lesions formation, neuritis, additional sensory and motor loss, and edema in the hands, feet, and face [25].
2. ***Type II (Erythema Nodosum Leprosum (ENL) Reactions***: This reaction only occurs in BL and LL forms and is distinguished by emergence of tender, erythematous, subcutaneous nodules seen on normal skin evidently. It is normally followed by systemic symptoms, such as fever, malaise, enlarged lymph nodes, anorexia, weight loss, arthralgia, and edema. It may also affect other organs like the testes, joints, eyes, and nerves [26, 27].

Pathogenesis

M. leprae replicates intracellularly, especially within skin **histocytes**, endothelial cells, and **Schwann cells** of nerves. Cell mediated immunity takes a major role in determining the response of the host to leprosy infection [5]. Schwann cells are important targets for *M. leprae,* leading to nerve injuries, demyelination of nerves, and consequent disabilities. The bacterium's binding to Schwann cells induces demyelination as well as loss of axonal conductance in Schwann cells [28].

Each leprosy manifestation type is accompanied by a characteristic profile of cell-mediated or humoral immune response [28] as shown in Fig. **4**.

LEPROSY MECHANISMS OF PATHOGENESIS

In the cell-mediated (T_h1) response of the TT pole, the elimination or containment of the organism in granulomas could be noticed whereas the unaffected humoral response at the LL (T_h2) pole allows the proliferation of mycobacteria within and around foamy macrophages. An unexpected displacement is seen in reversal reactions toward the T_h1 pole from the BT, BB, or BL state and ultimately result to irreversible nerve damage (neuritis). Erythema nodosum leprosum (ENL) reactions take place in BL or LL leprosy patients and display a rise in both cell-mediated and humoral responses to M. leprae. ENL is associated with the systemic release of TNF and IL-4, a brisk polymorphonuclear leukocyte (PMN) influx, and antigen-antibody (Ag/Ab) complex deposition. The mechanism of nerve damage is unclear but may involve immune injury due to release of inflammatory cytokines or activity of cytotoxic T cells, ischemia due to edema within the perineural sheath, apoptosis, or demyelination [28].

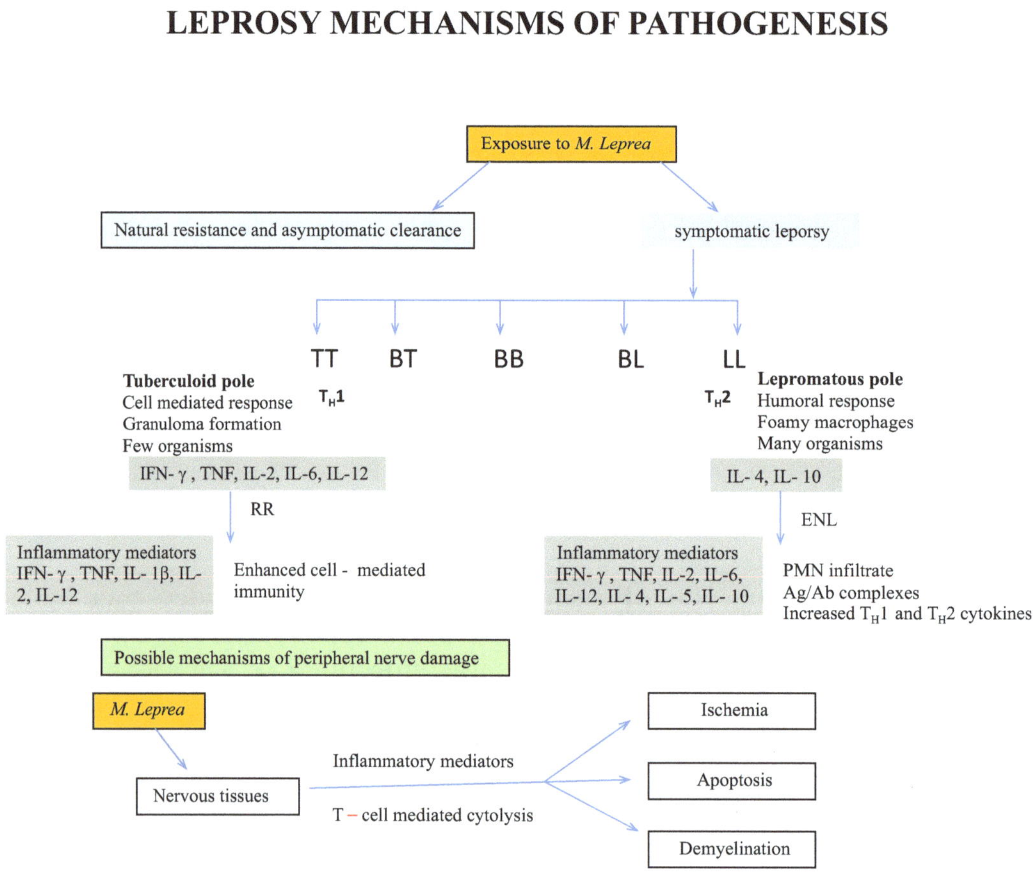

Fig. (4). Pathogenesis in leprosy.

Diagnosis

Early diagnosis and treatment prevent nerve damage and disability it causes [29].

Lepromin Skin Test: This clinical test determines the type of leprosy in a patient.

An extract of *M. leprae* is injected intradermally and is followed 48 hours later in those whom a cell-mediated immune response against organism exist [5].

Lab Diagnosis:

1. Microscopy: Smear made from scraping of skin, ear lobes, and patches, nodules *etc.* can be stained by modified Ziehl Neelsen stain method using 5% sulphuric acid and examined. The living bacilli stain uniformly as a strong rod; whereas dead bacilli are fragmented and granular. On the basis of the number of *M. leprae* and their morphology, two indices, which are helpful in evaluating the infection amount, viability of the organisms and following the progress of the patient, namely bacteriological index (BI) and morphological index (MI) can be determined. The former describes the bacterial loads whereas the latter is determined by counting the solid-staining acid-fast rods number [5].

According to WHO, **logarithmic index of biopsies (LIB),** a reliable index of the bacillary content of a lesion, is used to evaluate the state of patients at the beginning of the treatment and to assess the progress as treatment continues [5].

2. Culture: *Mycobacterium leprae* is a slow growing pathogen with doubling time of 14 days. It has not yet been successfully cultured *in vitro*, but it can be cultured in the laboratory by injection into the foot pads of mice or nine-banded armadillo [5].

3. Molecular Diagnosis: As a means of leprosy diagnosis, Polymerase Chain Reaction (PCR) can be used. Not only to skin samples, PCR has been used also to specimens such as skin smears, nerves, urine, oral or nasal swabs, blood, and ocular lesions [30 - 37]. Different sequences were used as targets for PCR, such as genes encoding the 36-kDa antigen [38], 18-kDa antigen [39], 65-kDa antigen [40], complex 85 [33], 16S rDNA [41], and the repetitive sequences [42] among other *M. leprae* genes.

Treatment and Current Drugs

MDT (multidrug therapy) should be used for curing leprosy. In 1981, a WHO Study Group recommended MDT treatment, with three drugs namely dapsone, rifampicin (Rifadin), and clofazimine (Lamprene) which helps in curing and averting the problems associated with the disease. 16 million people affecting from leprosy have been cured in the last two decades. Since 1995, WHO provides free medical care for all leprosy patients which was previously funded by the Nippon Foundation. Since 2000, the treatment is provided through an agreement with Novartis and will continue until 2020. Treatment depends on the type of leprosy. Daily regimen with dapsone and monthly regimen with rifampicin for six months is recommended in case of paucibacillary patients (Table **2**) while for multi-bacillary cases, daily treatment with dapsone and clofazimine along with monthly medication with rifampicin for 12 months is recommended (Table **3**) [43].

Dapsone (bacteriostatic or weakly bactericidal against *M. leprae*) was used as an exclusive treatment for curing leprosy for many years until widespread resistant strains appeared. Combination medication therapy has helped to slow or prevent the resistance development. A single dose of combination therapy including **rifampicin** (600 mg), **ofloxacin** (400 mg), and **minocycline** (100 mg) has been used to cure single lesion paucibacillary leprosy (Table **4**). Under the direction of WHO, Blister pack medication kits containing medications for 28 days have been provided for both paucibacillary leprosy and multibacillary leprosy. For single lesion paucibacillary leprosy, the blister pack kit contains the necessary medication for one-time administration of the 3 drugs [44].

WHO recommended following treatment regimens [44]:

Table 2. 6-month regimen for Paucibacillary (PB) Leprosy.

–	**Dapsone**	**Rifampicin**
Adults (50 – 70 kg)	100 mg Given daily	600 mg Given once a month under supervision
Child (10 – 14 years)[a]	50 mg Given daily	450 mg Given once a month under supervision

[a] Adjust dose appropriately for child less than 10 years. For example, dapsone 25 mg daily and rifampicin 300 mg given once a month under supervision.

Table 3. 12-month regimen for Multibacillary (MB) Leprosy.

–	**Dapsone**	**Rifampicin**	**Clofazimine**	
Adults (50 – 70 kg)	100 mg Given daily	600 mg Given once a month under supervision	50 mg Given daily	300 mg Given once a month under supervision
Child (10 - 14 years)[b]	50 mg Given daily	450 mg Given once a month under supervision	50 mg Given every other day	150 mg Given once a month under supervision

[b] Adjust dose appropriately for child less than 10 years. For example, dapsone 25 mg daily, rifampicin 300 mg given once a month under supervision, clofazimine, 50 mg given twice a week, and clofazimine 100 mg given once a month under supervision.

Table 4. Single Lesion Paucibacillary (SLPB) Leprosy (one-time dose of 3 medications taken together).

–	**Rifampicin**	**Ofloxacin**	**Minocycline**
Adults (50 – 70 kg)	600 mg	400 mg	100 mg

(Table 4) cont.....

–	Rifampicin	Ofloxacin	Minocycline
Child (10 - 14 years)[c]	300 mg	200 mg	50 mg

[c] Not recommended for pregnant women or children less than 5 years.

Dapsone

Dapsone is also known as **diaminodiphenyl sulfone** (**DDS**) [45]. It is commonly used for treatment of leprosy in combination with rifampicin and clofazimine [46]. This drug has been found effective in curing pneumocystis pneumonia and toxoplasmosis, acne, dermatitis herpetiformis, and various other skin lesions [47]. Dapsone can be administered both topically and by mouth [48]. Its application for treatment of leprosy started in 1945 [47].

Dapsone is included in the WHO's List of Essential Medicines [49]. Side effects may be severe such as decrease in blood cells, red blood cell breakdown especially in those individuals with glucose-6-phosphate dehydrogenase deficiency (G-6-PD), or hypersensitivity [46], nausea and loss of appetite [48], liver inflammation, and many types of skin rashes [46].

Pharmacokinetics

Dapsone is absorbed slowly after oral administration as the maximum plasma drug concentrations are reached at about 4 hours with an absorption half-life of 1.1 hours. The half-life of elimination of dapsone is around 30 hours. Within the therapeutic ranges, dapsone shows linear pharmacokinetics. Dapsone is about 70% to 90% protein bound while its monoacetylated metabolite MADDS is almost completely protein bound. At steady state (reached after 7-14 daily doses of 100 mg of dapsone), plasma drug concentration is about 150 times greater than the minimum inhibitory concentration (MIC) for *M. leprae* in blood of mice at any time. The volume of distribution of dapsone is assumed to be 1.5 L/kg. It is distributed in most of the tissues, but *M. leprae* living in Schwann cells of the nerves might be unaffected. It can cross the placenta. It is excreted in breast milk and saliva and self- metabolised. Dapsone, some MADDS and their hydroxylated metabolites, are found in urine, partly conjugated as N-glucuronides and N-sulphates. Simultaneous administration of rifampicin with dapsone decreases the half-life of the latter by a factor of about 2 and lowers its plasma, skin and nerve concentrations notably. Pyrimethamine, a medication used to treat toxoplasmosis, lowers the peak serum concentrations of dapsone. Haematological side effects below the daily dose of 100 mg are shown. Dapsone's therapeutic serum concentration ranges from 0.5 to 5 mg/L. Alcoholic liver disease decreases the protein binding capacity of dapsone while coeliac disease and dermatitis herpetiformis may delay its oral absorption. In case of severe leprosy, the extent of absorption is reported to be affected [50].

Clofazimine

Clofazimine, sold under the brand name **Lamprene**, is used to treat leprosy together with rifampicin and dapsone. The drug is specifically used for multibacillary (MB) leprosy and leprosy reaction type II, erythema nodosum leprosum. The drug has a marked anti-inflammatory effect [52]. It is included in the WHO's List of Essential Medicines [53]. It is taken orally and it was first accepted medically in the United States in 1986 [54].

Common side effects include abdominal pain, diarrhoea, itchiness, dry skin, and changes in skin colour [51], swelling of the gastrointestinal tract lining, increased blood sugar level and sensitivity to the sun [52]. It is not clear if it can be used during pregnancy [51]. Clofazimine is a phenazine dye [51] and works by preferentially binding to the bacterial DNA, thereby blocking the DNA replicates and inhibiting bacterial proliferation. The drug increases activity of bacterial phospholipase A2, which leads to release and accumulation of lysophospholipids [55, 56], therefore, being toxic and inhibiting bacterial proliferation [57, 58]. Clofazimine is also a functional inhibitor of acid sphingomyelinase (FIASMA) [59]. Swiss pharmaceutical company Novartis launched clofazimine in 1969 under the brand name Lamprene. Moreover, Novartis was granted FDA approval of clofazimine in December 1986 as an orphan drug (a pharmaceutical agent used for diagnosis, prevention or treatment of rare life- threatening diseases) [60].

Pharmacokinetics

Oral absorption of clofazimine is slow and dose-dependent but its faecal excretion increases with dose. A plasma half-life of around 10 days has been shown in single and multiple-doses studies. Bioavailability of the drug is more when given with food. The maximum plasma concentration is reached at 4 to 8 hours after the drug is given with breakfast. The drug is assumed to circulate in protein-bound form after absorption. The special features of clofazimine metabolism are slow and uneven distribution and prolonged retention in the tissues. Urinary excretion of clofazimine and its metabolites is around 1% of the dose. Clofazimine crosses placental barrier and is excreted into breast milk in significant amounts. The drug does not cross the blood-brain barrier. Small amount of the drug is excreted in sebum and sweat [55, 61].

Rifampicin

Rifampicin, also known as rifampin, is used to treat bacterial infections, including tuberculosis, *Mycobacterium avium* complex (a pulmonary pathogen that affects individuals who are immune compromised such as from AIDS, hairy cell leukemia, immunosuppressive chemotherapy), leprosy, and Legionnaires' disease. It may be taken either orally or intravenously. It is among the rifamycin group of antibiotics [62]. Common side effects include nausea, vomiting, diarrhoea, loss of appetite, red or orange colour of urine, sweat, and tears, hepatic problems or allergic reactions. Although, its safety for use in pregnancy is not clear, it is recommended for treatment of active tuberculosis during pregnancy. It works by inhibiting transcription [63].

Rifampicin was discovered in 1965 and marketed in Italy in 1968. It was approved in the United States in 1971 [64 - 66]. It is included in the WHO's List of Essential Medicines [53]. It is available as a generic medication [63]. Rifampicin is produced by the soil bacterium *Amycolatopsis rifamycinica* [65]. Rifampicin inhibits bacterial DNA-dependent RNA synthesis by inhibiting bacterial DNA-dependent RNA polymerase [67].

Pharmacokinetics

Oral doses of rifampicin are absorbed easily in the gastrointestinal tract as it has ester functional group which gets quickly hydrolysed in bile in presence of high pH and substrate specific esterases. The bioavailability of the drug is more when given before meals. The maximum plasma concentrations of the drug are reached at 1-2 hours. The drug binds to plasma proteins to about 80% to 90% and is found in saliva, cerebrospinal fluid, and breast milk. The drug is almost deacetylated after about 6 hours from its administration. Moreover, Desacetyl rifampicin, its major metabolite, also shows antimycobacterial activity in tuberculosis. This drug induces its own metabolism as well as that of several drugs including dapsone and steroids [68].

Ofloxacin

It is a fluoroquinoline antibiotic useful for the treatment of a number of bacterial infections such as pneumonia, cellulitis, urinary tract pneumonia, prostatis, plague and certain types of infectious diarrhoea [69, 70]. It is taken either orally or intravenously. It can be used in the treatment of multidrug resistant tuberculosis and leprosy, along with other medications [71]. It works by interfering with the bacterial DNA replication [69]. Common side effects include vomiting, diarrhoea, headache, rash, tendon rupture, numbness due to nerve damage, seizures, and psychosis [69]. Since, its safety for use in pregnancy is not clear, use in pregnancy is not recommended [72]. Ofloxacin was patented in 1980 and approved for medical use in 1985 [73]. It is included in the WHO's List of Essential Medicines, the most effective and safe medicines needed in a health system [74].

Ofloxacin is a broad spectrum antibiotic. It inhibits cell division of bacteria by inhibiting DNA gyrase, a type II topoisomerase, and topoisomerase IV [75].

Pharmacokinetics

The drug is given at a daily dose of 400 mg. It is rapidly absorbed and reached a maximum serum concentration of 2.9 µg/mL after 2 hours of its administration. It has a serum half-life of 7 hours and excreted unchanged through urine. Approximately, 32% of the drug in plasma is protein bound in the body. Major side effects reported are nausea, diarrhoea, gastrointestinal complaints and central nervous system complaints such as insomnia, headache, dizziness and hallucinations [76]. Hypersensitivity reactions to ofloxacin are found in the form of mild non-specific skin rashes [77].

Minocycline

Minocycline is a broad spectrum tetracycline. It is a bacteriostatic antibiotic having long half-life. Minocycline, being the most lipid-soluble of the tetracycline-class antibiotics, can penetrate into the prostate and brain. Common side effects include diarrhoea, upset stomach, dizziness, mouth sores, headache, vomiting, sleep disorders, and sensitivity to light [78]. It is commonly used for the treatment of acne vulgaris [79] and other skin infections like methicillin- resistant *Staphylococcus aureus* [80] as well as Lyme disease [81].

Patented in 1961, minocycline came into commercial use in 1971 [82]. It is not a naturally occurring antibiotic, but was synthesized semi-synthetically from natural tetracycline antibiotics by Lederle Laboratories in 1966, and marketed under the brand name *Minocin* [83].

Pharmacokinetics

Minocycline is metabolized by the liver and has poor urinary excretion and is the only tetracycline having significant activity against *M. Leprae*. The reason may be due to its high lipid soluble content enabling to cross the mycobacterial cell wall [84, 85]. The standard dose is 100 mg daily at which the maximum serum concentrations of 2-4 µg/ml (mean 1.84 µg/ml) are reached within 2 hours of administration of 0.2 µg/ml for *M. leprae*. The half-life of elimination reported is 11-23 hours. The drug is less powerful than rifampicin in giving bactericidal effect to *M. leprea* [84]. It binds reversibly to the ribosomal 30s sub-unit, blocking the binding of aminoacyl tRNA to the mRNA ribosomal complex, thereby inhibiting protein synthesis. Some of its side effects include teeth discolouration in infants and children, occasional skin pigmentation, various gastrointestinal complaints, and central nervous system toxicity. There has been a report of the occurrence of hepatitis or systemic lupus in patients treated with minocycline for acne [86].

Other Anti-Leprosy Drugs

Clathiromycin

Clarithromycin, related to erythromycin structurally, is a semisynthetic macrolide antibiotic. It has a better pharmacokinetic profile than erythromycin. It inhibits protein synthesis of bacteria by binding to 50s ribosomal sub-unit. It is administered as a dosage of 500 mg daily to leprosy patients and is reported to kill 99% of *M. leprae* by 58 days. It is readily absorbed from the gastrointestinal tract and undergoes rapid biodegradation into active 14-hydroxy (R) metabolite which is mainly excreted in the urine along with the parent compound. Its peak serum concentration and its 14-hydroxy metabolite obtainable with single oral doses of the drug are dose proportional. The peak concentration of the drug, 1 μg/ml is reached 1-4 hours after a 500 mg dose. The half-life of elimination is 6-7 hours. Common side effects include nausea, diarrhoea, dyspepsia, abdominal pain and headache [85].

Ansamycins

The new derivatives or analogues of rifampicin, also known as ansamycins, is more effective than rifampicin itself. The first ansamycin, Rifabutin or LM 427, exhibited more potency than rifampicin against *M. Tuberculosis.* There are reports of rifabutin to be potent against rifampicin resistant strains of *M. tuberculosis* in mice. The minimal inhibitory concentration is much lower than that for rifampicin in *M. leprae* from lepromatous leprosy patients [87].

R-76-1 (isobutylpiperazinyl rifampicin SV) and DL 473 (Rifapentine) have been reported to be more effective in *M. lepraemurium* cultures (a causative agent of feline leprosy) and against *M. leprae* in mice [88]. A longer half-life (of rifapentine) together with the greater intrinsic activity (rifabutin and R-76-1) against *M. leprae* makes them very attractive as components of intermittent therapy. But their utility in MDT remains unclear so far and the action of these ansamycins against *M. leprae* rifampicin-resistant strains has not yet proved [89].

Rifabutin (LM 427), a spiropiperidyl derivative of rifamycin S, is more lipid soluble drug than rifampicin. After single dose administration, it has relatively low oral bioavailability of about 20%. The maximum blood concentrations reach 2.5 - 3 hours after oral administration of the drug which is low compared to those levels with equivalent doses of rifampicin. Its serum half-life is relatively long almost 45 hours, but average plasma concentration remains comparatively low after repeated standard doses administration due to very large volume of distribution of the drug [90]. Rifabutin is more active against M avium-M intracellulare complex *in vitro.* It has similar action against M tuberculosis as rifampicin. However, due to its lower concentration at equivalent doses, its action *in vivo* is less seen [91].

The other drugs that have been reported for anti *M. leprae* activity are fusidic acid, combination of amoxicillin with potassium clavulanate, brodimoprim, thiacetazone and desoxy fructoserotonin.

CONCLUDING REMARKS

The Leprosy Act of 1898 with the view to institutionalise people affected from the disease was enacted by British India. After the widespread availability of MDT medications, the same Act was repealed in 1983. The National Leprosy Elimination Programme, formerly known as the National Leprosy Control Programme, converts its motives from just close observation to the treatment of people affected with leprosy in 1983. Our country, India still reports for more than half of the disease burden of the world [92].

From the WHO reports acquired from 138 countries, the predominance of leprosy registered in 2015 was 176176 cases which accounts for 0.2 cases per 10000 people [1]. The number of diseases affected cases reported globally was 215656 in 2013, 213899 in 2014 and 211973 in 2015. Over 16 million leprosy affected people have been given MDT treatment since the past 20 years [93].

In India, the local governments and NGOs have given community-based rehabilitation to some extent as the distinctive character provided by the society is found useful to reintegration, and models of self-management. It is reported to be successful by the collective agency independent of NGOs and government support [94]. In order to create universal awareness and acknowledge that it can be prevented, treated and cured, World Leprosy Day is celebrated on the last Sunday of January every year throughout the world. It was initiated by the renowned French philanthropist and writer, Raoul Follereau in 1954 [95].

The "Global Leprosy Strategy 2016-2020: Accelerating towards a leprosy free world" was started by WHO in 2016. Its main goal is to regenerate efforts to have control over leprosy and its difficulties to mankind, especially to the disease affected children developing countries. It gives importance the requirement of sustaining proficiency and increase the number of skilled leprosy staff. Moreover, it emphasises to promote the active participation of affected persons in leprosy services and reduce visible difficulties as well as negative stigmatization accompanied with the disease. It also encourages for revived engagement by political leaders and promoted commitment among partners while giving the need of research and improved data collection and analysis of the disease [96].

CONSENT FOR PUBLICATION

Not applicable.

CONFLICT OF INTEREST

The author confirms that this chapter contents have no conflict of interest.

ACKNOWLEDGEMENTS

K. Shaheen would like to thank Department of Sciences & Technology, Govt. Of India for providing the DST INSPIRE fellowship with sanction no. DST/INSPIRE Fellowship/2014/195; Department of Science & Technology, Ministry of Science & Technology, Government of India, New Delhi 110016.

DSN would like wish to thank Department of Biotechnology (DBT), Govt. of India for sponsoring the host laboratory under the scheme "Establishment of State Biotech Hubs" (BT/04/NE/2009)

REFERENCES

[1] https://www.webmd.com/skin-problems-and-treatments/guide/leprosy-symptoms-treatmentshistory#1.

[2] DNA of Jesus-Era Shrouded Man in Jerusalem Reveals Earliest Case of Leprosy. 2009.

[3] Fine PEM. Global leprosy statistics: A cause for pride, or frustration? Lepr Rev 2006; 77(4): 295-7. [PMID: 17343216]

[4] Hansen GHA. Investigations concerning the etiology of leprosy. Norsk Magazin for Lægevidenskaben 1874; 4: 1-88.

[5] https://microbeonline.com/introduction-transmission-pathogenesis-and-lab-diagnosis-of--eprosy-hansens-disease/.

[6] McMurray DN. Mycobacteria and NocardiaBaron S; et al Baron's Medical Microbiology. (4th ed.). Univ of Texas Medical Branch 1996; p. ISBN 0-9631172-1-1.

[7] Meredith A, Del Pozo J, Smith S, Milne E, Stevenson K, McLuckie J. Leprosy in red squirrels in Scotland. Vet Rec 2014; 175(11): 285-6. [http://dx.doi.org/10.1136/vr.g5680] [PMID: 25234460]

[8] Avanzi C, Del-Pozo J, Benjak A, *et al.* Red squirrels in the British Isles are infected with leprosy bacilli. Science 2016; 354(6313): 744-7. [http://dx.doi.org/10.1126/science.aah3783] [PMID: 27846605]

[9] Hastings RC, Gillis TP, Krahenbuhl JL, Franzblau SG. Leprosy. Clin Microbiol Rev 1988; 1(3): 330-48. [http://dx.doi.org/10.1128/CMR.1.3.330] [PMID: 3058299]

[10] Rastogi N, Legrand E, Sola C. The mycobacteria: An introduction to nomenclature and pathogenesis. Rev - Off Int Epizoot 2001; 20(1): 21-54.

[http://dx.doi.org/10.20506/rst.20.1.1265] [PMID: 11288513]

[11] Gutierrez MC, Supply P, Brosch R. Pathogenomics of mycobacteria. Genome Dyn 2009; 6: 198-210. [http://dx.doi.org/10.1159/000235772] [PMID: 19696503]

[12] Cole ST, Eiglmeier K, Parkhill J, *et al.* Massive gene decay in the leprosy bacillus. Nature 2001; 409(6823): 1007-11. [http://dx.doi.org/10.1038/35059006] [PMID: 11234002]

[13] Han XY, Seo YH, Sizer KC, *et al.* A new Mycobacterium species causing diffuse lepromatous leprosy. Am J Clin Pathol 2008; 130(6): 856-64. [http://dx.doi.org/10.1309/AJCPP72FJZZRRVMM] [PMID: 19019760]

[14] Han XY, Sizer KC, Thompson EJ, *et al.* Comparative sequence analysis of Mycobacterium leprae and the new leprosy-causing Mycobacterium lepromatosis. J Bacteriol 2009; 191(19): 6067-74. [http://dx.doi.org/10.1128/JB.00762-09] [PMID: 19633074]

[15] https://www.emedicinehealth.com/leprosy/article_em.htm#what_is_leprosy.

[16] Smith DS. Leprosy: Overview. eMedicine. Infect Dis 2008.

[17] Singh N, Manucha V, Bhattacharya SN, Arora VK, Bhatia A. Pitfalls in the cytological classification of borderline leprosy in the Ridley-Jopling scale. Diagn Cytopathol 2004; 30(6): 386-8. [http://dx.doi.org/10.1002/dc.20012] [PMID: 15176024]

[18] Ridley DS, Jopling WH. Classification of leprosy according to immunity. A five-group system. Int J Lepr Other Mycobact Dis 1966; 34(3): 255-73. [PMID: 5950347]

[19] Chemotherapy of leprosy for control programmes. World Health Organ Tech Rep Ser 1982; 675: 1-33. [PMID: 6806990]

[20] Bhat RM, Prakash C. Leprosy: An overview of pathophysiology. Interdiscip Perspect Infect Dis 2012; 2012181089. [http://dx.doi.org/10.1155/2012/181089] [PMID: 22988457]

[21] Fajardo TT. Indeterminate leprosy: A 3 year study, clinical observations. Int J Lepr 1971; 39: 94-5.

[22] Fajardo TT. Indeterminate leprosy: A five year study, clinical observations. Int J Lepr 1973; 41: 576.

[23] Sehgal VN, Tuli SM, Dube B. Leprotic nerve abscesses in northern India. Int J Lepr Other Mycobact Dis 1967; 35(1): 60-4. [PMID: 4290019]

[24] Sehgal VN, Srivastava G. Status of histoid leprosy-a clinical, bacteriological, histopathological and immunological appraisal. J Dermatol 1987; 14(1): 38-42. [http://dx.doi.org/10.1111/j.1346-8138.1987.tb02993.x] [PMID: 3301948]

[25] Lienhardt C, Fine PEM. Type 1 reaction, neuritis and disability in leprosy. What is the current epidemiological situation? Lepr Rev 1994; 65(1): 9-33. [http://dx.doi.org/10.5935/0305-7518.19940002] [PMID: 8201838]

[26] Sarno EN, Grau GE, Vieira LMM, Nery JA. Serum levels of tumour necrosis factor-alpha and interleukin-1 β during leprosy reactional states. Clin Exp Immunol 1991; 84(1): 103-8. [PMID: 2015700]

[27] Khanolkar-Young S, Rayment N, Brickell PM, *et al.* Tumour necrosis factor-alpha (TNF-alpha) synthesis is associated with the skin and peripheral nerve pathology of leprosy reversal reactions. Clin Exp Immunol 1995; 99(2): 196-202. [http://dx.doi.org/10.1111/j.1365-2249.1995.tb05532.x] [PMID: 7851011]

[28] Rambukkana A, Zanazzi G, Tapinos N, Salzer JL. Contact-dependent demyelination by Mycobacterium leprae in the absence of immune cells. Science 2002; 296(5569): 927-31. [http://dx.doi.org/10.1126/science.1067631] [PMID: 11988579]

[29] U.S. Department of Health and Human Services, Health Resources and Services Administration. (n.d.). National Hansen's disease (leprosy) program. Retrieved from "Archived copy". Archived from the original on 2011-02-10. Retrieved 2013-05-12.

[30] Jardim MR, Antunes SL, Santos AR, *et al.* Criteria for diagnosis of pure neural leprosy. J Neurol 2003; 250(7): 806-9.
[http://dx.doi.org/10.1007/s00415-003-1081-5] [PMID: 12883921]

[31] Santos AR, De Miranda AB, Sarno EN, Suffys PN, Degrave WM. Use of PCR-mediated amplification of Mycobacterium leprae DNA in different types of clinical samples for the diagnosis of leprosy. J Med Microbiol 1993; 39(4): 298-304.
[http://dx.doi.org/10.1099/00222615-39-4-298] [PMID: 8411091]

[32] Almeida EC, Martinez AN, Maniero VC, *et al.* Detection of Mycobacterium leprae DNA by polymerase chain reaction in the blood and nasal secretion of Brazilian household contacts. Mem Inst Oswaldo Cruz 2004; 99(5): 509-11.
[http://dx.doi.org/10.1590/S0074-02762004000500009] [PMID: 15543415]

[33] Martinez AN, Britto CF, Nery JA, *et al.* Evaluation of real-time and conventional PCR targeting complex 85 genes for detection of Mycobacterium leprae DNA in skin biopsy samples from patients diagnosed with leprosy. J Clin Microbiol 2006; 44(9): 3154-9.
[http://dx.doi.org/10.1128/JCM.02250-05] [PMID: 16954241]

[34] Shamsi FA, Chaudhry IA, Moraes MO, Martinez AN, Riley FC. Detection of Mycobacterium leprae in ocular tissues by histopathology and real-time polymerase chain reaction. Ophthalmic Res 2007; 39(2): 63-8.
[http://dx.doi.org/10.1159/000099375] [PMID: 17287607]

[35] de Wit MY, Douglas JT, McFadden J, Klatser PR. Polymerase chain reaction for detection of Mycobacterium leprae in nasal swab specimens. J Clin Microbiol 1993; 31(3): 502-6.
[PMID: 8458942]

[36] Caleffi KR, Hirata RD, Hirata MH, Caleffi ER, Siqueira VL, Cardoso RF. Use of the polymerase chain reaction to detect Mycobacterium leprae in urine. Braz J Med Biol Res 2012; 45(2): 153-7.
[http://dx.doi.org/10.1590/S0100-879X2012007500011] [PMID: 22286535]

[37] Rosa FB, Souza VC, Almeida TA, *et al.* Detection of Mycobacterium leprae in saliva and the evaluation of oral sensitivity in patients with leprosy. Mem Inst Oswaldo Cruz 2013; 108(5): 572-7.
[http://dx.doi.org/10.1590/S0074-02762013000500006] [PMID: 23903971]

[38] Kampirapap K, Singtham N, Klatser PR, Wiriyawipart S. DNA amplification for detection of leprosy and assessment of efficacy of leprosy chemotherapy. Int J Lepr Other Mycobact Dis 1998; 66(1): 16-21.
[PMID: 9614835]

[39] Scollard DM, Gillis TP, Williams DL. Polymerase chain reaction assay for the detection and identification of Mycobacterium leprae in patients in the United States. Am J Clin Pathol 1998; 109(5): 642-6.
[http://dx.doi.org/10.1093/ajcp/109.5.642] [PMID: 9576586]

[40] Plikaytis BB, Gelber RH, Shinnick TM. Rapid and sensitive detection of Mycobacterium leprae using a nested-primer gene amplification assay. J Clin Microbiol 1990; 28(9): 1913-7.
[PMID: 2229372]

[41] Martinez AN, Lahiri R, Pittman TL, *et al.* Molecular determination of Mycobacterium leprae viability by use of real-time PCR. J Clin Microbiol 2009; 47(7): 2124-30.
[http://dx.doi.org/10.1128/JCM.00512-09] [PMID: 19439537]

[42] Adams LB, Pena MT, Sharma R, *et al.* Insights from animal models on the immunogenetics of leprosy: A review. Mem Inst Oswaldo Cruz 107 2012; p. 197–208.
[http://dx.doi.org/10.1590/S0074-02762012000900028]

[43] Suzuki K, Akama T, Kawashima A, Yoshihara A, Yotsu RR, Ishii N. Current status of leprosy: Epidemiology, basic science and clinical perspectives. J Dermatol 2012; 39(2): 121-9. [http://dx.doi.org/10.1111/j.1346-8138.2011.01370.x] [PMID: 21973237]

[44] Leprosy WHO. 2009-08-01. Archived from the original on 2010-02-09. Retrieved 2010-01-31.

[45] Thomas L. Lemke Foye's Principles of Medicinal Chemistry. Lippincott Williams & Wilkins 2008; 1142. Archived from the original on 2016-03-04.

[46] Dapsone. The American Society of Health-System Pharmacists Archived from the original on 2001. Retrieved Jan 12, 2015

[47] Zhu YI, Stiller MJ. Dapsone and sulfones in dermatology: Overview and update. J Am Acad Dermatol 2001; 45(3): 420-34. [http://dx.doi.org/10.1067/mjd.2001.114733] [PMID: 11511841]

[48] Joel E. Gallant Johns Hopkins HIV Guide 2012. Jones & Bartlett Publishers 2008; 193. Archived from the original on 2016-03-04.

[49] WHO Model List of Essential Medicines (19th List) (PDF). World Health Organization. April 2015. Archived (PDF) from the original on 13 December 2016. Retrieved 8 December 2016.

[50] Zuidema J, Hilbers-Modderman ES, Merkus FWHM. Clinical pharmacokinetics of dapsone. Clin Pharmacokinet 1986; 11(4): 299-315. [http://dx.doi.org/10.2165/00003088-198611040-00003] [PMID: 3530584]

[51] Clofazimine. The American Society of Health-System Pharmacists. Archived from the original on 20 December 2016. Retrieved 8 December 2016.

[52] WHO Model Formulary 2008 (PDF). World Health Organization. 2009; 132. ISBN 9789241547659. Archived (PDF) from the original on 13 December 2016. Retrieved 8 December 2016.

[53] WHO Model List of Essential Medicines (19th List) (PDF). World Health Organization. April 2015. Archived (PDF) from the original on 13 December 2016. Retrieved 8 December 2016.

[54] Clofazimine. International Drug Price Indicator Guide. 2016. Retrieved 8 December 2016.

[55] Arbiser JL, Moschella SL. Clofazimine: A review of its medical uses and mechanisms of action. J Am Acad Dermatol 1995; 32(2 Pt 1): 241-7. [http://dx.doi.org/10.1016/0190-9622(95)90134-5] [PMID: 7829710]

[56] Morrison NE, Marley GM. The mode of action of clofazimine DNA binding studies. Int J Lepr Other Mycobact Dis 1976; 44(1-2): 133-4. [PMID: 945233]

[57] Dennis EA. Phospholipases. P D Boyer (ed) the enzymes. 3rd ed., Lipid enzymology. Academic Press, Inc., New York. 1983; 16: p. 307-353.

[58] Kagan VE. Tocopherol stabilizes membrane against phospholipase A, free fatty acids, and lysophospholipids. Ann N Y Acad Sci 1989; 570: 121-35. [http://dx.doi.org/10.1111/j.1749-6632.1989.tb14913.x] [PMID: 2698101]

[59] Kornhuber J, Muehlbacher M, Trapp S, *et al.* Identification of novel functional inhibitors of acid sphingomyelinase. PLoS One 2011; 6(8)e23852. [http://dx.doi.org/10.1371/journal.pone.0023852] [PMID: 21909365]

[60] https://reference.medscape.com/drug/clofazimine-342661.

[61] Venkatesan K. Clinical pharmacokinetic considerations in the treatment of patients with leprosy. Clin Pharmacokinet 1989; 16(6): 365-86. [http://dx.doi.org/10.2165/00003088-198916060-00003] [PMID: 2661102]

[62] Rifampicin. Santa Cruz Biotechnology Product Block. Santa Cruz Biotechnology. 2014; (CAS 13292-46-1). Archived from the original on 27 November 2014. Retrieved 14 November 2014.

[63] Rifampin. The American Society of Health-System Pharmacists. 2015. Archived from the original on 2015-09-07. Retrieved Aug 1, 2015.

[64] Sensi P. History of the development of rifampin. Rev Infect Dis 1983; 5 (Suppl. 3): S402-6. [http://dx.doi.org/10.1093/clinids/5.Supplement_3.S402] [PMID: 6635432]

[65] Oxford Handbook of Infectious Diseases and Microbiology. OUP Oxford. 2009; 56. Archived from the original on 2015-11-24.

[66] McHugh, Timothy D. Tuberculosis: Diagnosis and treatment. Wallingford, Oxfordshire: CAB International 2011; p. 219.

[67] Calvori C, Frontali L, Leoni L, Tecce G. Effect of rifamycin on protein synthesis. Nature 1965; 207(995): 417-8.
[http://dx.doi.org/10.1038/207417a0] [PMID: 4957347]

[68] Acocella G. Clinical pharmacokinetics of rifampicin. Clin Pharmacokinet 1978; 3(2): 108-27. [http://dx.doi.org/10.2165/00003088-197803020-00002] [PMID: 346286]

[69] Calvori C, Frontali L, Leoni L, Tecce G. Effect of rifamycin on protein synthesis Nature 2016; 207(995): 417–8.

[70] British National Formulary. BNF 69 (69 ed). British Medical Association. 2015; 409: p. 757-782.

[71] WHO Model Formulary 2008 (PDF). World Health Organization. 140. Archived (PDF) from the original on 13 December 2008.

[72] Ofloxacin Use During Pregnancy | Drugs.com . www.drugs.com 2016. Archived from the original on 28 December 2016. Retrieved 28 December 2016.

[73] Fischer Janos. Ganellin, C. Robin. Analogue-based Drug Discovery. John Wiley & Sons 2006. Archived from the original on 2016-12-29.

[74] WHO Model List of Essential Medicines (19th List) (PDF). World Health Organization. April 2015. Archived (PDF) from the original on 13 December 2016. Retrieved 8 December 2016.

[75] Drlica K, Zhao X. DNA gyrase, topoisomerase IV, and the 4-quinolones. Microbiol Mol Biol Rev 1997; 61(3): 377-92.
[PMID: 9293187]

[76] Jacobson RR. Needed research in chemotherapy of leprosy related to the individual patient. Int J Lepr Other Mycobact Dis 1996; 64(4) (Suppl.): S16-20.
[PMID: 9030119]

[77] Girdhar BK. Fluoroquinolones and their adverse effects. Indian J Lepr 1993; 65(1): 69-79.
[PMID: 8463726]

[78] Nonaka K, Nakazawa Y, Kotorii T. Effects of antibiotics, minocycline and ampicillin, on human sleep. Brain Res 1983; 288(1-2): 253-9.
[http://dx.doi.org/10.1016/0006-8993(83)90101-4] [PMID: 6661620]

[79] Strauss JS, Krowchuk DP, Leyden JJ, *et al.* Guidelines of care for acne vulgaris management. J Am Acad Dermatol 2007; 56(4): 651-63.
[http://dx.doi.org/10.1016/j.jaad.2006.08.048] [PMID: 17276540]

[80] Rogers RL, Perkins J. Skin and soft tissue infections. Prim Care 2006; 33(3): 697-710. [http://dx.doi.org/10.1016/j.pop.2006.06.005] [PMID: 17088156]

[81] Bernier C, Dréno B. [Minocycline]. Ann Dermatol Venereol 2001; 128(5): 627-37.
[PMID: 11427798]

[82] Fischer J. Ganellin, C Robin Analogue-based Drug Discovery . John Wiley & Sons 2006; p. 489. [http://dx.doi.org/10.1002/3527608001]

[83] Redin GS. Antibacterial activity in mice of minocycline, a new tetracycline. Antimicrob Agents

Chemother 1966; 6: 371-6.
[PMID: 5985260]

[84] Gelber RH. Activity of minocycline in Mycobacterium leprae-infected mice. J Infect Dis 1987; 156(1): 236-9.
[http://dx.doi.org/10.1093/infdis/156.1.236] [PMID: 3298454]

[85] Jacobson RR. Needed research in chemotherapy of leprosy related to the individual patient. Int J Lepr Other Mycobact Dis 1996; 64(4) (Suppl.): S16-20.
[PMID: 9030119]

[86] Jamet P, Traore I, Husser JA, Ji B. Short-term trial of clofazimine in previously untreated lepromatous leprosy. Int J Lepr Other Mycobact Dis 1992; 60(4): 542-8.
[PMID: 1299709]

[87] Hastings RC, Richard VR, Jacobson RR. Ansamycin activity against rifampicin-resistant Mycobacterium leprae. Lancet 1984; 1(8386): 1130.
[http://dx.doi.org/10.1016/S0140-6736(84)92549-2] [PMID: 6144865]

[88] Ji BH, Chen JK, Lu XZ, *et al.* Antimycobacterial activities of two newer ansamycins, R-76-1 and DL 473. Int J Lepr Other Mycobact Dis 1986; 54(4): 563-77.
[PMID: 3546547]

[89] Girdhar BK. Fluoroquinolones and their adverse effects. Indian J Lepr 1993; 65(1): 69-79.
[PMID: 8463726]

[90] https://www.sciencedirect.com/topics/pharmacology-toxicology-and-pharmaceutical-science/vo-ume-of-distribution.

[91] Skinner MH, Blaschke TF. Clinical pharmacokinetics of rifabutin. Clin Pharmacokinet 1995; 28(2): 115-25.
[http://dx.doi.org/10.2165/00003088-199528020-00003] [PMID: 7736687]

[92] Gussow Z. Leprosy, Racism, and Public Health. Boulder, Colorado: Westview Press 1989.

[93] http://www.who.int/lep/diagnosis/en/.

[94] Staples J. Communities of the afflicted: Constituting leprosy through place in South India. Med Anthropol 2014; 33(1): 6-20.
[http://dx.doi.org/10.1080/01459740.2012.714021] [PMID: 24383749]

[95] https://www.timeanddate.com/holidays/world/world-leprosy-day.

[96] McMenamin, Dorothy. Leprosy and stigma in the South Pacific: A region-by-region history with first person accounts. Jefferson, N.C.: McFarland 2011. Archived from the original on 2016-05-19.

CHAPTER 9

Silk Protein Sericin: Structure, Secretion, Composition and Antimicrobial Potential

Shamjetshabam Babeeta Chanu*, **Sanjenbam Kunjeshwori Devi** and **Laishram Rupachandra Singh**

Protein Biochemistry Laboratory, Department of Biochemistry, Manipur University, Manipur, India

Abstract: Silk sericin is a glycoprotein which surrounds and keeps two fibroin filaments together. It is produced in the middle silk gland during the fifth instar of the larval stage of the silkworm. During the process of degumming, sericin is removed from the silk cocoon. This waste sericin has been discovered to have a wide variety of applications as antioxidant, antityrosinase, wound healing, anti-wrinkle agents, *etc*. Sericin from various silk cocoons was also found to have antimicrobial activity against several fungal and bacterial pathogens. Sericin with antimicrobial activities can be used in various applications such as in the preparation of wound healing gels, and the treatment of fabrics for medicinal purposes. A particular study showed the application of sericin as a coating material on polyester or polyamide fibres, to be used as media for air filters. It reduces the free radicals in the filter media and contamination of fungi and bacteria, thus helping in purifying the polluted air. Hence, the biodegradable and biocompatible nature of silk protein sericin makes it a potentially promising substitute of various antibiotics and certain other harmful antimicrobial agents that we use in our daily life.

Keywords: Antibacterial, Antifungal, Antimicrobial, Silk, Sericin.

INTRODUCTION

Lepidopteran insects belonging to the families *Saturnidae* and *Bombycidae* spin silk fibers. The silkworms can be classified as mulberry and non-mulberry. *Bombyx mori* silkworm is the only mulberry silkworm. Non-mulberry silkworms are wild, heterogeneous and have a relatively wide distribution throughout the world. These silkworms can be broadly classified into two major categories; temperate and tropical. Temperate or oak tasar silkworms are found in China (*Antheraea pernyi*), Japan (*A. yamamai*), and North East India (*A. roylei, A. frithi,*

* **Corresponding Author Shamjetshabam Babeeta Chanu:** Protein Biochemistry Laboratory, Department of Biochemistry, Manipur University, Manipur, India; Tel.: +91 897 4356 250; E-mail: pakpis@gmail.com

K. Tamreihao, Saikat Mukherjee and Debananda S. Ningthoujam (Eds.)
All rights reserved-© 2019 Bentham Science Publishers

A. pernyi, and *A. proylei*), while tropical tasar silkworm *A. mylitta* is mostly confined to central India [1].

Silkworms, during pupation, spin the cocoons to protect the inactive pupae. The silk proteins: sericin and fibroin, are synthesized by silk gland cells and are stored in the lumen of the glands. Silkworm produces the silk proteins sericin and fibroin during the fifth instar of the larval stage. These two proteins are the main structural component of the silk cocoon. Fibroin is the main structural protein constituting about 70% of the total cocoon while sericin is a glycoprotein which adheres the fibroin proteins. It contributes about 20-30% of the total cocoon [2].

Sericin naturally is hydrophilic and amorphous. It helps in maintaining the structural integrity of the cocoon. During the degumming process of the silk textile industry, sericin is removed as waste from fibroin to make silk fibres more lustrous, soft, smooth, white, and dyeable [3]. The global discarded sericin constitutes approximately 50,000 tons out of the 1 million tons of fresh cocoons annually [4]. Sericin is mostly discarded in wastewater. This generates a high chemical and biological oxygen demand as well as contamination of water and environment [5].

Silk sericin which was considered to be a waste product in the silk industry is now found to have important biochemical functions such as inhibitory effects on tumor progression, and antioxidant and antityrosinase activities [6, 7]. Silk protein sericin of *Bombyx mori* is one of the most researched proteins. It has been shown to be useful as a degradable biopolymer for making functional membranes, fibres, and fabrics. An *in vivo* study of sericin as a dietary source in rats has shown that it reduces serum cholesterol and triglycerides, thus helping in preventing atherosclerosis [8]. Its high fibre content causes increased excretion of fecal nitrogen thus exhibits anti-constipation effect [9]. Because of its nature, sericin can be used in food, cosmetic and pharmaceutical products as well as for biomaterials manufacture [10]. Hence, the use of biodegradable and biocompatible sericin has a great potential in the development of novel anti-infective agents, for application as effective bioactive compounds in treating the drug-resistant pathogens, especially in developing countries such as China, India, and Brazil where sericulture is practiced.

Secretion of Silk Proteins

During the larval stage in the lifecycle of a silkworm, the silk gland synthesizes silk proteins. The silk gland consists of a pair of tubular labial structure which extends laterally to the digestive tract. The silk gland is constituted of three parts which are differentiated on the basis of morphology and function (Fig. **1**). The posterior silk gland (PSG), which is about 15 cm long and constituted of 500 secretory cells synthesizes the fibroin protein. The middle silk gland (MSG), which is about 7 cm long and constituted of 300 secretory cells synthesizes the sericin protein. The last part is the anterior silk gland (ASG); it is about 2 cm long and is constituted by about 250 cells which have no secretory functions. It functions as the excretory duct, excreting the silk proteins synthesized by the middle silk gland (MSG) and posterior silk gland (PSG). Silk protein secretion occurs in the 5th instar of the larval development stage of the silkworm [11 - 13].

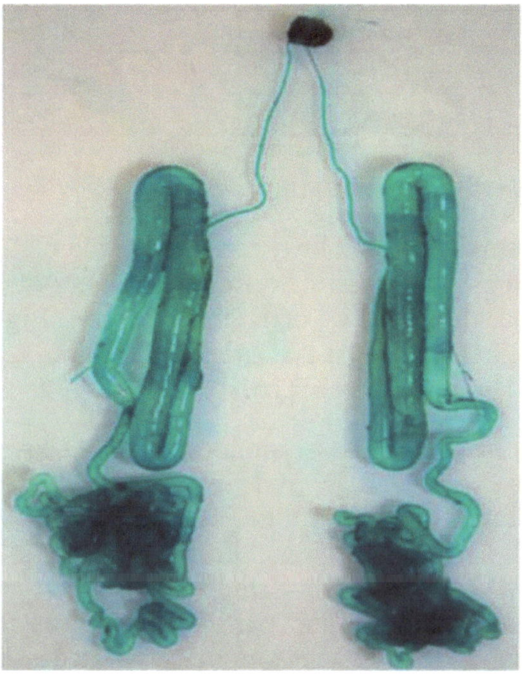

Fig. (1). Structure of *Bombyx mori* silk gland stained with 1% light green showing Anterior Silk Gland (ASG), Middle Silk Gland (MSG) and Posterior Silk Gland (PSG) (Adapted with permission from Kunz *et al.* [41]).

The fibroin is secreted with 15% protein in solution form in the PSG; it then migrates into the MSG where it is surrounded by sericin. The cells of the glandular epithelium gradually absorb water from the protein solution, reducing it to a gel with 30% protein. When the protein is excreted from the ASG, excess water and ions are absorbed gradually, converting the protein gel into a solid filament, thus converting the soluble silk proteins into insoluble silk fibers [14].

The silk cocoon is mainly composed of the two proteins; fibroin and sericin. Many non-protein components such as carbohydrates, salts, wax, flavonoids and other derivatives are also associated with cocoons (Table **1**) [15].

Table 1. Composition of *Bombyx mori* silk cocoon [40].

Component	%
Fibroin	70-80
Sericin	20-30
Wax matter	0.4-0.8
Carbohydrates	1.2-1.6
Inorganic matter	0.7
Pigment	0.2
Total	100

Structure and Composition of Sericin

Silk is a continuous strand of two brins of fibroin filaments which are adhered together with the glue-like protein sericin. Silk fibroin of *Bombyx mori* is constituted of three proteins: Heavy or High (H) chain, Light or Low (L) chain, and a glycoprotein P25. The size of the H chain, L chain, and P25 is around 350 kDa, 26kDa, and 30 kDa, respectively [16].

In silk fibre, the fibroin protein is surrounded by three layers of sericin protein layer, namely Sericin A, Sericin B, and Sericin C. Sericin A is located in the outermost layer, Sericin B in the middle and Sericin C is the innermost sericin protein adjacent to the fibroin protein. Sericin A is soluble in warm water. It contains around 17.2% nitrogen with serine, threonine, glycine and aspartic acid as major amino acids. Sericin B contains around 16.8% nitrogen and an additional amino acid tryptophan. Sericin C is insoluble in warm water. It contains around 16.6% nitrogen and all amino acids of Sericin A and Sericin B and an additional amino acid, proline [17].

Structurally, sericin is a globular protein consisting of random coil and β-sheets. Random coil conformation is found more in the soluble form. In hot water (50-60 °C or higher), protein adopts its soluble form. At lower temperatures, the solubility is reduced and the random coil structure is converted into β-sheets, resulting in the formation of a gel [19 - 21]. Sericin is highly hydrophilic with a molecular weight that ranges from 20 to 400 kDa. Macromolecule of hydrophilic character is composed of 18 amino acids with strong polar groups such as hydroxyl, carboxyl, and amino groups (Table **2**) [22], capable of forming crosslink, copolymerization, and combination with other polymers [23]. The organic portion is composed of 46.5% carbon, 31% oxygen, 16.5% nitrogen, and 6% hydrogen [24]. These unique properties enable sericin function as antioxidant, moisturizing, healing, antimicrobial, ultraviolet radiation protector, and antitumor agents [6, 10, 18, 25].

Table 2. Amino acid composition of *Bombyx mori* sericin [6].

Amino Acids	Molar Percent
Asp	17.8
Thr	8.0
Ser	31.0
Glu	4.4
Pro	0.4
Gly	19.1
Ala	3.8
Cys	<0.05
Val	3.1
Met	<0.05
Ile	0.4
Leu	0.8
Tyr	3.3
Phe	0.2
His	1.0
Lys	2.7
Arg	3.9

Antimicrobial Potential of Sericin

Silk sericins from various cocoon sources are found to have antimicrobial properties. The antimicrobial activities of the silk sericin depend on the types of silkworm and also on the method of extraction.

Silk sericin extracted in hot water (80 °C for 30 mins) from the cocoon of mulberry silkworm *Bombyx mori* was found to have antimicrobial activity against *Micrococcus luteus*. The antimicrobial activity increases with the increase in sericin concentration [26, 27]. Sericin was also extracted by boiling cocoons in sodium carbonate and sodium bicarbonate solution for 60 mins and precipitated using ethanol. The ethanol precipitated sericin displays antibacterial activity against *Staphylococcus aureus* and *Escherichia coli* [28].

Silk sericin from Eri silkworm (*Samia ricini*), which is a non-mulberry silkworm exhibits antibacterial activity against *Staphylococcus aureus* and *Escherichia coli*.

The sericin from the cocoon of Eri silkworm was extracted by two methods: boiling in distilled water for 60 minutes and boiling in 0.25% Na_2CO_3 for 90 minutes. The aqueous extract of sericin was more potent against *Staphylococcus aureus* while the 0.25% Na_2CO_3 extract was more potent against *Escherichia coli*. The antibacterial activity was also found to increase with the increase in sericin concentration [29]

Tasar sericin from Indian tropical tasar silkworm *Antheraea mylitta* displays antibacterial activity against *Staphylococcus aureus* and *Escherichia coli,* and antifungal activity against *Candida albicans* and *Aspergillus flavus* [30].

Interaction Mechanism

Several studies have shown that the antibacterial activity of sericin is due to its polycationic nature in acidic condition, which allows it to interact with the negatively charged bacterial cell membranes (lipopolysaccharides and proteins of the microbes). The interaction disrupts the permeability of the cell wall, inducing leakage of intracellular components and ultimately killing the cell [31 - 33]. Some studies demonstrated that the low molecular weight sericin could have directly penetrated the bacterial cells and form a complex with the anionic materials inside the cell, thereby, disrupting the normal physiological activities and ultimately killing the bacteria [34]. This may be one of the major factors for hot water extracted sericin to have antimicrobial activity since this method causes hydrolysis of sericin resulting in lowering the molecular weight [35].

The interaction of sericin with *E. coli* was also studied using Inverted Fluorescence Microscopy (IFM), Scanning Electron Microscopy and Transmission Electron Microscopy (TEM). The study suggested that there is a direct adhesion of sericin molecules on the surface of *E. coli* cells. Treatment of sericin induces membrane blebbing in *E. coli* cells, which is a typical mode of action of antibacterial peptides and proteins. TEM analysis confirmed that cytoplasm shrinkage was accompanied by the blurring of the membrane wall boundaries. Amino acids serine, aspartic acid, and glycine present in sericin molecules might induce membrane blebbing of *E. coli* cells [36].

Eri sericin was also shown to inhibit the process of cell division and cell growth. It also induces membrane dysfunction in *E. coli* and *S. aureus* [29].

Applications of Sericin having Antimicrobial Activity

Silk sericin having antimicrobial activity can be used as antimicrobial agents against infections. They can be used in the preparation of medicines for wound healing, and as components for the treatment of fabrics and polluted air. They can even be used in the synthesis of nanoparticle composites which have great biomedical applications as antimicrobial agents and in wound healing.

Wound Healing

Sericin based hydrogels are shown to have higher wound healing potential than traditional hydrogels. This is due to the fact that sericin has antibacterial activity, thus preventing the wound from bacterial infection and accelerating the wound healing process. The *in vivo* results also showed that sericin-based hydrogel could promote cell proliferation and accelerate the formation of granulation and neovessels [36].

Treatment of Fabrics

Cotton fabric coated with 2% sericin increased the tensile strength and reduced the number of spores of *Micrococcus luteus* [27]. It was reported that sericin-coated fabric showed good bactericidal activity against *Escherichia coli* and *Staphylococcus aureus* [28]. In a particular study, the influence of sericin and sericin based TiO_2 nanocomposite with and without polycarboxylic acid cross-linking agents treated on the cotton fabric was studied. It was found that fabrics treated with nanocomposites of sericin exhibit antibacterial activity against *Staphylococcus aureus* and *Escherichia coli* which are the major causes of nosocomial infections. It also does not significantly affect the breaking strength of the fabrics [37]. The results indicated that sericin could be used in the treatment of fabrics for use in medicinal purposes such as surgical fabrics, medical bandages used in wound dressing, diapers and diaper liners, *etc.*

The composite nanofibres prepared with chitosan and sericin (ratio of 2.5:1) showed antibacterial activity against *Escherichia coli* and *Bacillus subtilis*. 3-(4,5-dimethylthiazol-2-yl)-2,5-diphenyltetrazolium bromide (MTT) assay of the nanocomposite fibers further showed that it is not cytotoxic to fibroblast cell lines and helps the proliferation of the cell line. The composite fiber can thus be used as a good wound dressing agent [38].

Air Pollution Abatement

Air filters coated with filter media possessing antibacterial and antifungal activity will prevent the filter from being a potent habitat for pathogenic microorganisms from polluted air. It was shown that nylon and polyester fibres coated with sericin could potentially inhibit the growth of *Micrococcus* sp. and also have potential antifungal activity. Moreover, silk sericin also possesses antioxidant potential which helps in scavenging the free radicals, thus, reducing the amount of free radical entry in the body and increasing the quality of the air filter [39].

Stabilizing Nanoparticle Composites

Nanoparticles have been widely used in various applications. They are mostly synthesized using organic solvent and toxic reducing agents [45, 46, 48]. Silver nanoparticles have a wide variety of applications but have limited stability under certain conditions [47]. Nanoparticles are also toxic to viruses, bacteria, fungi and human cells [44]. Hence, there is a need for synthesizing nanoparticles that display higher stability and low toxicity to human cells, but exhibit higher toxicity to pathogens so that they can be used in various applications.

A novel, simple, one-step method to prepare sericin silver nanoparticle composite *in situ* in solution has been developed. Silk sericin capped nanoparticles are synthesized in alkaline condition. Silver nanoparticles have also been synthesized on the surface of sericin gel. Sericin served as the reductant of silver ion, dispersant, and stabilizer of the prepared sericin silver nanoparticle composite [42, 43, 49].

The sericin based nanoparticles are found to have long-term stability, effective antibacterial activity, and good biocompatibility. Sericin based silver nanoparticles have low cytotoxicity compared to the silver nanoparticle. They could inhibit and even kill many Gram-positive and Gram-negative bacteria *viz.*, MRSA, *S. aureus*, *B. subtilis*, *P. aeruginosa*, *A. baumannii* and, *E. coli,* thus, overcoming the problem of instability of silver nanoparticles in bacteria-rich environments [42, 43].

CONCLUDING REMARKS

Antibiotics extracted from bioactive microorganisms and some synthetic compounds are the most widely used antimicrobial agents for treating infectious diseases. But the growing trend of antibiotic resistance of pathogens has caused a serious alarm in the use of antibiotics as effective anti-infective agents. Synthetic antibiotics have adverse effects on human health because of bio-incompatibility. Hence, there is a need to search for novel, safe, less toxic, effective, biocompatible, environmentally safe, and cost-effective compounds for treating antibiotic-resistant pathogenic strains. Sericin protein which is a waste product of the silk industry is biocompatible and biodegradable. Hence, with further research sericin and sericin-based materials could have promise as potent antimicrobial agents in the future.

CONSENT FOR PUBLICATION

Not applicable.

CONFLICT OF INTEREST

The authors confirm that this chapter contents have no conflict of interest.

ACKNOWLEDGEMENTS

SBC acknowledges the support of the University Grant Commission (UGC), New Delhi in the form of a research project (MRP-MAJOR-BIOC-2013-22857) that facilitated the writing of this article.

REFERENCES

[1] Kundu SC, Kundu B, Talukdar S, *et al.* Invited review nonmulberry silk biopolymers. Biopolymers 2012; 97(6): 455-67.
[http://dx.doi.org/10.1002/bip.22024] [PMID: 22241173]

[2] Zhaoa HP, Fenga XS, Yua SW, Cuib WZ, Zou FZ. Mechanical properties of silkworm cocoons. Polymer (Guildf) 2005; 46: 9192-201.
[http://dx.doi.org/10.1016/j.polymer.2005.07.004]

[3] Gupta D, Agrawal A, Rangi A. Extraction and characterization of silk sericin. Indian J Fibre Text Res 2012; 39(4): 364-72.

[4] Gulrajani ML. Sericin: a bio-molecule of value. Proceedings of the Souvenir 20th Congress of the International Sericulture Commission. 21-9.

[5] Fabiani C, Pizzichini M, Spadoni M, Zeddita G. Treatment of waste water from silk degumming processes for protein recovery and water reuse. Desalination 1996; 105(1-2): 1-9.
[http://dx.doi.org/10.1016/0011-9164(96)00050-1]

[6] Kato N, Sato S, Yamanaka A, Yamada H, Fuwa N, Nomura M. Silk protein, sericin, inhibits lipid peroxidation and tyrosinase activity. Biosci Biotechnol Biochem 1998; 62(1): 145-7.
[http://dx.doi.org/10.1271/bbb.62.145] [PMID: 9501526]

[7] Zhaorigetu S, Sasaki M, Watanabe H, Kato N. Supplemental silk protein, sericin, suppresses colon tumorigenesis in 1,2-dimethylhydrazine-treated mice by reducing oxidative stress and cell proliferation. Biosci Biotechnol Biochem 2001; 65(10): 2181-6.
[http://dx.doi.org/10.1271/bbb.65.2181] [PMID: 11758907]

[8] Kato N, Iwami K. Resistant protein; its existence and function beneficial to health. J Nutr Sci Vitaminol (Tokyo) 2002; 48(1): 1-5.
[http://dx.doi.org/10.3177/jnsv.48.1] [PMID: 12026181]

[9] Ghosh S, Rao RS, Nambiar KS, Haragannavar VC, Augustine D, Sowmya SV. Sericin, a dietary additive: Mini review. J Med Radiol Pathol Surg 2017; 4: 13-7.
[http://dx.doi.org/10.15713/ins.jmrps.89]

[10] Wu JH, Wang Z, Xu SY. Preparation and characterization of sericin powder extracted from silk industry wastewater. Food Chem 2007; 103(4): 1255-62.
[http://dx.doi.org/10.1016/j.foodchem.2006.10.042]

[11] Mondal M, Trivedy K, Kumar SN. The silk proteins, sericin and fibroin in silkworm, Bombyx mori Linn.,—a review. CJES 2007; 5(2): 63-76.

[12] Dhawan S, Gopinathan KP. Cell cycle events during the development of the silk glands in the mulberry silkworm Bombyx mori. Dev Genes Evol 2003; 213(9): 435-44.
[http://dx.doi.org/10.1007/s00427-003-0343-7] [PMID: 12883881]

[13] Sorour J, Larik O, Ramadan A, Shalaby A, Osman S. Anatomical, histological and electron microscopy studies on the salivary glands of larvae of *Spodoptera littoralis* Boids. (Lep.Noctuidae).

Zool Jahrb Abt Anat Ontogenie Tiere 1990; 120: 251-71.

[14] Akai H. The structure and ultrastructure of the silk gland. Experientia 1983; 39(5): 443-9. [http://dx.doi.org/10.1007/BF01965158]

[15] Liu X, Zhang KQ. Silk fiber—molecular formation mechanism, structure-property relationship and advanced applications Oligomerization of Chemical and Biological Compounds. IntechOpen 2014; p. 3.

[16] Wang HY, Wang YJ, Zhou LX, Zhu L, Zhang YQ. Isolation and bioactivities of a non-sericin component from cocoon shell silk sericin of the silkworm Bombyx mori. Food Funct 2012; 3(2): 150-8. [http://dx.doi.org/10.1039/C1FO10148J] [PMID: 22101964]

[17] Kimura K, Oyama F, Ueda H, Mizuno S, Shimura K. Molecular cloning of the fibroin light chain complementary DNA and its use in the study of the expression of the light chain gene in the posterior silk gland of Bombyx mori. Experientia 1985; 41(9): 1167-71. [http://dx.doi.org/10.1007/BF01951711] [PMID: 2995115]

[18] Shaw JTB, Smith SG. Amino-acids of silk sericin. Nature 1951; 168(4278): 745. [http://dx.doi.org/10.1038/168745a0] [PMID: 14882336]

[19] Aramwit P, Kanokpanont S, De-Eknamkul W, Srichana T. Monitoring of inflammatory mediators induced by silk sericin. J Biosci Bioeng 2009; 107(5): 556-61. [http://dx.doi.org/10.1016/j.jbiosc.2008.12.012] [PMID: 19393558]

[20] Kataoka K. The solubility of sericin in water. Nippon Sanshigaku Zasshi 1977; 46(3): 227-30.

[21] Zhu LJ, Yao J, Youlu L. Structural transformation of sericin, a dissolved from cocoon layer in hot water. Zhejiang Nongye Daxue Xuebao 1998; 24(3): 268-72.

[22] Zhu LJ, Arai M, Hirabayashi K. Sol-gel transition of sericin. Nippon Sanshigaku Zasshi 1996; 65(4): 270-4.

[23] Zhang YQ. Applications of natural silk protein sericin in biomaterials. Biotechnol Adv 2002; 20(2): 91-100. [http://dx.doi.org/10.1016/S0734-9750(02)00003-4] [PMID: 14538058]

[24] Dash BC, Mandal BB, Kundu SC. Silk gland sericin protein membranes: fabrication and characterization for potential biotechnological applications. J Biotechnol 2009; 144(4): 321-9. [http://dx.doi.org/10.1016/j.jbiotec.2009.09.019] [PMID: 19808068]

[25] Rajput SK, Kumar M. Sericin—a unique biomaterial. IOSR JPTE 2015; 2(3): 29-35.

[26] Aramwit P, Keongamaroon O, Siritientong T, Bang N, Supasyndh O. Sericin cream reduces pruritus in hemodialysis patients: a randomized, double-blind, placebo-controlled experimental study. BMC Nephrol 2012; 13: 119. [http://dx.doi.org/10.1186/1471-2369-13-119] [PMID: 23006933]

[27] Jassim KN, Al-Saree OJ. Study of the antimicrobial activity of silk sericin from silkworm bombyx mori. Iraqi J Community Med 2010; 23(2): 130-3.

[28] Rajendran R, Balakumar C, Sivakumar R, Amruta T, Devaki N. Extraction and application of natural silk protein sericin from Bombyx mori as antimicrobial finish for cotton fabrics. J Textil Inst 2012; 103(4): 458-62. [http://dx.doi.org/10.1080/00405000.2011.586151]

[29] Senakoon W, Nuchadomrong S, Sirimungkararat S, Senawong T, Kitikoon P. Antibacterial action of eri (samia ricini) sericin against *Escherichia coli* and *staphylococcus aureus*. AJFAI 2009; pp. 222-8.

[30] Iqbal S, Ahamad M, Vootla SK. Extraction and evaluation of antimicrobial potential of Antheraea mylitta silk sericin. IJRSR 2018; 9,1(C): 23019-22.

[31] Helander IM, Nurmiaho-Lassila EL, Ahvenainen R, Rhoades J, Roller S. Chitosan disrupts the barrier

properties of the outer membrane of gram-negative bacteria. Int J Food Microbiol 2001; 71(2-3): 235-44.
[http://dx.doi.org/10.1016/S0168-1605(01)00609-2] [PMID: 11789941]

[32] Lim SH, Hudson SM. Application of a fiber-reactive chitosan derivative to cotton fabric as an antimicrobial textile finish. Carbohydr Polym 2004; 56: 227-34.
[http://dx.doi.org/10.1016/j.carbpol.2004.02.005]

[33] Shahidi F, Arachchi JKV, Jeon YJ. Food applications of chitin and chitosans. Trends Food Sci Technol 1999; 10: 37-51.
[http://dx.doi.org/10.1016/S0924-2244(99)00017-5]

[34] Shi L, Zhao Y, Zhang X, Su H, Tan T. Antibacterial and anti-mildew behavior of chitosan/nano-TiO2 composite emulsion. Korean J Chem Eng 2008; 25: 1434-8.
[http://dx.doi.org/10.1007/s11814-008-0235-7]

[35] Oh H, Lee JY, Kim MK, Um IC, Lee KH. Refining hot-water extracted silk sericin by ethanol-induced precipitation. Int J Biol Macromol 2011; 48(1): 32-7.
[http://dx.doi.org/10.1016/j.ijbiomac.2010.09.008] [PMID: 20875446]

[36] Xue R, Liu Y, Zhang Q, *et al.* Shape change and interaction mechanism of Escherichia coli treated by sericin and sericin-based hydrogel for wound healing. Appl Environ Microbiol 2016; 82(15): 4663-72.
[http://dx.doi.org/10.1128/AEM.00643-16] [PMID: 27235427]

[37] Doakhan S, Montazer M, Rashidi A, Moniri R, Moghadam MB. Influence of sericin/TiO_2 nanocomposite on cotton fabric: part 1. Enhanced antibacterial effect. Carbohydr Polym 2013; 94(2): 737-48.
[http://dx.doi.org/10.1016/j.carbpol.2013.01.023] [PMID: 23544628]

[38] Zhao R, Li X, Sun B, *et al.* Electrospun chitosan/sericin composite nanofibers with antibacterial property as potential wound dressings. Int J Biol Macromol 2014; 68: 92-7.
[http://dx.doi.org/10.1016/j.ijbiomac.2014.04.029] [PMID: 24769088]

[39] Sarovart S, Sudatis B, Meesilpa P, Grady BP, Magaraphan R. The use of sericin as an antioxidant and antimicrobial for polluted air treatment. Rev Adv Mater Sci 2003; 5: 193-8.

[40] Gulrajani ML. Degumming of silk; In Silk dyeing printing and finishing. Department of Textile Technology, IIT, New Delhi 1988 63.

[41] Kunz RI, Brancalhão RMC, Ribeiro LFC. Natali MRM. Silkworm Sericin: Properties and Biomedical Applications. BioMed Res Int 2016; 1-19.
[http://dx.doi.org/10.1155/2016/8175701]

[42] He H, Tao G, Wang Y, *et al. In situ* green synthesis and characterization of sericin-silver nanoparticle composite with effective antibacterial activity and good biocompatibility. Mater Sci Eng C 2017; 80: 509-16.
[http://dx.doi.org/10.1016/j.msec.2017.06.015] [PMID: 28866194]

[43] Aramwit P, Bang N, Ratanavaraporn J, Ekgasit S. Green synthesis of silk sericin-capped silver nanoparticles and their potent anti-bacterial activity. Nanoscale Res Lett 2014; 9(79): 1-7.

[44] You C, Han C, Wang X, *et al.* The progress of silver nanoparticles in the antibacterial mechanism, clinical application and cytotoxicity. Mol Biol Rep 2012; 39(9): 9193-201.
[http://dx.doi.org/10.1007/s11033-012-1792-8] [PMID: 22722996]

[45] Iravani S, Korbekandi H, Mirmohammadi SV, Zolfaghari B. Synthesis of silver nanoparticles: chemical, physical and biological methods. Res Pharm Sci 2014; 9(6): 385-406.
[PMID: 26339255]

[46] Cai R, Tao G, He H, *et al.* One-step synthesis of silver nanoparticles on polydopamine-coated sericin/polyvinyl alcohol composite films for potential antimicrobial applications. Molecules 2017; 22(5): 1-14.
[http://dx.doi.org/10.3390/molecules22050721] [PMID: 28468293]

[47] Kumar R, Münstedt H. Silver ion release from antimicrobial polyamide/silver composites. Biomaterials 2005; 26(14): 2081-8.
[http://dx.doi.org/10.1016/j.biomaterials.2004.05.030] [PMID: 15576182]

[48] Solomon SD, Bahadory M, Jeyarajasingam AV, Rutkowsky SA, Boritz C. Synthesis and study of silver nanoparticles. J Chem Educ 2007; 84: 322-5.
[http://dx.doi.org/10.1021/ed084p322]

[49] Tao G, Liu L, Wang Y, *et al.* Characterization of silver nanoparticle in situ synthesis on porous sericin gel for antibacterial application. J Nanomater 2016; 1-8.

CHAPTER 10

Understanding the Realm of Antibiotics: Mechanisms of Action and Their Applications as Anti-infective Agents

Laishram Jaya Devi[1,*], **Rakhi Khunjanmayum**[1], **Roshan Singh Asem**[1], **Elangbam Shanta Singh**[1], **Sumita Banerjee**[2] and **Debananda S. Ningthoujam**[1]

[1] *Advanced Level State Biotech Hub (AdL- SBT Hub), Department of Biochemistry, Manipur University Canchipur 795003, India*

[2] *Department of Oral Pathology and Microbiology, Regional Institute of Medical Sciences (RIMS), Imphal, Manipur 795004, India*

Abstract: Human beings and the microbial world have co-existed and maintained a symbiotic balance; providing a protective and stabilizing effect on the body as resident microbes. Pathogenic bacteria invade and grow in human tissues causing diseases and damaging the body. They represent a major problem threatening the health of humans, sometimes leading to death. This stimulated the scientists to find new solutions to many diseases by clarifying the interactions of antibacterial compounds with the biological medium. The use of antibiotics protects the body from pathogenic microorganisms, however, there are also some side effects. Proper characterization and adequate understanding of the mode of action of antibiotics are, therefore, an indispensable necessity. Examining the mechanism of action of the various antibiotics illustrates how they are effective against pathogenic microorganisms with minimal selectively. The mechanism of action of antibiotics occurs in the cell wall or within the cell of pathogens where it may block the synthesis or break down the cell wall, block catabolic energy-supplying mechanisms or anabolic protein synthesizing processes. Hence, in this chapter, the classification of antibiotics, their mode of action, application and, how antibiotics are used as anti-infective agents will be discussed.

Keywords: Actinomycete, Antibiotics, Antibacterial drug, Anti-infective agents, Bacteriostatic, Inflammation, Nucleic acid synthesis, Protein synthesis, Ribosomes.

* **Corresponding author Laishram Jaya Devi:** Advanced Level State Biotech Hub (AdL- SBT Hub), Department of Biochemistry, Manipur University Canchipur 795003, India; Tel: +91 986 2639 460; E-mail: abejaya@gmail.com

K. Tamreihao, Saikat Mukherjee and Debananda S. Ningthoujam (Eds.)
All rights reserved-© 2019 Bentham Science Publishers

INTRODUCTION

The term antibiotic was derived from the word "antibiosis" which literally means "against life". An antibiotic or an antibacterial compound, is a drug which issued to treat and prevent bacterial infections [1, 2]. They may either inhibit the growth or kill the bacteria [3]. Several antibiotics are also effective against fungi and protozoans. However, some are toxic to humans and animals even when prescribed in therapeutic range. They are not effective against viruses such as viruses that cause common cold or influenza and may be harmful when taken inappropriately.

Sometimes the antibiotic is broadly referred to any substance which is used against microbes. However, in medical term, they are refer to those produced naturally whereas, non-antibiotic antibacterial drugs (such as sulfonamides and antiseptics) are fully synthetic. In the past, antibiotics were considered as organic compounds produced by single microorganism, which are detrimental to other microorganisms. As a result of this notion, antibiotic was considered as a secondary metabolite produced by a microorganism, or of biological origin which at low concentrations can suppress the growth of other microorganisms. However, this definition has been modified in modern times, to include antimicrobial metabolites that are also produced partly or wholly through synthetic means. Those antibiotics which are able to completely kill other bacteria are known as bactericidal, while those inhibit the growth are termed bacteriostatic.

Discovery

With the discovery of antibiotics, the pharmaceutical industry was drastically revolutionised in the 20th century. On the other hand, their effectiveness and easy access have led to overuse; prompting target pathogens to develop resistance [4 - 8]. Before the early part of 20th century, human depends primarily on medicinal folklore to treat the infections cause by pathogenic microorganisms. They use the mixtures of plants having antimicrobial properties in order to treat the disease [9]. Many ancient cultures including the ancient Egyptians and ancient Greeks, used selected molds and plant materials to treat infections [10, 11].

In the late 1880s, in Germany, Paul Ehrlich initiated synthetic antibiotic chemotherapy for the development of antibacterial compounds [12]. Ehrlich noted that certain dyes can colour animal, human and bacterial cells. After high throughput screening of various dyes on many organisms, he discovered first synthetic antibacterial Salvarsan, in 1907, also known as arsphenamine [12 - 14]. Prontonsil, the first sulphonamide and the first systemically active antibacterial drug was developed by a research team led by Gerhard Domagk in 1932 or 1933 at the Bayer Laboratories of the IG Farben conglomerate in Germany [15 - 17].

Domagk received Nobel Prize in Physiology or Medicine for this discovery in 1939 [18]. As a result of subsequent developments, many previously fatal bacterial infections can now be treated successfully.

Classification of Antibiotics

Antibiotics can be classified into various categories:

Activity Against Gram-positive Bacterial Infection

Antibiotics used for treating infectious disease caused by Gram-positive bacteria include Tetracycline, Vancomycin, Chloramphenicol, Penicillin, Rifampicin, Gentamicin, Erythromycin, Clindamycin, Daptomycin, and Teicoplanin [19].

Vancomycin

Vancomycin, a glycopeptide antibiotic was extracted in the year 1956 from actinobacteria *Streptomyces orientalis* [20]. It is used for treating the intricated skin infections, blood stream infections, endocarditis, bone and joint infections, and meningitis caused by methicillin–resistant *Staphylococcus aureus* (MRSA). The clinical use of vancomycin became widespread in 1958 with the emergence of penicillinase-producing staphylococci. This drug is used in the United States for the treatment of serious Gram-positive infections, particularly MRSA [21].

Tetracycline

Benjamin Duggar discovered tetracycline in 1945 from a soil bacterium of the genus *Streptomyces* [22]. They exhibit a broad-spectrum antimicrobial activity however, their general usefulness reduced with the onset of antibiotic resistance [23]. They are inexpensive antibiotics used extensively in the prophylaxis and therapy of human and animal infections, and also at subtherapeutic levels as growth promoters in animal feed. Collectively, tetracyclines are known as “derivatives of polycyclic naphthacene carboxamide” [24, 25]. Chlortetracycline (Aureomycin) was the first compound among this class to be purified. The compound of this class have four hydrocarbon rings and they are known with the suffix–cycline. Based on the method of synthesis, tetracyclines are grouped into different generations. Compound obtained by direct biosynthesis are called First generation members which include Tetracycline, Chlortetracycline, Demeclocycline and Oxytetracycline. Antibiotics such as Doxycycline, Lymecycline, Meclocycline, Methacycline, Minocycline, and Rolitetracycline are considered as Second generation members because they are derivatives of semi-synthesis. Third generation member are obtained from total synthesis which include Tigecycline [26]. The mechanism of action of Tetracycline target is to target the bacterial ribosomes. They disrupt the elongation of polypeptide chains during protein synthesis and also inhibit amino acyl-tRNA binding [22, 27]. Some of the organisms targeted by tetracycline are *Haemophilus influenza* (*H. influenzae*), *Streptococcus pneumonia, etc*. Antibiotics included in the tetracycline group are sold under the trade name (OraceaTR), (AdoxaTR), (AtridoxTR) [28].

Chloramphenicol

Chloramphenicol was discovered after being isolated from *Streptomyces venezuelae* in 1947. It is an old antimicrobial agent that is rarely used today. Earlier, the antibiotic was used to treat conjunctivitis, ear infection, meningitis, plague, cholera, and typhoid fever [29].

Penicillin

Penicillin, one of the first and still one of the most widely used antibiotic agents derived from the mold *Penicillium* was discovered in 1929 by Alexander Fleming [30]. Penicillin G was the first to be produced amongst this group of antibiotics and was originally discovered and isolated from the fungus *P. notatum* by Alexander Fleming. Penicillin is used in the treatment of throat infections, meningitis, syphilis, and various other infections. The chief side effects of penicillin are hypersensitivity reactions, including skin rash, hive, swelling, anaphylaxis, or allergic shock. They are diverse group of compounds containing a nucleus of 6-aminopenicillanic acid (lactam plus thiazolidine) ring and other ring side chains [31]. This class of Penicillin include Penicillin G, Penicillin V, Oxacillin (dicloxacillin), Methicillin, Nafcillin, Ampicillin, Amoxicillin, Carbenicillin, Piperacillin, Mezlocillin, and Ticarcillin [32]. Some of the antibiotics of Penicillin are Streptomycin, aminopenicillins, antipseudomonal penicillin, and β-lactamase inhibitors. *Staphylococci, Streptococci, Clostridium, Neisseria* and *Listeria genera, H. influenzae, N. gonorrhoea, E. coli etc*. are those organisms targeted by this group of antibiotics [33]. Streptomycin prevents formation of initiation complex by insertion of improper amino acids. Novobiocin inhibits DNA gyrase by binding the ATP binding site in the ATPase subunit [34, 33]. Amoxicillin inhibit Penicillin binding proteins(PBPs) by mimicking the natural D-alanyl-D-alanine substrate [35]. They are sold under the trade name (Amoxil^{TR}), (Moxatag^{TR}), (Larotid^{TR}) [34, 35]. Due to the presence of beta lactam ring in Penicillin group of drugs, they are also called beta lactam antibiotics (Figs. **1** & **2**) [36]. This beta lactam ring is sensitive towards some bacteria and can be hydrolyzed by beta lactamases (enzymes produced by gram positive and gram negative bacteria). They are bactericidal in action and also inhibit cell wall synthesis [34].

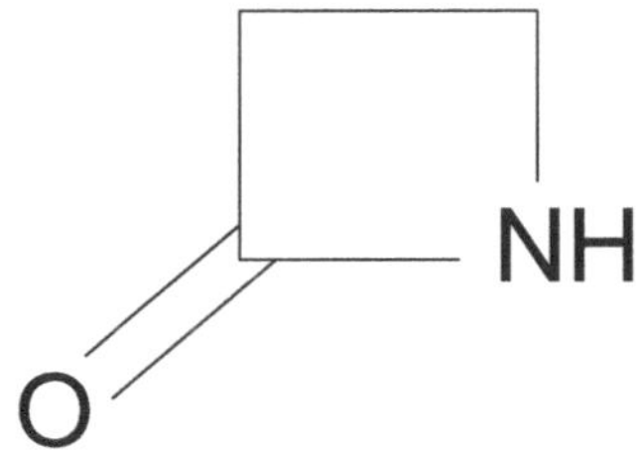

Fig. (1). Structure of Beta-lactam.

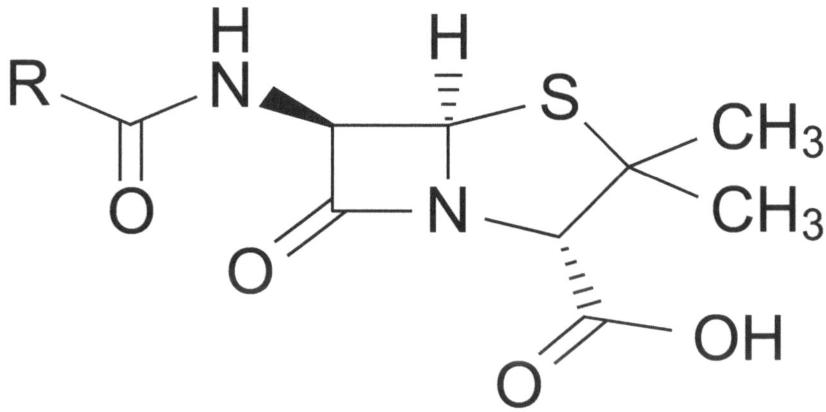

Fig. (2). Core structure of Penicillin.

Rifampicin

Rifampicin is a semi synthetic antibiotic produced from *Streptomyces mediterranei*. Rifampicin is a broad-spectrum antibiotic having activity against several *Mycobacterium* species. In susceptible organisms, it forms a stable complex with the enzyme by inhibiting DNA-dependent RNA polymerase activity, and suppressing the initiation of RNA synthesis. Rifampicin acts on both intracellular and extracellular organisms and is bactericidal in action [37]. It is used to treat tuberculosis, Mycobacterium avium complex, leprosy, and Legionnaire's disease.

Gentamicin

Gentamicin was discovered in 1963 [38]. The drug is under the antibiotics aminoglycoside [39], purified from *Micromonospora purpurea*. It is necessary for the treatment of pelvic inflammatory disease, pneumonia bone infections, meningitis, endocarditis, urinary tract infections, and sepsis. This antibiotic can be given intravenously, intramuscularly or topically. It is bacteriostatic in nature.

Erythromycin

Erythromycin is produced by *Saccharopolyspora erythraea* in 1952 [40, 41]. It belongs to the class of macrolide antibiotics. Other antibiotics in this class include azithromycin (Zithromax, Zmax) and clarithromycin (Biaxin). It is used in the treatment of pelvic inflammatory disease, skin infections, respiratory tract infections, syphilis and Chlamydia infections and to improve delayed stomach emptying [40]. Sometimes during pregnancy, it is used to prevent Group B Streptococcal infection in the newborn [42].

Clindamycin

It was first synthesized in 1966 or 1967 [43, 44] and belongs to the lincosamide group of antibiotics. It is used in the treatment of anaerobic, Staphylococcal and Streptococcal infections which was accepted by the US Food and Drug Administration (FDA). It is sold under the drug name Cleocin. This drug inhibits bacterial protein synthesis by binding to the 23SrRNA of the 50S subunit of the ribosome [45]. Clindamycin is applied in the treatment of pneumonia, pelvic inflammatory disease, strep throat, middle ear infections, endocarditis and bone or joint infections and acne as well as malaria treatment and against MRSA [46]. Clindamycin ointment can be applied to the skin or in the vagina [47, 48].

Daptomycin

A cyclic lipopeptide antibiotic obtained from the soil saprotroph Roseosporus [49]. It is a new type of antibacterial antibiotic. It is a cyclic, branched, anionic lipopeptide antibiotic and used for Gram-positive bacterial infection, including vancomycin-resistant Enterococci and MRSA [50].

Teicoplanin

The activity of Teicoplanin is very much similar to that of vancomycin [51]. This antibiotic is necessary for the treatment of Gram-positive bacteria viz., *Enterococcus faecalis* and MRSA and also in prophylaxis. It is marketed under the trade name Targocid by Sanofi-Aventis and Ticocin by Cipla (India) [52].

Activity Against Gram-Negative Bacterial Infection

Ampicillin

It was discovered in 1958 and had come into use commercially in 1961 [53, 54]. This drug is used to treat meningitis, urinary tract infections, respiratory tract infections, salmonellosis, and endocarditis [55]. In new born baby, it is used to prevent group B Streptococcal infection [55]. Ampicillin is necessary for treatment of the middle ear, sinuses, stomach and intestines, bladder and kidney, meningitis, endocarditis, and uncomplicated gonorrhea [56].

Olfloxacin

In 1980, Ofloxacin was patented and it was approved for use in medical treatment in 1985 [57]. The drug is a broad-spectrum antibiotic and is used for the treatment of pneumonia, bronchitis, gonococcal infection and diarrhoea.

Cefazolin

Cefazolin was patented in 1967 and in 1971 it had come into use commercially [58]. It is used for treating a wide variety of bacterial infections. Cefazolin are also used before and during certain surgeries to prevent infection. Cefazolin is available under the following brand names: Kefzol and Ancef and necessary for the treatment of pneumonia, cellulitis, urinary tract infections, joint infection, endocarditis, and biliary tract infections [59, 60]. It is used for the prevention of group B Streptococcal disease before surgery and during delivery and also given intramuscular or intravenously [61].

Ceftazidime / Clavulanic Acid

Ceftazidime is commercially sold under the brand names Fortaz. It was patented in the year 1978 and use commercially in 1984 [62], It is also a broad spectrum antibiotic which is necessary for the treatment of infections caused in urinary tract, brain, lungs, and abdomen. It is used for pneumonia, joint infections, sepsis, urinary tract infections, meningitis, malignant otitis externa, and vibrio infection [63].

Cefuroxime

Cefuroxime was first marketed in 1978 as Zinacef, synthesised by Glaxo, now GlaxoSmithKline. In October 1983 the drug received approval from the U.S. Food and Drug Administration [64], and sold in the brand name Ceftin [65]. It is necessary for the treatment of gonorrhea, throat infections, sinus infections and Lyme disease.

Cotrimaxozole

It is a combination of two antifolate agents: one-part trimethoprim to five parts sulfamethoxazole. It is used to treat MRSA skin infections, urinary tract infections, respiratory tract infections, travelers' diarrhea, and cholera [66]. It is used for the treatment and prevention of pneumocystis pneumonia and toxoplasmosis for those people suffering from HIV/AIDS [67]. It can be given by mouth or intravenous.

Antibiotic Classification Based on Chemical and Molecular Structure

β-lactams

These members contain a 1-nitrogen ring and 3-carbon that is highly reactive and interfere with synthesis of proteins essential for bacterial cell wall synthesis (Figs. **1**, **2**). The β-lactam antibiotics are able to bind to penicillin-binding protein (PBP), and interfere in the synthesis of peptidoglycan resulting to lysis and cell death [68]. β-lactam class of antibiotic includes Penicillin, Cephalosporins (Fig. **3**), Monobactams (Fig. **4**), and Carbapenems (Fig. **5**).

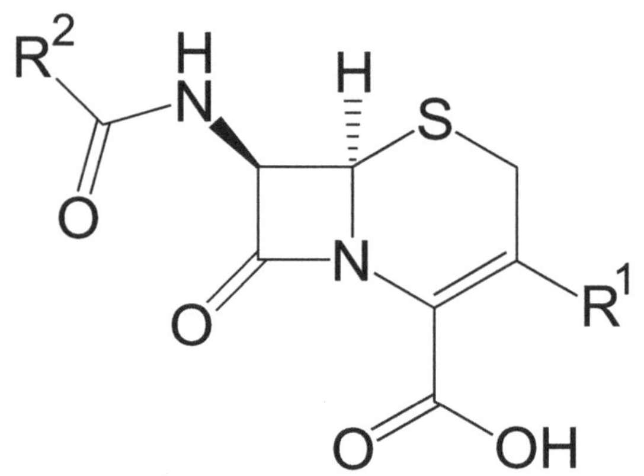

Fig. (3). Structure of Cephalosporin.

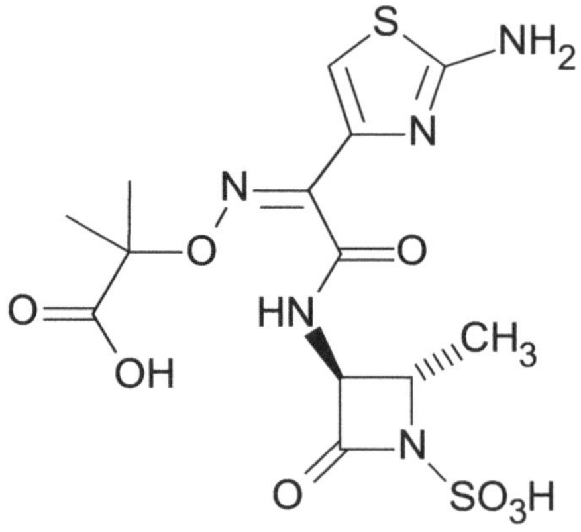

Fig. (4). Structure of Monobactam.

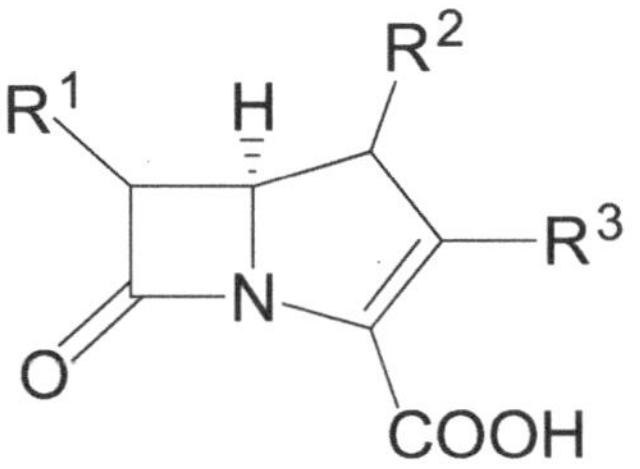

Fig. (5). Structure of Carbapenem.

Cephalosporins

These antibiotics is very much similar in their structure and mode of action to that of penicillin. In 1945, Guiseppe Brotzu isolated the first member of this group of antibiotics from the fungus *Cephalosporium acremonium*. It contains 7-aminocephalosporanic acid nucleus and side chain containing 3, 6- dihydro-2 H-1, 3- thiazane rings. They are used in the treatment of diseases arising from Penicillinase-producing Methicillin-susceptible Staphylococci and Streptococci, *Proteus mirabilis*, some *Escherichia coli*, *Klebsiella pneumonia*, *Haemophilus influenza*, *Enterobacter aerogenes* and some Neisseria [69]. They have a variety of side chains which enable them to get attach to different penicillin-binding proteins (PBPs) in order to circumvent blood brain barrier, resist breakdown by penicillinase producing bacterial strains and ionize to facilitate entry into Gram-negative bacterial cells [70].

Monobactams

It is produced by *Chromobacterium violaceum* and was first reported by Skyes and co-workers [71]. Monobactams, a β-lactam antibiotic where ring of monobactams stand alone but is not fused to another ring [72, 73]. Aztreonam is the only commercially available monobactam antibiotic which are active against aerobic Gram-negative bacteria viz., *Neisseria* and *Pseudomonas* and are used to treat septicemia, pneumonia, and urinary tract infections. They are uneffective against Gram-positive bacteria or anaerobes [74].

Carbapenems

It is known as the 4:5 fused ring lactam of penicillins having a double bond between C-2 and C-3 but with the substitution of carbon for sulfur at C-1 [75]. They are β-lactamantibiotics having a broad spectrum activity against many Gram positive and Gram negative aerobic and anaerobic organisms. Mechanism of action of Carbapenems is similar to that of β-lactam antibiotic and cephalosporins. Carbapenems have fused β-lactam ring structure exhibiting resistant to most β-lactamases are produced by bacteria inactivating penicillin [76]. This carbapenems resist the hydrolytic action of β-lactamase enzyme and possess abroad spectrum activity against Gram positive and Gram negative bacteria. They are known as "antibiotics of last resort" [77]. Examples of carbapenem include: a) Imipenem – a broad spectrum antibiotic which is effective against both aerobic and anaerobic pathogens, b) Meropenem– a broad spectrum antibiotic effective against non-fermentative Gram negative bacilli; c) Ertapenem – a broad spectrum antibiotic having limited activity against non- fermentative Gram negative bacilli [78].

Macrolides

In 1952, J.M. McGuire isolated the antibiotic from the fungus *Saccharopolyspora erythraea* which was formerly known as *Streptomyces erythraeus* [79]. They are characterized by 14-, 15-, or 16- membered macrocyclic lactose rings having unusual deoxy sugars L-cladinose and D-desosamine attached. They exhibit a broad spectrum activity which are often used for those patients allergic to penicillin [79]. They either kill or inhibits protein synthesis of pathogenic microorganisms. Macrolides (Fig. **6**) have a tendency to build up in the body because the liver is able to recycle it into the bile and also have the capacity to cause inflammation. Examples include Azithromycin, Erythromycin, and Clarithromycin [80].

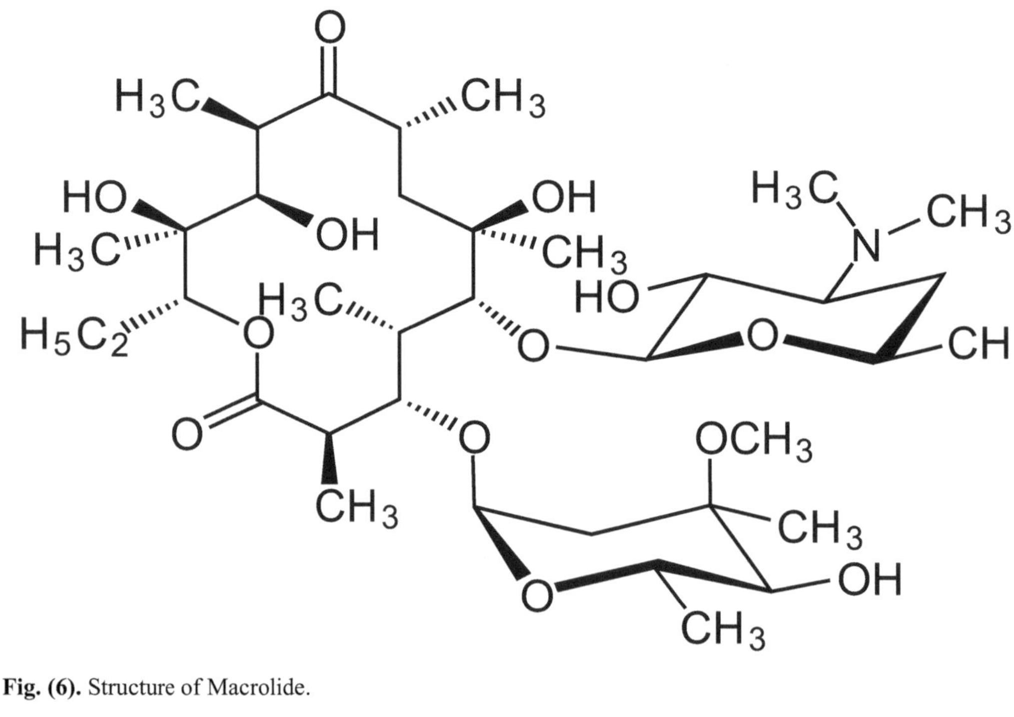

Fig. (6). Structure of Macrolide.

Tetracyclines

Details of tetracycline (Fig. **6**) have already discussed earlier.

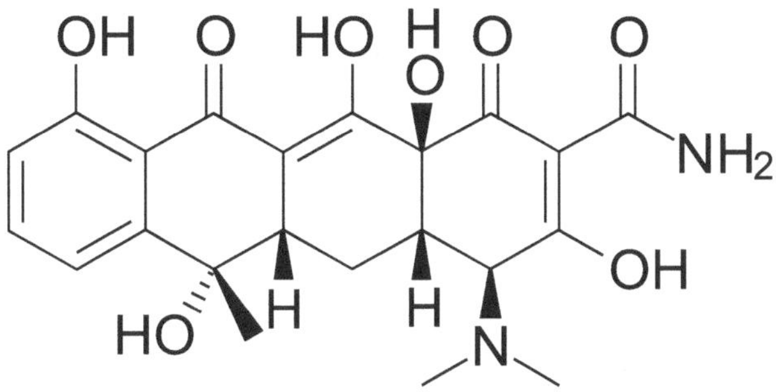

Fig. (7). Structure of Tetracycline.

Quinolones

It was first discovered by scientists involving in search of antimalarial drugs as Nalidixic acid derivatives. In the early sixties, during the development of quinine, Nalidixic acid was discovered as an impurity. They disrupt the replication and transcription process in bacteria. Quinolones (Fig. **8**) and naphthyridones are developed from quinolones including ofloxacin, ciproxacin, cinoxacin, norfloxacin, temafloxacins, parfloxacin, enoxacin, nalidixic acid, *etc* [81]. It consists of two rings whereas, recent generations of quinolones possess an added ring structure enabling them to extend their antimicrobial activity spectrum to some bacteria, particularly anaerobic bacteria that were otherwise resistant to quinolone. Members include ciprofloxacin, floxacin, and levofloxacin [81]. Modifications in the basic structure of quinolones are reported to have improved their bioavailability, spectrum of activity and potency and enhances their performance to treat urinary, systemic and respiratory tract infections [71].

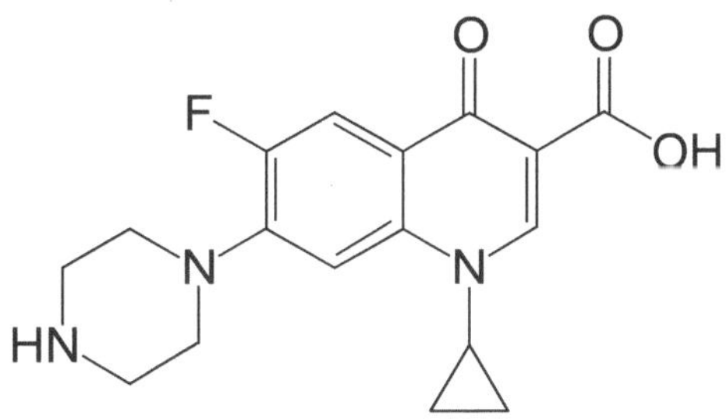

Fig. (8). Structure of Quinolones.

Aminoglycosides

Streptomycin was the first drug to be discovered among this group of antibiotics. It has been widely used against *Mycobacterium tuberculosis*, the causal agent of tuberculosis. Their structure consists of 3-amino sugars connected by glycosidic bonds and are produced by Actinomycetes. They exhibit a broad spectrum of antibacterial activity and have the capacity to bind to one of the ribosomal subunits thereby inhibiting the protein synthesis in bacteria [82 - 84]. They are effective against aerobic Gram negative bacteria. Streptomycin, the oldest known aminoglycoside (Fig. **9**), is used to treat tuberculosis, bubonic plague and tularemia [85]. But streptomycin was found to be highly toxic, so scientists are trying to find new type of aminoglycosides which is effective against bacteria, but less toxic to humans and this led to discovery of different type of antibiotics including Neomycin, Gentamicin, Tobramycin and Amikacin, Kanamycin, Dibekacin, and Netilmicin [86]. Gentamicin is less toxic which is widely used for infections caused by Gram negative rods (*Escherichia*, *Pseudomonas*, *Shigella* and *Salmonella* species). Tobramycin, in particular, is used to treat *Pseudomonas* species infections in cystic fibrosis patients [87].

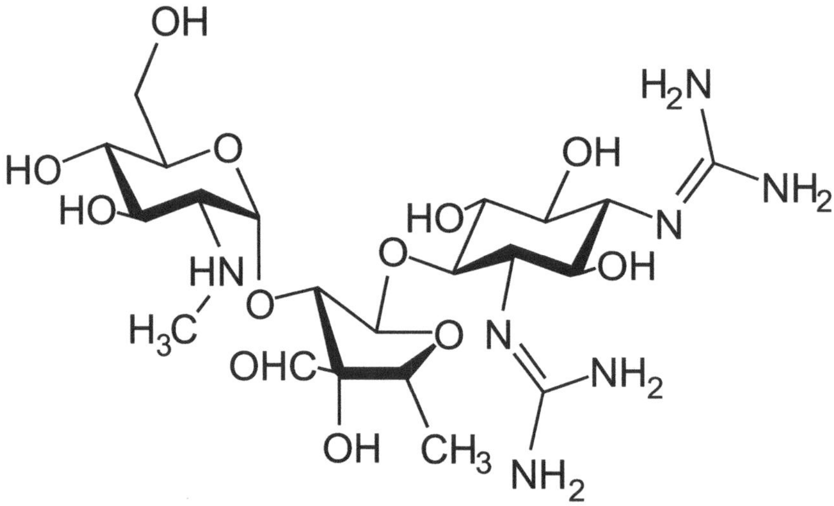

Fig. (9). Structure of Aminoglycoside.

Sulphonamides

Sulphonamides were the first group of antibiotics which are used in medicine and veterinary practice [88]. They are synthetic antimicrobial agents which contain the sulphonamide group (Fig. **10**) [89]. They have the property to inhibit Gram negative bacteria such as *Klebsiella*, *Nocardia*, *Salmonella*, *E. coli*, *Shigella*, and *Enterobacter*, *Chlamydia trachomatis* and some Protozoa. These antibiotics are used to treat tonsillitis, septicaemia, bacillary dysentery, meningococcal meningitis, and some urinary tract infections [88].

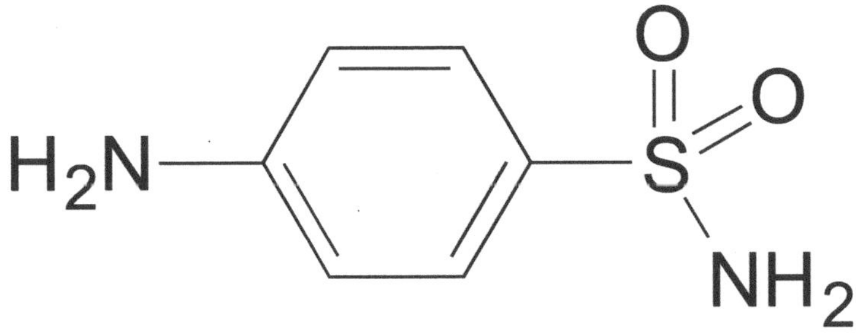

Fig. (10). Structure of Sulphonamide.

Glycopeptides

Glycopeptides (Fig. **11**) antibiotics were originally extracted as natural products but the last 20 years, it had been emerged as semi-synthetic derivatives with the improved in activity and pharmacokinetic properties [90, 91]. Naturally, glycopeptides are made of a cyclic peptide of 7 amino acids, to which 2 sugars are bound, that is why it is name as glycopeptides [92].

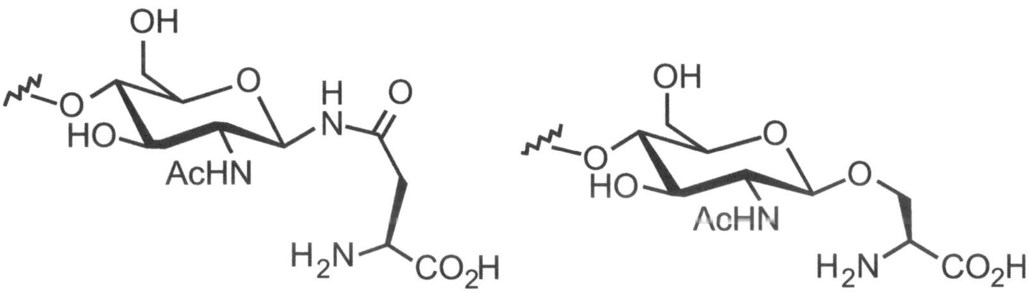

Fig. (11). (**a**) GlcNac-β-Ser (**b**) GlcNAc-β-Asn.

Oxazolidinones

They are a group of synthetic antibiotics. Linezoid, the first member to be synthesized was approved in the year 2000. Oxazolidinones (Fig. **12**) binds to the P site of the ribosomal 50S subunit thereby inhibiting protein synthesis [93, 94]. They have a broad spectrum activity against Gram positive bacteria including methicillin and vancomycin-resistant *Staphylococci*, vancomycin-resistant *Enterococci*, penicillin-resistant *Pneumococci*, and anaerobes [94]. Linezoid is used to treat respiratory tract and skin infections caused by Gram positive bacterial pathogens [95]. Oxazolidinones are also used in preventing the surgical infections as they can easily penetrate and accumulate in the tissue including bone, lung, vegetations (plant-like growth in tissues), haematoma and cerebrospinal fluid [94].

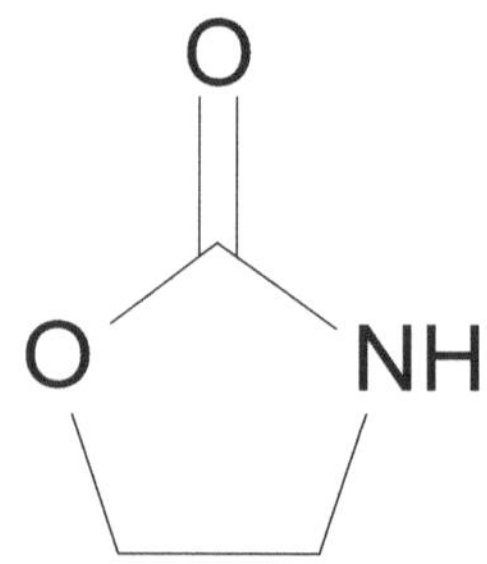

Fig. (12). 12 Structure of Oxazolidinones.

Peptide Groups

Peptide groups are divided into two types of antibiotics; Type 1: Non-Ribosomally and Type 2: Ribosomally. Type 1 includes Vancomycin, teicoplanin, streptogramin, colimycin, antitumor antibiotic bleomycin, polymixin, and Type 2 includes defensins, bacteriocins *etc* [96]. They inhibit protein and peptidoglycan synthesis [97]. Peptide group of antibiotics target *Staphylococcus aureus*, fungi, viruses *etc* [98]. Polymyxins, the peptide antibiotics, disrupt the structure of bacterial cell membrane [99].

Antibiotic Classification Based on Function

Antibiotics act by disrupting various molecular targets within bacteria and cell membrane, preventing growth or initiating killing. The most common targets of antibiotics are shown (Fig. **13**).

The modes of action of antibiotics are as follows: i) Inhibition of cell wall synthesis ii) Inhibition of membrane function iii) Inhibition of nucleic acid synthesis iv) Inhibition of protein synthesis v) Blockage of key metabolic pathways [100, 101].

Inhibition of Cell Wall Synthesis

Drugs like penicillins, carbapenems, and cephalosporins are able to block the cross-linking of peptidoglycan units thereby inhibiting the peptide bond formation catalysed by PBPs [102]. Most antibiotics belonging to the glycopeptides antibiotics such as vancomycin inhibit bacterial growth by inhibiting the synthesis of peptidoglycan (PG) by binding themselves to PG units, as well as blocking transglycosylase and transpeptidase activity [90].

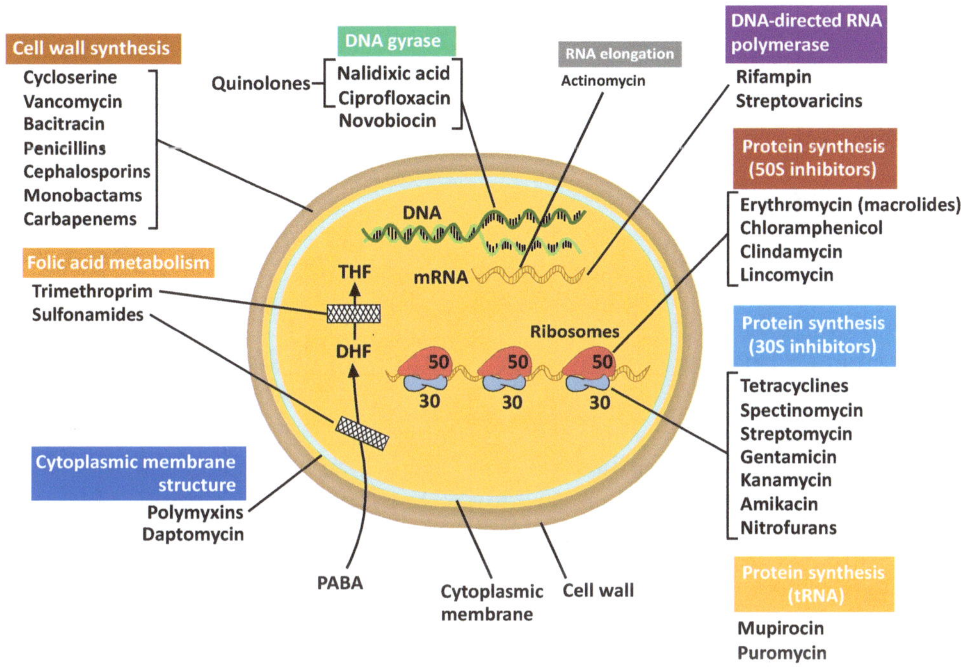

Fig. (13). Antibiotics and target sites in the cell (Adapted with permission from Pearson Prentice Hall, Inc [102]).

Inhibition of Membrane Function

These classes of antibiotics damage cell membranes of bacteria due to differences in the types of lipids in their cell membranes. For example, Daptomycin depolarizes calcium-dependent membrane, and leads to the cessation of macromolecular synthesis and disruption of the cellular membrane in bacteria [103]. The polymyxins possess a positively charged molecules and are attracted to the negatively charged bacteria. It binds to the cell membrane, alters its structure and increase the permeability thereby disrupting the osmotic balance causing leakage of cellular molecules, inhibition of respiration, and increased water uptake leading to cell death [104].

Inhibition of Nucleic Acid Synthesis

The synthesis of nucleic acids is very essential in the metabolic pathways. Antibiotics interfere in synthesis of nucleic acid by blocking replication or stopping transcription [105]. For example, quinolone group of antibiotics binds and interfere in the normal functioning of helicase enzyme thereby, disrupting in unwinding DNA. This action ultimately truncates the process of DNA replication and repair amongst susceptible bacteria [106]. Antibiotics inhibiting nucleic acid synthesis also target topoisomerase II and topoisomerase IV of bacteria by disrupting the activities of these enzymes adversely affecting RNA polymerase thereby preventing RNA synthesis. Quinolones are antagonistic to both Gram positive and Gram negative bacteria [107].

Inhibition of Protein Synthesis

The type of drugs that inhibits protein synthesis are included under the broadest classes of antibiotics and can be divided into two subclasses: the 50S inhibitors and 30S inhibitors. The 50S ribosome inhibitors antibiotics include erythromycin, chloramphenicol, clindamycin, lincomycin, and linezolid [108, 109]. Inhibition of 50S ribosome is done by physically blocking either the initiation phase or the elongation phase of protein synthesis where the incoming amino acid is linked up with the growing nascent peptide chain [110 - 112]. Examples of antibiotics that block initiation of protein translation are members of Oxazolidinones [110], while macrolides such as lincosamide and streptogramin block protein synthesis by inhibiting the elongation phase of mRNA translation [111, 112]. These latter groups of antibiotics are therefore reportedly ineffective when elongation has progressed beyond a critical length [113]. The 30S ribosome-inhibitors principally work by blocking the access of aminoacyl-tRNAs to the ribosome. Antibiotics include tetracycline, streptomycin, spectinomycin, *etc* [114, 115]. Inhibition of some proteins at the 50S ribosomes have also been reported [116].

Blockage of Key Metabolic Pathways

Some antibiotics like sulphonamides and trimethoprim have been shown to resemble a microbial substrate needed for cellular metabolism of bacteria. This deception causes bacterial enzymes to attach themselves to the antibiotic rather than the normal substrate. In particular, sulphonamides act like tetrahydrofolate which is required for the synthesis of folic acid in bacterial cells [100]. Folic acid is vital in the metabolism of nucleic acid and amino acids; therefore, sulphonamides ultimately disrupt the production of nucleic acids (DNA and RNA) and amino acids, as they mimic substrates required for folic acid metabolism [100].

Actinobacteria as Prolific Producer of Antibiotics

Actinobacteria are soil-dwelling, Gram positive bacteria that have the property of producing several secondary metabolites. Secondary metabolites include antitumor (*e.g.*, doxorubicin and bleomycin), antifungals (*e.g.*, amphotericin B and nystatin), immunosuppressives (*e.g.*, FK-506 and rapamycin), insecticides (*e.g.*, spinosyn A and avermectin B), and herbicides (*e.g.*, phosphinotricin). In particular, 80% of antibiotics are obtained from the genus *Streptomyces* and rare actinobacteria, such as *Actinomadura* [117]. *Streptomyces* members are filamentous bacteria that grow in various ecosystems even at harsh conditions by forming a spore [118]. Soil is the main niche which were isolated and identified as prolific producers of effective bioactive compounds other than antibiotics such as antivirals, anticancers, anti-hypertensives, and immunosuppressives [119, 120]. Genome sequence surveys on various actinobacteria especially *Streptomyces* species indicate that each bacterium is able to produce about 10-fold more secondary metabolites than the wild type [121, 122]. The major groups of antibiotics we discussed earlier such as tetracyclines, amino glycosides, macrolides, chloramphenicol, ivermectin, rifamycins are produced by *Streptomyces* species.

Some of the Important Antibacterial Drugs Produced by Actinomycetes

Tigecycline is a semi-synthetic product of chlorotetracycline isolated from *Streptomyces aureofaciens* and is composed of 9-tert-butyl-glycylamido derivative of minocycline. It showed antibacterial activity typical of other tetracyclines, but with potent activity against tetracycline-resistant organisms [123].

Everolimus is an orally active 40-O-(2-hydroxyethyl) derivative of rapamycin extracted from *Streptomyces hygroscopicus*. It exhibits immunosuppressive effect by blocking growth factor interleukin-2 (IL-2) and interleukin-5 (IL-5) mediated proliferation of hematopoietic (T cells and B cells) and non-hematopoietic (vascular smooth muscle cells) cells thereby inhibiting p70 S6 kinase. This leads to arrest of the cell cycle at the G1/S phase [124].

Daptomycin is a cyclic lipopeptide antibacterial agent obtained from *Streptomyces roseosporus*. The antibiotic is used to treat complicated skin and skin structure infections (cSSSIs). It binds to bacterial cell membranes thereby disrupting the membrane potential leading to blocking replication, transcription, and translation [125].

Amrubicin hydrochloride is a completely synthetic 9-aminoanthracycline, a derivative of doxorubicin obtained from *Streptomyces peucetius*. The antibiotic showed activity comparable to that of doxorubicin on transplanted animal tumours, including P388 leukemia, sarcoma 180. Lewis lung carcinoma, and more potent antitumor activity against human tumour xenografts of breast, lung and gastric cancer [126].

Pimecrolimus is a novel analog of ascomycin extracted from *Streptomyces hygroscopicus*. It blocks T-cell activation through pimecrolimus-macrophilin complex thereby preventing the dephosphorylation of the cytoplasmic component of the nuclear factor of activated T cells (NF-AT). This drug is used to treat inflammatory skin diseases such as allergic contact dermatitis and atopic dermatitis [121].

Gemtuzumabozogamicin is a drug of calicheamicin bound to anti-CD33 monoclonal antibody. The calicheamicins (also known as the LL-E3328 antibiotics) is extracted from *Micromonospora echinospora.* It is released by cleaving the covalent link between the monoclonal antibody and calicheamicin by the lysosomes in the cells. Calicheamicin is a hydrophobic member of the enediyne family of DNA-cleaving antibiotics used for treating patients with acute myeloid lymphoma [127].

Multidrug-Resistant Organisms and their Future Challenges

Multidrug-resistant organisms (MDROs)are bacteria that have become resistant to many broad spectrum antibiotics that are currently available. They are found mainly in hospitals and long-term care facilities. They are effective to those people who are older or very ill, and can cause severe infections [128].

Common multidrug-resistant organisms include:

- Vancomycin-Resistant *Enterococci* (VRE)
- Methicillin-Resistant *Staphylococcus aureus* (MRSA)
- Extended-spectrum β-lactamase (ESBLs) produced by Gram negative bacteria
- Multidrug-Resistant Gram negative rods (MDR GNR) bacteria include *Enterobacter species*, *E.coli*, *Klebsiella pneumoniae*, *Acinetobacter baumannii*, *Pseudomonas aeruginosa*. The infections caused by Multidrug-resistant organisms includes: bloodstream, lungs, urinary tract, wounds, skin, and surgical site.

Methicillin Resistant Staphylococcus Aureus (MRSA)

In 1968, MRSA was first isolated in the United States. By the early 1990s, 20-25% of *S. aureus* were isolated from hospitalized patients. In 1999, more than 50% of *S. aureus* were isolated from patients in ICUs in the National Nosocomial Infection Surveillance (NNIS) system, and in 2003, 59.5% of *S. aureus* isolates in NNIS ICUs were MRSA [129].

Vancomycin-Resistant Enterococcus (VRE)

From 1990 to 1997, the prevalence of VRE in enterococcal isolates from hospitalized patients increased from less than 1% to approximately 15%. In 1999

VRE accounted for almost 25% of *Enterococcus* isolates in NNIS ICUs and 28.5% in 2003 [130].

NOBLE ANTIBIOTICS AND CONCLUDING REMARKS

Researchers from University of Illinois purified a new class of antibiotics known as odilorhabdins (ODLs). These kinds of antibiotics are obtained from symbiotic bacteria which are found in soil-dwelling nematode worms that colonize insects for food. Nosopharm and their researchers found that ODLs target a unique site on the bacterial ribosome. Maxime Gualtieri, chief scientific officer and co-founder of Nosopharm, said that ODL compounds cured mice infected with several pathogenic bacteria which had a demonstrated activity against both Gram negative and Gram positive pathogens, notably including carbapenem-resistant *Enterobacteriacae* [131]. In the late 1940s, a powerful compound called teixobactin was newly discovered. This antibiotic was isolated from the newly discovered soil bacterium Eleftheria terrae, using a device called the isolation chip (iChip) [132]. Teixobactin has been found to be an extremely potent antibiotic capable of working against the gram-positive group of microbes, including bacteria that cause tuberculosis (*Mycobacterium tuberculosis*), lobar pneumonia (*Streptococcus pneumoniae*), strep throat and rheumatic fever (*Streptococcus pyogenes*), severe diarrhoea (*Clostridium difficile*), anthrax (*Bacillus anthracis*), as well as *Staphylococcus aureus*, the bacterium that causes toxic shock syndrome and methicillin-resistant (MRSA) infections [133]. Teixobactin is being fast-tracked into preclinical development studies [134]. Unfortunately, teixobactin does not have any effect on gram-negative bacteria. Therefore, teixobactin will not be available to fight such dangerous illnesses as cholera (*Vibrio cholerae*), plague (*Yersinia pestis*), and gonorrhea (*Neisseria gonorrhoeae*), or infections from pathogenic strains of the common bacteria *E. coli* and *Pseudomonas aeruginosa* [135].

CONSENT FOR PUBLICATION

Not applicable.

CONFLICT OF INTEREST

The authors confirm that this chapter contents have no conflict of interest.

ACKNOWLEDGEMENTS

The authors wish to thank Department of Biotechnology (DBT), Govt. of India for sponsoring the host laboratory under the scheme "Establishment of State Biotech Hubs" (BT/04/NE/2009).

REFERENCES

[1] Antibiotics". NHS. 5 June 2014. Retrieved 17 January 2015.

[2] Factsheet for experts. European Centre for Disease Prevention and Control. Retrieved 21 December 2014.

[3] Chemical Analysis of Antibiotic Residues in Food. John Wiley& Sons, Inc. 2012; pp. 1-60.

[4] Gualerzi CO, Brandi L, Fabbretti A, Pon CL. Antibiotics: Targets, Mechanisms and Resistance. John Wiley & Sons 2013; p. 1. [http://dx.doi.org/10.1002/9783527659685]

[5] UK study warns of threat of antibiotics overuse, lack of new drugs". CCTV America. 19 May 2016. Retrieved 12 June 2016.

[6] Antibiotics being incorrectly prescribed in Australian nursing homes, prompting superbug fears". ABC Australia. 10 June 2016. Retrieved 12 June 2016.

[7] Superbugs could kill more people than cancer, report warns". CBS News. 19 May 2016. Retrieved 12 June 2016.

[8] Brooks M. Public Confused About Antibiotic Resistance, WHO Says. Medscape Multispeciality 2015.

[9] Lindblad WJ. Considerations for determining if a natural product is an effective wound-healing agent. Int J Low Extrem Wounds 2008; 7(2): 75-81. [http://dx.doi.org/10.1177/1534734608316028] [PMID: 18483011]

[10] Forrest RD. Early history of wound treatment. J R Soc Med 1982; 75(3): 198-205. [PMID: 7040656]

[11] Wainwright M. Moulds in ancient and more recent medicin. Mycologist 1989; 3(1): 21-3. [http://dx.doi.org/10.1016/S0269-915X(89)80010-2]

[12] Calderon CB, Sabundayo BP. Antimicrobial Classifications: Drugs for Bugs.Antimicrobial Susceptibility Testing Protocols. Columbia, MO: CRC Press. Taylor & Frances group 2007.

[13] Limbird LE. The receptor concept: a continuing evolution. Mol Interv 2004; 4(6): 326-36. [http://dx.doi.org/10.1124/mi.4.6.6] [PMID: 15616162]

[14] Bosch F, Rosich L. The contributions of Paul Ehrlich to pharmacology: a tribute on the occasion of the centenary of his Nobel Prize. Pharmacology 2008; 82(3): 171-9. [http://dx.doi.org/10.1159/000149583] [PMID: 18679046]

[15] Goodman LS, Gilman A. The Pharmacological Basis of Therapeutics. New York: Macmillan 1941.

[16] The Nobel Prize in Physiology or Medicine , Paul Erlich – Biography, 1908.

[17] Wright PM, Seiple IB, Myers AG. The evolving role of chemical synthesis in antibacterial drug discovery. Angew Chem Int Ed Engl 2014; 53(34): 8840-69. [http://dx.doi.org/10.1002/anie.201310843] [PMID: 24990531]

[18] Aminov RI. A brief history of the antibiotic era: lessons learned and challenges for the future. Front Microbiol 2010; 1: 134. [http://dx.doi.org/10.3389/fmicb.2010.00134] [PMID: 21687759]

[19] Antibiotics for Gram-Positive BacterialInfection: Vancomycin, Teicoplanin,Quinupristin/Dalfopristin, Oxazolidinones, Daptomycin, Telavancin, and CeftarolineMichael D. Nailor, PharmDa,b,c, Jack D. Sobel, MDc,*. Med Clin North Am 2011; 95: 723-42. [http://dx.doi.org/10.1016/j.mcna.2011.03.011] [PMID: 21679789]

[20] Pfeiffer RR. Structural features of vancomycin. Rev Infect Dis 1981; 3 (Suppl.): S205-9. [http://dx.doi.org/10.1093/clinids/3.Supplement_2.S205] [PMID: 7342283]

[21] Moellering RC Jr. Vancomycin: a 50-year reassessment. Clin Infect Dis 2006; 42(1) (Suppl. 1): S3-4. [http://dx.doi.org/10.1086/491708] [PMID: 16323117]

[22] Sánchez AR, Rogers RS III, Sheridan PJ. Tetracycline and other tetracycline-derivative staining of the teeth and oral cavity. Int J Dermatol 2004; 43(10): 709-15. [http://dx.doi.org/10.1111/j.1365-4632.2004.02108.x] [PMID: 15485524]

[23] Stein GE, Craig WA. Tigecycline: a critical analysis. Clin Infect Dis 2006; 43(4): 518-24. [http://dx.doi.org/10.1086/505494] [PMID: 16838243]

[24] Perdue BE, Standiford HC. Tetracyclines.Antimicrobial Therapy and Vaccines. Baltimore: Williams and Wilkins 1999; p. 981.

[25] Colton B, McConeghy KW, Schreckenberger PC, Danziger LH. I.V. minocycline revisited for infections caused by multidrug-resistant organisms. Am J Health Syst Pharm 2016; 73(5): 279-85. [http://dx.doi.org/10.2146/ajhp150290] [PMID: 26896499]

[26] Fuoco D. Classification framework and chemical biology of tetracycline-structure-based drugs. Antibiotics (Basel) 2012; 1(1): 1-13. [http://dx.doi.org/10.3390/antibiotics1010001] [PMID: 27029415]

[27] Medical News Today. Antibiotics: How do antibiotics work? MediLexicon International Ltd. Bexhill-on-sea UK. 2015.

[28] Sánchez AR, Rogers RS III, Sheridan PJ. Tetracycline and other tetracycline-derivative staining of the teeth and oral cavity. Int J Dermatol 2004; 43(10): 709-15. [http://dx.doi.org/10.1111/j.1365-4632.2004.02108.x] [PMID: 15485524]

[29] Jensen T, Pedersen SS, Garne S, Heilmann C, Høiby N, Koch C. Colistin inhalation therapy in cystic fibrosis patients with chronic Pseudomonas aeruginosa lung infection. J Antimicrob Chemother 1987; 19(6): 831-8. [http://dx.doi.org/10.1093/jac/19.6.831] [PMID: 3301785]

[30] McGeer A, Fleming CA, Gree K, Low DE. Antimicrobial resistance in Ontario: Are we making progress? Laboratory Proficiency Testing Program Newsletter 2001; 293: 1-2.

[31] Zahner H, Maas W. Biology of Antibiotics. New York: Springer-Verlag, 1972. [http://dx.doi.org/10.1007/978-1-4613-9373-3]

[32] BoundlessAntibiotic Classifications. Boundless microbiology https://www.boundless.com/microbiology/textbooks/boundless-microbiology-textbook/antimicrobial-drugs-13/overvi-w-of-antimicrobial-therapy-153/antibiotic-classifications-775-4905/.Accessed2016.

[33] Walsh TJ, Standiford HC, Reboli AC, *et al.* Randomized double-blinded trial of rifampin with either novobiocin or trimethoprim-sulfamethoxazole against methicillin-resistant Staphylococcus aureus colonization: prevention of antimicrobial resistance and effect of host factors on outcome. Antimicrob Agents Chemother 1993; 37(6): 1334-42. [http://dx.doi.org/10.1128/AAC.37.6.1334] [PMID: 8328783]

[34] https://www.healthline.com/health/amoxicillin-oral-tablet.

[35] https://www.medicinenet.com/amoxicillin/article.htm.

[36] Kleinkauf H, von Döhren H. Peptide antibiotics, beta-lactams, and related compounds. Crit Rev Biotechnol 1988; 8(1): 1-32. [http://dx.doi.org/10.3109/07388558809150536] [PMID: 3063387]

[37] Gilman. Goodman and Gilman's The Pharmacological Basis of Therapeutics, 9th ed, p1160.

[38] "Gentamicin sulphate",The American Society of Health-System Pharmacists. 2015.

[39] Pucci.Handbook of antibiotic discovery and development (2011) 2012. Dougherty Thomas, Michael J, Weinstein Marvin J, Eds. 2016; 238.

[40] "Erythromycin", The American Society of Health-System Pharmacists. 2015.

[41] Vedas JC. Biosynthesis: polyketides and vitamins. 2000.

[42] Camilleri , Parkman HP, Shafi MA, Abell TL, Gerson L. Clinical guideline: management of gastroparesis. The American Journal of Gastroenterology 2013; 108(1): 18-37. [PMID: 23147521]

[43] Formulary N. Neonatal Formulary: Drug Use in Pregnancy and the First Year of Life.John Wiley & Sons. 2014; p. 162.

[44] Smieja M. Current indications for the use of clindamycin: A critical review. Can J Infect Dis 1998; 9(1): 22-8. [http://dx.doi.org/10.1155/1998/538090] [PMID: 22346533]

[45] https: // www.drugbank.ca.

[46] Daum RS. Clinical practice. Skin and soft-tissue infections caused by methicillin-resistant Staphylococcus aureus. N Engl J Med 2007; 357(4): 380-90. [http://dx.doi.org/10.1056/NEJMcp070747] [PMID: 17652653]

[47] Clindamycin Hydrochloride. The American Society of Health System Pharmacists 2015.

[48] Leyden James J. Hidradenitis suppurativa. Berlin: Springer 2016; p. 152.

[49] Thorne GM, Adler J. Daptomycin: a novel lipopeptide antibiotic. Clin Microbiol Newsl 2002; 24: 33-40. [http://dx.doi.org/10.1016/S0196-4399(02)80007-1]

[50] Tally FP, DeBruin MF. Development of daptomycin for gram-positive infections. J Antimicrob Chemother 2000; 46(4): 523-6. [http://dx.doi.org/10.1093/jac/46.4.523] [PMID: 11020247]

[51] Lundstrom TS, Sobel JD. Antibiotics for gram-positive bacterial infections: vancomycin,teicoplanin, quinupristin/dalfopristin and linezolid. In: Kaye D, editor.Philadelphia; WB Saunders Co. Infect Dis Clin North Am 2000;14(2):463–74.

[52] Reynolds PE. Structure, biochemistry and mechanism of action of glycopeptide antibiotics. Eur J Clin Microbiol Infect Dis 1989; 8(11): 943-50. [http://dx.doi.org/10.1007/BF01967563] [PMID: 2532132]

[53] Fischer J, Ganellin RC. Analogue-based Drug Discovery. John Wiley & Sons 2016; p. 490.

[54] Ravina E. The evolution of drug discovery: from traditional medicines to modern drugs. 1st ed. Weinheim: Wiley-VCH 2011; p. 262.

[55] "Ampicillin". The American Society of Health-System Pharmacists. 2015.

[56] https: // www.rxlist.com.

[57] Fischer J, Ganellin RC. Analogue-based Drug Discovery. John Wiley & Sons 2006; p. 500. [http://dx.doi.org/10.1002/3527608001]

[58] Fischer J, Ganellin RC. Analogue-based Drug Discovery. John Wiley & Sons 2006; p. 493. [http://dx.doi.org/10.1002/3527608001]

[59] International Drug Price Indicator Guide. 2014.

[60] Hamilton R. Tarascon Pocket Pharmacopoeia 2015 Deluxe Lab-Coat Edition. Jones & Bartlett Learning 2015; p. 84.

[61] "Cefazolin Sodium". The American Society of Health-System Pharmacists. 2016.

[62] Fischer J, Ganellin RC. Analogue-based Drug Discovery. John Wiley & Sons 2006; p. 495. [http://dx.doi.org/10.1002/3527608001]

[63] "Ceftizimide" The American Society of Health-System Pharmacists. 2016.

[64] "Cefuroxime medical facts from". Drugs.com.

[65] http://www.covispharma.ch/assets/pdf/covis-pharma-acquires-portfolio-of-drugs-from-glaxosmithkline.pdf.

[66] https://medlineplus.gov/druginfo/meds/a684026.html.

[67] http://www.aidsmap.com/Cotrimoxazole-iSeptrini/page/1731332/.

[68] Heesemann J. [Mechanisms of resistance to beta-lactam antibiotics]. Infection 1993; 21(1) (Suppl. 1): S4-9.
[http://dx.doi.org/10.1007/BF01710336] [PMID: 8314292]

[69] Pegler S, Healy B. In patients allergic to penicillin, consider second and third generation cephalosporins for life threatening infections. BMJ 2007; 335(7627): 991.
[http://dx.doi.org/10.1136/bmj.39372.829676.47] [PMID: 17991982]

[70] Cephalosporins Abraham E. Drugs 1987; 4(2): 1-4.

[71] Etebu E, Arikekpar I. Antibiotics: Classification and mechanisms of action with emphasis on molecular perspectives. Int J App Microbio Biotech Res 2016; 4: 90-101.

[72] Bonner DP, Sykes RB. Structure activity relationships among the monobactams. J Antimicrob Chemother 1984; 14(4): 313-27.
[http://dx.doi.org/10.1093/jac/14.4.313] [PMID: 6389473]

[73] Sykes RB, Bonner DP. Discovery and development of the monobactams. Rev Infect Dis 1985; 7(4) (Suppl. 4): S579-93.
[http://dx.doi.org/10.1093/clinids/7.Supplement_4.S579] [PMID: 3909315]

[74] Sykes RB, Cimarusti CM, Bonner DP, *et al.* Monocyclic β-lactam antibiotics produced by bacteria. Nature 1981; 291(5815): 489-91.
[http://dx.doi.org/10.1038/291489a0] [PMID: 7015152]

[75] https://www.sciencedirect.com/topics/medicine-and-dentistry/carbapenem.

[76] Papp-Wallace KM, Endimiani A, Taracila MA. BonomoRA. Antimicrobial agents and chemotherapy. Am SocMicrobiol 2011; 55(11): 4943-60.

[77] Torres JA, Villegas MV, Quinn JP. Current concepts in antibiotic-resistant gram-negative bacteria. Expert Rev Anti Infect Ther 2007; 5(5): 833-43.
[http://dx.doi.org/10.1586/14787210.5.5.833] [PMID: 17914917]

[78] Brink AJ, Feldman C, Grolman DC, *et al.* Appropriate use of the carbapenems. S Afr Med J 2004; 94(10 Pt 2): 857-61.
[PMID: 15566108]

[79] Moore D. Antibiotic Classification and Mechanism , http://www.orthobullets.com /basic-science/9059/ antibiotic-classification-and-mechanism [Accessed on September, 1 2016];

[80] Hamilton-Miller JM. Chemistry and biology of the polyene macrolide antibiotics. Am Soc Microbiol 1973; 37(2): 166-96.

[81] Domagala JM. Structure-activity and structure-side-effect relationships for the quinolone antibacterials. J Antimicrob Chemother 1994; 33(4): 685-706.
[http://dx.doi.org/10.1093/jac/33.4.685] [PMID: 8056688]

[82] Peterson LR. Currently available antimicrobial agents and their potential for use as monotherapy. Clin Microbiol Infect 2008; 14(6) (Suppl. 6): 30-45.
[http://dx.doi.org/10.1111/j.1469-0691.2008.02125.x] [PMID: 19040464]

[83] Takano M, Okuda M, Yasuhara M, Hori R. Cellular toxicity of aminoglycoside antibiotics in G418-sensitive and -resistant LLC-PK1 cells. Pharm Res 1994; 11(5): 609-15.
[http://dx.doi.org/10.1023/A:1018999423464] [PMID: 8058626]

[84] Bar-Nun S, Shneyour Y, Beckmann JS. G-418, an elongation inhibitor of 80 S ribosomes. Biochim

Biophys Acta 1983; 741(1): 123-7.
[http://dx.doi.org/10.1016/0167-4781(83)90018-0] [PMID: 6193810]

[85] Talaro KP, Chess B. Foundations in microbiology. 8th ed., New York: McGraw Hill 2008.

[86] Gilbert DN. Aminoglycosides.Principles and practice of infectious diseases. 4th ed. New York, N.Y.: Churchill Livingstone 1995; pp. 279-306.

[87] Gilbert D. Aminoglycosides.Mandell, Douglas, and Bennett's principles and practice of infectious diseases. 5th ed. Philadelphia: Churchill Livingstone 2000; pp. 307-36.

[88] Eyssen HJ, Van den Bosch JF, Janssen GA, Vanderhaeghe H. Specific inhibition of cholesterol absorption by sulfaguanidine. Atherosclerosis 1971; 14(2): 181-92.
[http://dx.doi.org/10.1016/0021-9150(71)90048-7] [PMID: 5118612]

[89] Henry RJ. The mode of action of sulfonamides. Bacteriol Rev 1943; 7(4): 175-262.
[PMID: 16350088]

[90] Kahne D, Leimkuhler C, Lu W, Walsh C. Glycopeptide and lipoglycopeptide antibiotics. Chem Rev 2005; 105(2): 425-48.
[http://dx.doi.org/10.1021/cr030103a] [PMID: 15700951]

[91] Van Bambeke F. Glycopeptides in clinical development: pharmacological profile and clinical perspectives. Curr Opin Pharmacol 2004; 4(5): 471-8.
[http://dx.doi.org/10.1016/j.coph.2004.04.006] [PMID: 15351351]

[92] Kang H-K, Park Y. Glycopeptide antibiotics: Structure and mechanism of action. J Bacteriol Virol 2015; 45(2): 67-78.
[http://dx.doi.org/10.4167/jbv.2015.45.2.67]

[93] Shinabarger DL, Marotti KR, Murray RW, *et al.* Mechanism of action of oxazolidinones: effects of linezolid and eperezolid on translation reactions. Antimicrob Agents Chemother 1997; 41(10): 2132-6.
[http://dx.doi.org/10.1128/AAC.41.10.2132] [PMID: 9333037]

[94] Bozdogan B, Appelbaum PC. Oxazolidinones: activity, mode of action, and mechanism of resistance. Int J Antimicrob Agents 2004; 23(2): 113-9.
[http://dx.doi.org/10.1016/j.ijantimicag.2003.11.003] [PMID: 15013035]

[95] Moellering RC. Linezolid: the first oxazolidinone antimicrobial. Ann Intern Med 2003; 138(2): 135-42.
[http://dx.doi.org/10.7326/0003-4819-138-2-200301210-00015] [PMID: 12529096]

[96] Kleinkauf H, von Döhren H. Peptide antibiotics, beta-lactams, and related compounds. Crit Rev Biotechnol 1988; 8(1): 1-32.
[http://dx.doi.org/10.3109/07388558809150536] [PMID: 3063387]

[97] Jensen T, Pedersen SS, Garne S, Heilmann C, Høiby N, Koch C. Colistin inhalation therapy in cystic fibrosis patients with chronic Pseudomonas aeruginosa lung infection. J Antimicrob Chemother 1987; 19(6): 831-8.
[http://dx.doi.org/10.1093/jac/19.6.831] [PMID: 3301785]

[98] Giroir BP, Quint PA, Barton P, *et al.* Preliminary evaluation of recombinant amino-terminal fragment of human bactericidal/permeability-increasing protein in children with severe meningococcal sepsis. Lancet 1997; 350(9089): 1439-43.
[http://dx.doi.org/10.1016/S0140-6736(97)06468-4] [PMID: 9371168]

[99] Vitale M, Scatassa ML, Cardamone C, *et al.* Staphylococcal food poisoning case and molecular analysis of toxin genes in Staphylococcus aureus strains isolated from food in Sicily, Italy. Foodborne Pathog Dis 2015; 12(1): 21-3.
[http://dx.doi.org/10.1089/fpd.2014.1760] [PMID: 25384106]

[100] Talaro KP, Chess B. Foundations in microbiology. 8th ed., New York: McGraw Hill 2008.

[101] Madigan MT, Martinko JM. Brock biology of microorganisms. 11th ed., Pearson Prentice Hall Inc.

2006.

[102] Josephine HR, Kumar I, Pratt RF. The perfect penicillin? Inhibition of a bacterial DD-peptidase by peptidoglycan-mimetic beta-lactams. J Am Chem Soc 2004; 126(26): 8122-3. [http://dx.doi.org/10.1021/ja048850s] [PMID: 15225046]

[103] Alborn WE Jr, Allen NE, Preston DA. Daptomycin disrupts membrane potential in growing Staphylococcus aureus. Antimicrob Agents Chemother 1991; 35(11): 2282-7. [http://dx.doi.org/10.1128/AAC.35.11.2282] [PMID: 1666494]

[104] Falagas ME, Rafailidis PI, Matthaiou DK. Resistance to polymyxins: Mechanisms, frequency and treatment options. Drug Resist Updat 2010; 13(4-5): 132-8. [http://dx.doi.org/10.1016/j.drup.2010.05.002] [PMID: 20843473]

[105] Gale E, Cundliffe E, Reynolds P, Richmond MH, Waring MJ. The molecular basis of antibiotic action. 1981.

[106] Chen CR, Malik M, Snyder M, Drlica K. DNA gyrase and topoisomerase IV on the bacterial chromosome: quinolone-induced DNA cleavage. J Mol Biol 1996; 258(4): 627-37. [http://dx.doi.org/10.1006/jmbi.1996.0274] [PMID: 8636997]

[107] Etebu E. Potential panacea to the complexities of polymerase chain reaction (PCR). Adv LifeSci Tech 2013; 13: 1-8.

[108] Douthwaite S. Interaction of the antibiotics clindamycin and lincomycin with Escherichia coli 23S ribosomal RNA. Nucleic Acids Res 1992; 20(18): 4717-20. [http://dx.doi.org/10.1093/nar/20.18.4717] [PMID: 1383931]

[109] Katz L, Ashley GW. Translation and protein synthesis: macrolides. Chem Rev 2005; 105(2): 499-528. [http://dx.doi.org/10.1021/cr030107f] [PMID: 15700954]

[110] Patel U, Yan YP, Hobbs FW Jr, *et al.* Oxazolidinones mechanism of action: inhibition of the first peptide bond formation. J Biol Chem 2001; 276(40): 37199-205. [http://dx.doi.org/10.1074/jbc.M102966200] [PMID: 11483595]

[111] Vannuffel P, Cocito C. Mechanism of action of streptogramins and macrolides. Drugs 1996; 51(1) (Suppl. 1): 20-30. [http://dx.doi.org/10.2165/00003495-199600511-00006] [PMID: 8724813]

[112] Menninger JR, Otto DP. Erythromycin, carbomycin, and spiramycin inhibit protein synthesis by stimulating the dissociation of peptidyl-tRNA from ribosomes. Antimicrob Agents Chemother 1982; 21(5): 811-8. [http://dx.doi.org/10.1128/AAC.21.5.811] [PMID: 6179465]

[113] Tenson T, Lovmar M, Ehrenberg M. The mechanism of action of macrolides, lincosamides and streptogramin B reveals the nascent peptide exit path in the ribosome. J Mol Biol 2003; 330(5): 1005-14. [http://dx.doi.org/10.1016/S0022-2836(03)00662-4] [PMID: 12860123]

[114] Hong W, Zeng J, Xie J. Antibiotic drugs targeting bacterial RNAs. Acta Pharm Sin B 2014; 4(4): 258-65. [http://dx.doi.org/10.1016/j.apsb.2014.06.012] [PMID: 26579393]

[115] Chopra I, Roberts M. Tetracycline antibiotics: mode of action, applications, molecular biology, and epidemiology of bacterial resistance. Microbiol Mol Biol Rev 2001; 65(2): 232-60. [http://dx.doi.org/10.1128/MMBR.65.2.232-260.2001] [PMID: 11381101]

[116] Epe B, Woolley P. The binding of 6-demethylchlortetracycline to 70S, 50S and 30S ribosomal particles: a quantitative study by fluorescence anisotropy. EMBO J 1984; 3(1): 121-6. [http://dx.doi.org/10.1002/j.1460-2075.1984.tb01771.x] [PMID: 6423382]

[117] Ehrlich J, Bartz QR, Smith RM, Joslyn DA, Burkholder PR. Chloromycetin, a new antibiotic from asoil actinomycete. Science 1947; 106(2757): 417.

[http://dx.doi.org/10.1126/science.106.2757.417] [PMID: 17737966]

[118] Ohnishi Y, Ishikawa J, Hara H, *et al.* Genome sequence of the streptomycin-producing microorganism *Streptomyces griseus* IFO 13350. J Bacteriol 2008; 190(11): 4050-60. [http://dx.doi.org/10.1128/JB.00204-08] [PMID: 18375553]

[119] Procópio RE, Silva IR, Martins MK, Azevedo JL, Araújo JM. Antibiotics produced by Streptomyces. Braz J Infect Dis 2012; 16(5): 466-71. [http://dx.doi.org/10.1016/j.bjid.2012.08.014] [PMID: 22975171]

[120] Singh V, Haque S, Singh H, *et al.* Isolation, screening,and identification of novel isolates of Actinomycetes from India for antimicrobial applications. Front Microbiol 2016; 7: 1921. [http://dx.doi.org/10.3389/fmicb.2016.01921] [PMID: 27999566]

[121] Al husnan LA, Alkahtani MDF. Molecular Identification of Streptomyces producing antibiotics and their antimicrobial activities. Ann Agric Sci 2016; 61: 251-5. [http://dx.doi.org/10.1016/j.aoas.2016.06.002]

[122] Silva MSC, de Carvaiho Santos-Ebinuma V, Lopes AM, de Oliveira Rangel-Yagui C. Dextransulfate/Triton X two-phase micellar systems as an alternative first purification step for clavulanic acid. Fluid Phase Equilib 2015; 399: 80-6. [http://dx.doi.org/10.1016/j.fluid.2015.04.026]

[123] Zhanel GG, Homenuik K, Nichol K, *et al.* The glycylcyclines: a comparative review with the tetracyclines. Drugs 2004; 64(1): 63-88. [http://dx.doi.org/10.2165/00003495-200464010-00005] [PMID: 14723559]

[124] Procópio RE, Silva IR, Martins MK, Azevedo JL, Araújo JM. Antibiotics produced by Streptomyces. Braz J Infect Dis 2012; 16(5): 466-71. [http://dx.doi.org/10.1016/j.bjid.2012.08.014] [PMID: 22975171]

[125] Fenton C, Keating GM, Curran MP. Daptomycin. Drugs 2004; 64(4): 445-55. [http://dx.doi.org/10.2165/00003495-200464040-00009] [PMID: 14969579]

[126] Singh V, Haque S, Singh H, *et al.* Isolation, screening,and identification of novel isolates of Actinomycetes from India for antimicrobial applications. Front Microbiol 2016; 7: 1921. [http://dx.doi.org/10.3389/fmicb.2016.01921] [PMID: 27999566]

[127] Weber T, Charusanti P, Musiol-Kroll EM, *et al.* Metabolic engineering of antibiotic factories: new tools for antibiotic production in actinomycetes. Trends Biotechnol 2015; 33(1): 15-26. [http://dx.doi.org/10.1016/j.tibtech.2014.10.009] [PMID: 25497361]

[128] www.sahealth.sa.gov.au/wps/wcm/.../multidrug.

[129] https://www.osha.gov/SLTC/etools/hospital/hazards/mro/mro.html.

[130] https://portal.ct.gov/DPH/.../Multidrug.

[131] Pantel L, Florin T, Dobosz-Bartoszek M, *et al.* Odilorhabdins, Antibacterial Agents that Cause Miscoding by Binding at a New Ribosomal Site. Mol Cell 2018; 70(1): 83-94.e7. [http://dx.doi.org/10.1016/j.molcel.2018.03.001] [PMID: 29625040]

[132] Nichols D, Cahoon N, Trakhtenberg EM, *et al.* Use of ichip for high-throughput in situ cultivation of "uncultivable" microbial species. Appl Environ Microbiol 2010; 76(8): 2445-50. [http://dx.doi.org/10.1128/AEM.01754-09] [PMID: 20173072]

[133] Bush K, Courvalin P, Dantas G, *et al.* Tackling antibiotic resistance. Nat Rev Microbiol 2011; 9(12): 894-6. [http://dx.doi.org/10.1038/nrmicro2693] [PMID: 22048738]

[134] Ling LL, Schneider T, Peoples AJ, *et al.* A new antibiotic kills pathogens without detectable resistance. Nature 2015; 517(7535): 455-9. [http://dx.doi.org/10.1038/nature14098] [PMID: 25561178]

[134] Ling LL, Schneider T, Peoples AJ, *et al.* A new antibiotic kills pathogens without detectable resistance. Nature 2015; 517(7535): 455-9.
[http://dx.doi.org/10.1038/nature14098] [PMID: 25561178]

[135] Wright G. Antibiotics: An irresistible newcomer. Nature 2015; 517(7535): 442-4.
[http://dx.doi.org/10.1038/nature14193] [PMID: 25561172]

CHAPTER 11

The Use of Medicinal Plants in the Treatment of Malaria

Ibemhal D. Asem[*], **Khullakpam Shaheen** and **Debananda S. Ningthoujam**

Department of Biochemistry, Manipur University, Imphal, Manipur-795003, India

Abstract: Malaria is an infectious disease. Many anti-malarial drugs have been introduced to eliminate malaria. Earlier, the major antimalarial drugs were natural products but in due course synthetic drugs have replaced them. Pursuing multiple strategies is needed for discovering new drugs for malaria. Global International Centers of Excellence for Malaria Research (ICEMR) network is conducting many research studies. The research activities include clinical studies for assessing antimalarial drug efficacies, drug susceptibilities of parasite isolates and determining resistance-mediating parasite polymorphisms. There are several approaches for the discovery of new drugs. The approaches should also focus on low cost and novel therapies. Currently, the available drugs are optimized in many ways using combination therapy and the discovery of compounds from plants. This chapter focuses on the available antimalarial medications, including both synthetic and natural products. The present chapter also highlights indigenous medicinal plants, which can be potentially used for the development of antimalarial drugs.

Keywords: Antimalarial medications, Malaria, Medicinal plants, Plasmodium.

INTRODUCTION

Malaria is one of the major infectious diseases in the world. It is commonly found in tropical countries. It is caused by the protozoa of the genus Plasmodium. In 2015, around 438,000 people died due to malaria among 214 million cases of malaria reported worldwide. Malaria is widely distributed in Africa, Asia, Middle East, Central South America, Hispaniola and Oceania. However, it was spread in Canada by travellers who used to travel to these endemic areas. Around 1 million Canadians are reported to travel to these places every year, resulting in 350 to 1000 annual malaria cases and 1 or 2 deaths per year. Earlier, people used to rely on plant extracts as drugs against malaria. Quinine remained as the major antimalarial drug for many years. However, from 1930's synthetic drugs started replacing the natural products. The synthetic drugs include 8-aminoquinoline

[*] **Corresponding author Ibemhal D. Asem:** Department of Biochemistry, Manipur University, Imphal, Manipur-795003, India; Tel: +91 961 2035 173; E-mail: ibemasem@gmail.com

K. Tamreihao, Saikat Mukherjee and Debananda S. Ningthoujam (Eds.)
All rights reserved-© 2019 Bentham Science Publishers

(*e.g.* primaquine), 4-aminoquinoline (*e.g.* chloroquine, amodiaquine) and inhibitors of folic acid synthesis (*e.g.* proguanil, primethamine) [1]. Malaria was expected to be eradicated worldwide in mid-1950s but the problem of *Plasmodium falciparum* resistance arose in the mid-1960s [2]. In the beginning only some strains of *P. falciparum* showed resistance to chloroquine, later, several strains of *P. falciparum* became multi-drug resistance. Today, drug resistant stains are widespread in S.E. Asia, S. America and E. Africa [1]. In addition, due to the increasing number of international travellers, malaria did not remain solely confined to the tropical countries instead started spreading to other countries [2]. For the management of malaria, there is an urgent need to discover new drugs. Besides, establishment of efficacy and development of safety measures for the use of traditional medicinal plants are also necessary. This chapter mainly focuses on medications for malaria and a comprehensive list of various medicinal plants used for the treatment of malaria.

Cause of Malaria

Malaria is a mosquito borne parasitic infection spread by Anopheles mosquito. Malarial parasites are single-celled microorganisms of the Plasmodium group. Malaria is mainly caused by 4 species of Plasmodium in humans. They are *P. falciparum*, *P. malariae*, *P. ovale* and *P. vivax*. Majority of the deaths are mainly caused by the *P. falciparum* infection [3, 4]. Although malaria caused by *P. malariae*, *P. ovale* and *P. vivax* is milder, it colonizes in liver and can cause chronic relapses [5]. In sub-Saharan Africa and Oceania, *P. falciparum* is particularly frequent while outside Africa, *P. vivax* is more common [6].

Signs and Symptoms

The typical symptoms of malaria are fever, tiredness, vomiting and headache. The severity of the disease may cause yellow skin, seizure, coma or death. The signs and symptoms appear after 8-25 days of infection. However, patients under antimalarial medication show delayed symptoms. Flu like symptom is shown by all patients suffering from malaria [7], which may resemble to gastroenteritis and viral diseases, etc [8]. Other symptoms may include shivering, joint pain, haemolytic anaemia, jaundice, haematuria, retinal damage and convulsion [3]. When malaria is caused by *P. vivax* and *P. ovale* paroxysm occurs every 2 days, which is known as tertian fever. Moreover, when caused by *P. falciparum*, there may be recurrent fever every 36-48 hours; while in some cases the fever may be less pronounced but is continuous [9]. *P. falciparum* malaria is often referred as falciparum malaria. It is the severest and the symptoms are shown after 9-30 days of infection [7]. Neurological symptoms are frequent in cerebral malaria individuals, which may include abnormal posturing, nystagmus, conjugate gaze palsy, seizure or coma [7]. Cerebral malaria is a severe form, which can involve encephalopathy. It causes whitening of retina (an important clinical sign for distinguishing malaria). Severe headache, enlargement of spleen and liver or both, low blood sugar and renal failure may also occur [7].

Serious complications of malaria may include respiratory distress development, which occur in 25% of adults and 40% of children. Besides, severe falciparum malaria can result acute distress syndrome in 5-25% of adults and 40% of children [10]. Malaria increases mortality when co-infection with HIV occurs [11]. Infection with both *P. falciparum* and *P. vivax* in pregnant women may cause abortion, stillbirth, infant mortality and low birth weight [12].

Life Cycle

Plasmodium parasite multiplies in red blood cells of humans and in the intestine of mosquitos. The female mosquito ingests blood from an infected person and when it feeds on another person, the infection is transmitted. Plasmodia have different life stages; sexual multiplication phase in the insect vector; an asexual multiplication phase occurring in the vertebrate host's tissue. It is then followed by the main phase of asexual multiplication in blood. The life cycle of Plasmodium occurring in humans comprises the exo-erythrocytic and erythrocytic stages and in mosquitos, the sporogonic cycle exists. Humans and other vertebrates play as an intermediate host for parasites and mosquitos [13].

Exo-erythrocytic Stages of Malaria Parasite in Human

In humans, the malaria infection begins by the injection of sporozoites into the blood. During a blood meal, the sporozoites are released into the blood by the vector mosquito. However, the number of sporozoites released may vary from dozens to thousands [13]. The duration of the appearance of the symptoms of malaria depends on the number of sporozoites. When the number of sporozoites is large, within a short incubation period, malarial symptoms appear. Sporozoites reach the liver through the circulation and thus in hepatocytes the asexual exo-erythrocytic schizogonic cycle starts. In the liver, the trophozoite initially appears as a mono-nucleated round body within the host cell's cytoplasm, which subsequently develops and multiplies asexually forming mature schizonts (parasite's multinucleated stage) and finally releases a number of merozoites. Mature schizonts have no pigment and occupy the entire cell cytoplasm (around 30-70 μm large). The length of schizogenic cycle of liver and the number of merozoites produced are species dependent. The number of merozoites production is approximately 2000 for *P. malariae*, 10,000 for *P. vivax/P. ovale* and for *P. falciparum* is up to 30,000 [14]. The pre-latent periods are 5.5, 8, 9 and 15 days for *P. falciparum*, *P. vivax*, *P. ovale* and P. malariae, respectively [13]. By the rupturing of matured schizont, merozoites are released into liver's sinusoids and then the merozoites infect red blood cells.

Biological Basis for Relapses

P. vivax and *P. ovale* determine a relapsing infection in malaria [13]. Some liver trophozoites undergo exo-erythrocytic schizogonic cycle and some remain in dormant stage. Those in dormant stage are known as hypnozoites. The dormant strain of *P. vivax* has a homogenous population of sporozoites, the latency of which can be 250 days or more. For the *P. vivax* strain which has a heterogonous population of sporozoites, relapses occur at intervals of 2 to 3 months for as long as up to 2 years [15].

Erythrocytic Stages of Malaria Parasite in Humans

This stage has several clinical importance. During this stage, diagnosis of the infection and identification of the species can be done. For each species, the duration of erythrocytic cycle varies. From the liver schizonts, merozoites are released into the blood [16]. To initiate the trophozoite stage, merozoites invade erythrocyte. As the parasite grows, expansion of the cytoplasm occurs within 12-24 hours and by the end of this phase, trophozoite is pigmented with large cytoplasm and a single nucleus. The nuclear division continues until a number of merozoites are produced. The number of merozoites of *P. falciparum*, *P. vivax* and P. *malariae* are 36, 24 and 12, respectively. By the end of this phase, erythrocytes are ruptured and the merozoites are released into blood stream, which results in typical malaria paroxysm. Schizogonic cycle continues until the process is inhibited. The inhibitor may be a specific immune response or chemotherapy. During the schizogonic cycle in the red blood cell, some merozoites differentiate into sexual gametocyte [13]. In the infection caused by *P. vivax*, *P. ovale* and *P. malariae*, gametocytes appear early in the third generation, and for *P. falciparum*, at least 10 generations are required for the appearance of gametophytes in blood [17].

The parasite's maturation in human blood begins in the form of a ring. The ring form in *P. falciparum* has variable size (diameter of the smallest is 1.2 μm). They tend to adhere to the erythrocyte's internal surface and the nucleus divides to form two chromatin dots. The cytoplasm then becomes fleshy with smaller vacuole and thus, the parasites disappear from the peripheral circulation. *P. vivax* and *P. ovale* ring forms have similar features. In *P. vivax* and *P. ovale*, trophozoites appear in peripheral circulation. During this phase, parasites mature, cytoplasm enlarges, amoeboid pseudopods appear and vacuole disappears. Besides, pigment, which is the product of hemoglobin catabolism becomes prominent. In addition, striplings are observed. *P. malariae* trophozoites are regular in shape with a small vacuole and abundant pigment but there is no stripling. The mature schizonts of *P. vivax* and *P. ovale* have numerous merozoites, which are arranged irregularly in the red blood cells, while in *P. malariae* small number of merozoites are arranged regularly around the central mass of pigment and there is no stripling. The gametocytes of *P. vivax*, *P. ovale* and *P. malariae* are similar to the late trophozoite morphologically; however, they present a matured parasite with abundant and un-agglomerated pigment [13]. The shape of *P. falciparum* gametocytes is like a typical banana. Male parasite's nuclear material is dispersed as it prepares for ex-flagellation while it is condensed in female parasite.

Sporogonic Cycle in Mosquito

For the production of egg, female mosquito ingests a blood meal [13]. Throughout the life of the mosquito, the cycle of blood meal and oviposition continues. This requires the contact of vertebrate host repeatedly permitting ingestion of malaria parasites, their multiplication, maturation and transmission to other individual host during the upcoming feedings.

During the blood meal, the sporogonic cycle begins, when a suitable species of Anopheles ingests the mature male and female gametocytes. Then, the gametocytes reach the insect mid-gut where the female gametocyte sheds the red blood cell. It remains as a macrogamete in the extracellular space freely. Whereas the nucleus of the male gametocyte divides producing 8 flagellated microgametes. They then leave the erythrocyte and reach the mid-gut where they fertilize to macrogametes. Within 18 hours from the blood meal, Zygote becomes elongated, slowly motile ookinete. Then, ookinete travels into peritrophic membrane and epithelium of the mid-gut and remains under the basal lamina of outer gut wall. Thereafter, 24-72 hours of the blood meal, the ookinete develops into oocyst, which is non-motile. In the beginning, the diameter of the oocyst is 6-8 µm with a thin wall and a single nucleus. On maturity, the oocyst reaches up to 40-60 µm in diameter. Then, the nucleus of the mature oocyst repeatedly divides forming around 10,000 new individual nuclei. Development of initial oocyst to maturation is dependent on parasite species and temperature. There is variation in the duration of attaining maturity, which may be from 7 to 30 days. Sporozoites are the product of mature oocyst. They are actively motile and are 10-15 µm in length and are narrow and curvy in shape. Sporozoites travel to the insect's haemocelomic space by leaving the cyst, passing the small perforations and while passing, they do not destroy the wall. When the mosquito feeds, the salivary fluid and the content of sporozoites are injected into the vertebrate host, which marks the beginning of another asexual replicative cycle.

Diagnosis

There are certain instances where laboratory diagnostic tests cannot be afforded. In such cases, a history of subjective fever is used which serves as an indication to treat malaria. The most preferred malarial diagnosis is microscopy in which microscopic examination of the blood is done. In some instances, as an alternative, even saliva and urine are used for investigation. Many modern techniques are available for the diagnosis of malaria (such as antigen tests or polymerase chain reactions). Two methods of parasitological diagnosis are used, light microscopy and immune chromatographic RDTs [18].

Antimalarial Medications

Antimalarial medications are developed for preventing and curing malaria. It may be used for individuals with suspected or confined infection, for the prevention of malarial infection in those individuals who have no immunity (malaria prophylaxis) and for those travelling to a malaria-endemic region as well as for intermittent preventive therapy (treatment in endemic regions).

Today, combination therapy is being used for the treatment of malaria for example Coartem. There are various advantages of combination therapy. These may include reducing the risk of treatment failure, reducing the risk of resistance development, enhancing convenience and reducing side effects. Before the onset of the treatment, patients, who are suspected for malaria should undergo several clinical tests. They may undertake microscopy that is confirmed by parasitological characterization or by undertaking rapid diagnostic experiments.

Quinine

Quinine was used for the treatment of malaria from a very early time, *i.e.* from 1600s. It is derived from the bark of cinchona (quina-quina tree). It was the first successful report on the use of a chemical compound for the treatment of infectious diseases [19]. Quinine was discovered accidentally. An Indian was lost in an Andean jungle, having high fever. He drank water from a pool of stagnant water. The water was bitter as quina-quina trees contaminated it. Then he thought he was poisoned but to his surprise, his fever was alleviated. Thus, from that accidental discovery, the villagers started using quina-quina bark extracts for the treatment of fever [20]. Quinine was introduced to Europe in 1638 by the Spanish Countess of Chinchon. She went to Peru and contracted a fever. Her fever was cured by the Bark of a tree. In her return to Spain, she brought the bark. Later, in 1742, in her honour, Carl Linnaeus, the Botanist called the tree "Cinchona" [21]. Before, 1820, dried fine powder of cinchona bark was mixed into a liquid (commonly wine was used) [22]. However, after 1820, the extraction of quinine from the tree bark was started. Thus, standard malarial treatment began by purified quinine replacing the bark of quinine [23]. Until 1920s, quinine was mainly used to treat malaria, later; several effective synthetic antimalarial drugs were introduced. Among them, chloroquine was the most important which was extensively used in the beginning of 1940s [24]. In late 1950s, there was development of resistance of *P. falciparum* to chloroquine. It was observed in some parts of Southeast Asia and South America. When resistance to chloroquine kept increasing, quinine began to play a major role in severe malarial treatment [24].

Quinine is a cinchona alkaloid of aryl alcohol group of drugs [22]. It is the form of a salt and different preparations are available for it (including hydrochloride, dihydrochloride, sulphate, bisulphate and gluconate salts). It has rapid schizonticidal action against intra-erythrocytic parasites. For *P. vivax* and *P. malariae*, it shows gametocytocidal property. Analgesic property is also a property of quinine. Quinine can be absorbed rapidly both orally and parenterally [25]. It is distributed in the body fluids. It is protein bound. The main protein to which quinine binds is alpha-1 glycoprotein. Its binding ability in plasma is dependent on the concentration and level of alpha-1 acid glycoprotein. The level of this protein is high in malaria patients, thus, binding of quinine to the protein is increased in them [26].

The common side effects of quinine are known as cinchonism, which include mild forms of tinnitus, slight hearing impairment (which is concentration dependent), reversible headache and nausea [27]. There are other symptoms when the side effects become severe. They may include vertigo, vomiting, abdominal pain, diarrhoea, marked auditory loss and visual symptoms (which may include loss of vision). Hypotension occurs when the drug is taken rapidly and venous thrombosis may occur following intravenous injections [22, 28]. Hypoglycemia is also a common side effect [26, 29], which is problematic to pregnant women [30]. Quinine treatment has other serious side effects including skin eruptions, asthma, thrombocytopenia, hepatic injury and psychosis [31].

Oral quinine is used for uncomplicated malaria [32, 33]. Higher cure rates are mainly observed when quinine is used in combination, *e.g.*, quinine in combination with sulphadoxine-pyrimethamine, tetracycline or clindamycin or artesunate [34, 35]. In some regions where there is high multi-drug resistance, artemisinin-based combination therapy (ACT) is used. In Brazil, artemether-lumefantrine (AL) has faster recovery time for those treated with quinine-doxycycline [36]. ACT has certain advantages *i.e.*, it has a very simple dosing system, better tolerance, etc. In addition, the risks of serious toxicity decreases with ACT. However, ACT is costly and less available in markets. Moreover, quinine is a relatively cheap drug. Recently, combinations of quinine and antibiotics (tetracycline or clindamycin) have been introduced. A combination of azithromycin is used especially for pregnant women and children (below 8 years).

The WHO recommends combination of quinine and clindamycin for malarial treatment in the first trimester of pregnancy [37]. Clindamycin is good in pregnancy as it is very safe for pregnancy [38] and during pregnancy; the pharmacokinetic properties remain unchanged [39]. Quinine and Clindamycin combination is highly effective against several multidrug resistant *P. falciparum* strains. In malarial multidrug resistant areas, ACT is better than oral quinine in the clearance of parasites as well as fever also. In Africa, quinine monotherapy is the most widely used malarial treatment in the first trimester of pregnancy and is also very safe for pregnancy [22]. It is a major public health concern, in those areas which are affected by both HIV and malaria. Only few studies have been reported where the role of quinine was evaluated in managing malaria-HIV infected populations.

The mechanism of action of quinine involves inhibition of hemozoin biocrytallization. Although, quinine as a blood schizonticidal agent is less effective and more toxic than chloroquine, it is very effective and widely used for acute cases of *P. falciparum*. There are areas where there is high level of resistance to chloroquine, mefloquine and combination of sulfa drug with pyrimethamine. In those areas, quinine is especially used. Quinine is also given in post-exposure treatment *i.e.*, to those individuals who are coming back from malaria endemic area. Neurological effects can also be seen because of the neurotoxic properties of the drug. Quinine mediates these actions by decreasing excitability of motor neuron end plates, which causes functional impairment of the 8 cranial nerve. This may result in confusion, delirium and coma. Patients' blood glucose levels are monitored for every 4-6 hours because quinine can cause hypoglycemia as it can stimulate the secretion of insulin. Extra care is needed for pregnant women while administering and monitoring the dose. Renal failure may occur due to repeated consumption or over-dosing. In addition, even death may be caused by the depression of respiratory system.

The two most common alkaloids related to quinine are quinimax and quinidine. They may be used in malaria treatment and prevention. Quinimax is a combination of four alkaloids; they are quinine, quinidine, cinchoine and cinchonidine. The combination of these four alkaloids has shown to be more effective than quinine in many studies. One direct derivative of quinine is quinidine. It is a diastereoisomer and has similar properties of anti-malaria to that of the parent compound. It is found in very severe cases. Warburg's tincture was developed by Carl Warbung in 1834. Quinine was a key ingredient of Warburg's tincture. It was a popular anti-malarial drug in the 19th century. In the beginning, it was sold secretly as a medicine but later it was appreciated by several eminent professionals in medicine. It was considered more superior than quinine. The formula of Warburg's tincture was published in the Lancet, in 1875 [40].

Chloroquine

Chloroquine, until recently, was the most widely used, least expensive, and best-tested drug for malaria treatment. It was the safest than other drugs available. It is more effective when it is used in combination with other antimalarial drugs [41]. It is a 4-aminoquinoline compound. Other popular drugs are chloroquine FNA, resochin and dawaquin. They are based on chloroquine phosphate nivaquine. The mechanism of action of chloroquine is complicated and remained unclear. Its mechanism of action may involve interfering the nucleic acids synthesis of the parasites or by forming chloroquine-haem or chloroquine-DNA complex. Chloroquine shows its action against all schizonts (except the strains and gametocytes of *P. falciparum* or *P. vivax*, which are resistant to chloroquine). When resistant becomes widespread, it is still useful because of its anti-pyretic and anti-inflammatory effect. There are no abortifacient and teratogenic effects of Chloroquine so far.

Amodiaquine

Amodiaquine is a 4-aminoquinolone drug, which is used in the treatment of malaria [42]. Its structure as well as mechanism of action is similar to chloroquine. Some patients prefer amodiaquine to chloroquine because it has less itching effect. One of the WHO recommended artemisinin-combination is amodiaquine with artesunate (ASAQ). There are certain combination therapies, which are not recommended such as the combination with sulfadoxine and pyrimethamine [37]. The side effects of amodiaquine include bradycardia, itching, nausea, vomiting and abdominal pain. In a few patients, blood and hepatic disorders were also observed.

Pyrimethamine

Pyrimethamine is used as combination therapy in the treatment of malaria. For example, pyrimethamine with sulfadoxine is used for uncomplicated malaria [43]. Pyrimethamine is very useful against chloroquine resistant strains of *P. falciparum*. Its mechanism of action involves stopping DNA replication, cell division and reproduction. It occurs by inhibiting parasite's hydrofolate reductase and thus, purine and pyrimidine synthesis are prevented. During the erythrocytic phase, it acts primarily on the schizonts. Currently, it is used with sulphonamide only.

Proguanil

Proguanil or chloroguanide is a biguanide. It is the synthetic derivative of pyrimidine, which was developed by a group of British Antimalarial researchers in 1945. It is administered in combination with another antimalarial medicine [44]. It has several mechanisms of action. The most important is intermediate formation of metabolite cycloguanil and thus, inhibition of the enzyme, dihydrofolate reductase of malaria. It is effective on *P. falciparum*, *P. vivax* and *P. ovale* primary tissue stages. It is not used in the prevention of relapses. It is not recommended for therapy in acute infection as its blood schizonticidal activity is weak. However, proguanil combined with atovaquone or chloroquine is also used. This combination is useful for prophylaxis. Proguanil-chloroquine combination does not provide protection against *P. falciparum* resistant strains. There are only few side effects of proguanil such as slight loss of hair slightly and mouth ulcer.

Sulfonamide

Sulfonamides are also often used in combination with trimethoprim and pyrimethamine. Sulfadoxine and sulfamethoxypyridazine are structural analogs of p-aminobenzoic acid (PABA). They compete with PABA by blocking the conversion of dihydrofolic acid. They are inhibitors of dihydropteroate synthetase enzyme during the pathway of tetrahydrofolate synthesis of malaria parasite. It acts on schizont stages of erythrocytic (asexual) cycle of parasite. Administration of a fixed dose of sulfadoxine-pyrimethamine can cure sensitive strains of malaria by producing synergistic effects

Mefloquine

Mefloquine is used as an antimalarial drug. It treats malaria by killing the casual organisms [45]. Mefloquine was developed during the Vietnam War for protection from those parasites which were resistant to drugs. It is related to quinine chemically. It is effective for *P. vivax*, *P. ovale* and *P. malariae* and the resistant strains of *P. falciparum*. It is also effective in acute therapy and in prophylaxis.

Atovaquone

Atovaquone is a quinine antimalarial drug. It is available as oral suspension [46]. It is also available in combination with proguanil and is commonly used in prophylaxis by travellers. In areas where drug resistance exists, atovaquone may be used [47]. It is used in developed countries to treat falciparum malaria.

Primaquine

Primaquine is an active 8-aminoquinoline. It is effective on the gametocytes of *P. falciparum*. In addition, it is also effective on the merozoites present in the blood stream and on the dormant hepatic forms (hypnozoites) of *P. vivax* and *P. ovale* [48]. It acts on relapsing malaria infections and in acute cases as well. The mechanism of its action is not known, however, it is believed to block oxidative metabolism of Plasmodia. There are a few significant side effects of primaquine such as nausea, vomiting, anorexia, cramps, weakness of chest, anaemia and abdominal pain. In addition, whenever over dosed, there may be occurrence of granulocytopenia.

Artemisinin and Derivatives

Artemisin is derived from *Artemisia annua*. It is an herb, which has been used for the treatment of fever for over 1000 years [49]. Artemesinin, an active compound extract from *Artemisia annua,* is still in used today. Artemesinin is proved useful for all multi-drug resistant *P. falciparum.* It is strictly controlled under the WHO guidelines. It can be given in combination with anti-malarial drug. Artemisinin has a rapid action. Treatment of acute patients with artemisinin shows improvement in 1-3 days. Semi-synthetic artemisinin derivatives are easier to use. Examples of semi-synthetic artemisinin derivatives are artesunate and artemether. There are a few side effects of artemesinin. They are nausea, headache, vomiting, abnormal bleeding, dark color of urine and itching. There are reports of some cardiac changes during a clinical trial.

Artemether is a methyl ether derivative of dihydroartemesinin [50]. Its mechanism of action is similar to artemesinin. As a hypnozoiticidal compound, it has some reduced ability but acts significantly in decreasing gametocyte carriage. Artesunate is a artemisinin-type drug and it is currently in frequent used. Artesunate is a hemisuccinate derivative of the active metabolite, dihydroartemidin. It is used in combination therapy, and has shown its effectiveness in cases of uncomplicated *P. falciparum*. Dihydroartemisinin is the least stable but the most effective artemisinin compound. It acts strongly against blood shizont and in the reduction of gametocyte transmission. It is used in cases of resistant and uncomplicated *P. falciparum.* No side effects of dihydroartemisinin used in combination with artesunate have been recorded.

Halofantrine

The drug, Halofantrine was developed by Walter Reed Army Institute of Research in the 1960s. Halofantrine is a phenanthrene methanol acting as a blood schizonticide. Halofantrine is effective against all *Plasmodium* and the mechanism of action is like other anti-malarial drugs. Halofantrine is effective against drug resistant parasites but due to its high cost, it is not commonly used. Halofantrine is not recommended during pregnancy and lactation, for small children and for those who have already taken mefloquine before. A relative of halofantrine is available namely lumefantrine, which is used in some combination therapy [51].

Doxycycline

Doxycycline is a tetracycline compound. It has been derived from oxytetracycline [52]. It is a bacteriostatic agent. It acts by inhibiting protein synthesis. As it is relatively effective and cheap, it is probably one of the mostly used antimalarial drug. There are many places where there is the existence of chloroquine resistant. In those places, for chemoprophylasis, doxycycline is primarily used. It has slow action against acute malaria. For monotherapy, doxycycline should not be used. When combined with quinine, it is used in the treatment of *P. falciparum* resistance. Doxycycline has some side effects. They are permanent enamel hypoplasia, depression of bone growth transiently, disturbances in gastrointestine and increase in photosensitivity. It has an effect on bone and tooth growth. Due to these reasons, it is not used in children below 8 years. Pregnant and lactating women and patients with hepatic dysfunction cannot use it.

Clindamycin

The action of Clindamycin against blood schizonticides is slow. It is a derivative of lincomycin [53] and is used in combination with quinine only. This combination is used against acute *P. falciparum* resistant infections. In addition, the combination is not used as prophylactic. It is more toxic than other antibiotic which can be alternatively used. Therefore, it is used in children who already had contraindication with tetracyclines. Some of the side effects of clindamycin are nausea, abdominal pains and cramps. However, such side effects can be alleviated by the intake of large quantities of water and food during the drug treatment. Commercially available drugs which are being used in the treatment of malaria are listed in Table **1** [54]

Medicinal Plants in Treatment of Malaria

Natural products have been used in the development of drugs for treating various human diseases. Antimalarial chemotherapy available is based on natural products. New leads may arise from medicinal plants. Biological chemical compounds are important source in the search and discovery of new antimalarial drugs. The WHO recommended artemisinin derived combination therapies to overcome single drug resistance [55]. The combination may be with artemether, artesunate-amodiaquine, artesunate-sulphdoxine-pyremethamine, artesunate-mefloquine, amodiquine-sulphdoxine-pyremethamine. Conventionally used antimalarial drugs are losing effectiveness rapidly. One main reason is the increase in parasite resistance. Thus, there is an increased demand for developing new antimalarial drugs [56]. Herbs were used for anti-malarial treatment earlier. There is a strong believe that plant products are the only alternative. They might be safer having better effectiveness [57].

Recently, many attempts for the isolation and characterization of numerous antimalarial metabolites from plants have been made. Considering the occurrence of resistance to malaria drugs, there is a need of extensive research for identifying medicinal plants and their metabolites against malaria. In addition, the production of new herbal malaria medicines is essential. There are several studies on medicinal plants, which reported that medicinal plants are reliable for the treatment of malaria as well as other dangerous diseases, which include artheroclerosis, diabetes, cancer, and gastrointestinal diseases [58]. Medicinal plants which have antiplasmodial activities and used in malaria treatments are listed in Table **2**. The crude extracts and natural compounds from medicinal plants have many anti plasmodial activities [59]. Furthermore, studies are encouraged on the use of traditional medicines in the treatment of malaria; this may lead to the discovery of new antimalarial phytomedicines.

Table 1. A list of medications available in the market.

Drug Name	Generic Name	Brand Name	Drug Class	Reference
Aralen	Chloroquine systemic	Aralen	Amebicides, antimalarial quinolines	[54]
Aralen Phosphate	Chloroquine systemic	Aralen Phsophate	Amebicides, antimalarial combinations	[54]
Artemether/ lumefantrine	Artemether/ lumefantrine systemic	Coartem	Antimalarial combinations	[54]
Atovaquone	Atovaquone systemic	Mepron	Miscellaneous antibiotics	[54]
Atovaquone/Proguanil	Atovaquone/Proguanil systemic	Malarone, Malarone pediatric	Antimalarial combinations	[54]
Cardioquin	Quinidine systemic	Cardioquin, Quinaglute, Quinalan, Quinidex Extentabs	Group I antiarrhythmics	[54]

(Table 1) cont.....

Drug Name	Generic Name	Brand Name	Drug Class	Reference
Chloroquine	Chloroquine systemic	Aralen Phosphate, Aralen Hydrochloride	Amebicides, antimalarial quinolines	[54]
Cleocin	Clindamycin systemic	Cleocin	Lincomycin derivatives	[54]
Cleocin HCl	Clindamycin systemic	Cleocin HCl, Cleocin Pediatric, Dalacin C Palmitate	Lincomycin derivatives	[54]
Cleocin Pediatric	Clindanycin systemic	Cleocin Pediatric	Lincomycin derivatives	[54]
Cleocin Phosphate	Clindanycin systemic	Cleocin Phosphate IV	Lincomycin derivatives	[54]
Clindamycin	Clindanycin systemic	Cleocin, Cleocin Pediatric, Cleocin HCl, Cleocin Phosphate	Lincomycin derivatives	[54]
Coartem	Artemether/ lumefantrine systemic	Coartem	Antimalarial combinations	[54]
Doryx	Doxycycline systemic	Acticlate, Adoxa, Alodox, Avidoxy, Doryx, Mondoxyne NL, Monodox, Morgidox, Oracea, Oraxyl, Targadox, Vibramycin	Tetracyclines, miscellaneous Antimalarial drugs	[54]
Doryx 100	Doxycycline systemic	Doryx 100	Tetracyclines, miscellaneous Antimalarial drugs	[54]
Doryx MPC	Doxycycline systemic	Adoxa, Adoxa Ck, Adoxa Pak, Adoxa TT, Doryx, Doryx MPC, Monodox, Oracca, Periostat, Vibramycin Calcium, Vibramycin Hyclate, Vibra-Tabs		[54]
Doxycycline	Doxycycline systemic	Doryx, Doryx 100, Doryx MPC, Monodox, Morgidox,, Occudox, Oraxyl, Vibra-Tabs, Vibramycin	Tetracyclines, miscellaneous Antimalarial drugs	[54]

(Table 1) cont.....

Drug Name	Generic Name	Brand Name	Drug Class	Reference
Hydroxy Chloroquine	Hydroxy Chloroquine systemic	Plaquenil	Artirheumatics, Antimalarial quinolines	[54]
Krintafel	Tafenoquine systemic		Antimalarial quinolines	[54]
Lariam	Mefloquine systemic	Lariam	Antimalarial quinolines	[54]
Malarone	Atovaquone/proguanil systemic	Malarone, Malarone Pediatric	Antimalarial combinations	[54]
Malarone Pediatric	Atovaquone/proguanil systemic	Malarone, Malarone Pediatric	Antimalarial combinations	[54]
Mefloquine	Mefloquine systemic	Lariam	Antimalarial quinolines	[54]
Mepron	Atovaquone systemic	Mepron	Miscellaneous antibiotics	[54]
Monodox	Doxycycline systemic	Acticlate, Adoxa, Alodox, Advidoxy, Doryx, Mondoxyne NL, Monodox, Morgidox, Oracea, Oraxyl, Targadox, Vibramycin	Tetracyclines, miscellaneous Antimalarial drugs	[54]
Morgidox	Doxycycline systemic	Acticlate, Adoxa, Alodox, Advidoxy, Doryx, Mondoxyne NL, Monodox, Morgidox, Oracea, Oraxyl, Targadox, Vibramycin	Tetracyclines, miscellaneous Antimalarial drugs	[54]
Ocudox	Doxycycline systemic		Tetracyclines, miscellaneous Antimalarial drugs	[54]
Oraxyl	Doxycycline	Acticlate, Adoxa, Alodox, Avidoxy, Doryx, Mondoxyne NL, Monodox, Morgidox, Oracea, Oraxyl, Targadox, Vibramycin	Tetracyclines, miscellaneous Antimalarial drugs	[54]
Plaquenil	Hydroxychloroquine systemic	Plaquenil, Quineprox	Antirheumatics, antimalarial quinolines	[54]
Primaquine	Phosphate systemic	Primaquine	Antimalarial quinolines	[54]

(Table 1) cont.....

Drug Name	Generic Name	Brand Name	Drug Class	Reference
Quin- G	Quinidine systematic	Quin- G	Group I antiarrhythmics	[54]
Quinidine	Quinidine systemic	Cardioquin, Quin-G, Quinidex Extentabs	Group I antiarrhythmics	[54]
Quinidex Extentabs	Quinidine systematic	Cardioquin, Quinaglute, Quinalan, Quinidex, Extentabs	Group I antiarrhythmics	[54]
Tafenoquine	Tafenoquine systematic	Arakoda, Krintafel	Antimalarial quinolines	[54]
Vibra-Tabs	Doxycycline systemic	Adoxa, Adoxa Ck, Adoxa Pak, Adoxa TT, Doryx, Doryx MPC, Monodox, Oracea, Periostat, Vibramycin Calcium, Vibramycin Hyclate, Vibra-Tabs	Tetracyclines, miscellaneous Antimalarial drugs	[54]
Vibramycin	Doxycycline systemic	Acticlate, Adoxa, Alodox, Advidoxy, Doryx, Mondoxyne NL, Monodox, Morgidox, Oracea, Oraxyl, Targadox, Vibramycin	Tetracyclines, miscellaneous Antimalarial drugs	[54]

Table 2. Medicinal plants having antiplasmodial activities and used in malaria treatment.

Family	Species Name	Plant Parts Used	Reference
Amaranthaceae	*Amaranthus spinosus*	Stembark	[60]
Amaranthaceae	*Uvariopsis congolana*	Leaves, stem	[61]
Annonaceae	*Polyalthia oliveri*	Stem bark	[61]
Annonaceae	*Enantia chlorantha*	Stem, Stem bark	[61]
Aphloiaceae	*Aphloiatheiforms*	Leaves, bark	[55]
Apiaceae	*Ferula oopoda*	Roots	[62]
Apiaceae	*Astrodaucus orientalis*	Aerial parts	[62]
Apocynaceae	*Picralima nitida*	Seeds	[63]
Ascleipiadaceae	*Caralluma tuberculata*	Aerial parts	[64]
Ascleipiadaceae	*Vernonia amygdalina*	Leaves	[65]
Asteraceae	*Psiadiaarguta*	Leaves	[55]

(Table 2) cont.....

Family	Species Name	Plant Parts Used	Reference
Asteraceae	*Centaurea bruguieriana*	Aerial parts	[62]
Asteraceae	*Centaurea golestanica*	Aerial parts	[62]
Boraginaceae	*Heliotropium zeylanicum*	Aerial parts	[64]
Buxaceae	*Buxus hyrcana*	Aerial parts	[62]
Caesalpiniaceae	*Cassia occidentalis*	Leaves	[65]
Capparaceae	*Boscia angustifolia*	Leaves	[66]
Crayophyllaceae	*Minuaritia lineata*	Aerial parts	[62]
Clusiaceae	*Croton zambesicus*	Roots	[67]
Clusiaceae	*Garcinia kola*	Stem bark	[65]
Clusiaceae	*Symphonia globulifera*	Leaves	[68]
Combretaceae	*Terminalia bentzoe L.*	Leaves	[55]
Cucurbitaceae	*Momordica foetida*	Shoots	[69]
Dilleniaceae	*Tefracera pogge*	Leaves	[65]
Euphorbiaceae	*Euphorbia hirta*	Whole parts	[65]
Euphorbiaceae	*Neoboutonia glabracens*	Leaves	[61]
Euphorbiaceae	*Croton zambesicus*	Stem bark	[61]
Euphorbiaceae	*Phyllantus niruri*	Whole plant	[65]
Fabaceae	*Glycyrrhi zaglabra*	Aerial parts	[62]
Fabaceae	*Erythrina fusca*	Stem bark	[70]
Fabaceae	*Stylosanthes erecta*	Aerial parts	[66]
Fabaceae	*Tetrapleura tetraptera*	Fruits	[71]
Geraniaceae	*Erodium oxyrrhnchum*	Aerial parts	[62]
Hypericaceae	*Harungana madagascariensis*	Stem bark, seeds	[68, 72]
Lamiaceae	*Otostegia persica*	Fruits, leaves	[62]
Lamiaceae	*Otostegia michauxii*	Aerial parts	[62]
Lamiaceae	*Perovskia abrotanoides*	Aerial parts	[62]
Loganiaceae	*Nuxia verticillata*	Leaves, bark	[55]
Loganiaceae	*Buddleja salviifolia*	Leaves, bark	[55]
Loganiaceae	*Strychnos angolensis*	Roots	[73]
Loganiaceae	*Strychnos cocculoides*	Leaves	[73]
Loganiaceae	*Strychnos gossweileri*	Roots	[73]
Loganiaceae	*Strychnos henningsii*	Leaves	[73]
Loganiaceae	*Strychnos johnsonii*	Stem	[73]
Loganiaceae	*Strychnos mellodora*	Leavers, stem, roots	[73]

(Table 2) cont.....

Family	Species Name	Plant Parts Used	Reference
Loganiaceae	*Strychnos scheffleri*	Leaves	[73]
Loganiaceae	*Strychnos variabilis*	Roots	[73]
Meliaceae	*Trichilia emetica*	Leaves	[66]
Mimosaceae	*Cylicodiscus gabunensis*	Stem bark	[74]
Mimosaceae	*Albizia zygia*	Stem bark	[68]
Moraceae	*Artocarpus communis*	Leaves	[61]
Nyctagynaceae	*Boerhaavia erecta*	Stem bark	[59]
Polygalaceae	*Securidaca longipedunculata*	Leaves	[66]
Rubiaceae	*Vangueriainfausta*	Bark, root	[75]
Rubiaceae	*Morindamorindoides*	Leaves	[65]
Sapindaceae	*Cardiospermum halicacabum*	Shoots	[69]
Solanaceae	*Licium shawii*	Aerial parts	[64]
Tamariacaceae	*Tamarix aralensis*	Aerial parts	[62]
Verbenaceae	*Lantana camara*	Leaves	[60]
Vitaceae	*Cissus quadrangulari*	Whole plant	[66]
Zingiberaceae	*Cucurma longa*	Rhizomes	[76]
Zingiberaceae	*Siphonochilus aethiopicus*	Rhizomes	[77]
Zingiberaceae	*Zingiber officinale*	Rhizomes	[76]

CONCLUDING REMARKS

This chapter has attempted to highlight antimalarial medications and medicinal plants, which are used for and associated with malaria treatment. Quinine plays an important role in malarial management. It is an alternative to artesunate, when artesunate is not available. ACT also acts as a good option as it has simple dosing system and the duration of treatment is short as well. Natural products are playing a dominant role in discovering leads; these leads may be used in antimalarial drugs development. On the other hand, conventional antimalarial drugs are losing effectiveness, as there is an increased problem of drug resistant malaria parasites. Therefore, there is always a need for developing and introducing novel drugs to treat malaria. They can be synthetic or natural products which are free from resistance problems. Efficacy and safety measures of traditional medicines should be validated. In addition, the active constituents of traditional medicines should be identified and reliable quality controls should be established.

CONSENT FOR PUBLICATION

Not applicable.

CONFLICT OF INTEREST

The authors confirm that the contents of this chapter have no conflict of interest.

ACKNOWLEDGEMENTS

The authors acknowledge the financial support granted under the DBT RA program, DBT, Govt. of India and Advanced Level State Biotech Hub to the Dept. of Biochemistry, Manipur University by DBT, Govt. of India.

REFERENCES

[1] Mojab F. Antimalarial natural products: A review. Avicenna J Phytomed 2012; 2(2): 52-62. [PMID: 25050231]

[2] Phillipson JD, O'Neill MJ. Antimalarial and amoebicidal natural products.Biologically Active Natural Products. Oxford: Clarendon Press 1987; pp. 49-64.

[3] Beare NA, Taylor TE, Harding SP, Lewallen S, Molyneux ME. Malarial retinopathy: A newly established diagnostic sign in severe malaria. Am J Trop Med Hyg 2006; 75(5): 790-7. [http://dx.doi.org/10.4269/ajtmh.2006.75.790] [PMID: 17123967]

[4] Sarkar PK, Ahluwalia G, Vijayan VK, Talwar A. Critical care aspects of malaria. J Intensive Care Med 2010; 25(2): 93-103. [http://dx.doi.org/10.1177/0885066609356052] [PMID: 20018606]

[5] Caraballo H, King K. Emergency department management of mosquito-borne illness: Mmalaria, dengue, and West Nile virus. Emerg Med Pract 2014; 16(5): 1-23. [PMID: 25207355]

[6] Arnott A, Barry AE, Reeder JC. Understanding the population genetics of *Plasmodium vivax* is essential for malaria control and elimination. Malar J 2012; 11: 14. [http://dx.doi.org/10.1186/1475-2875-11-14] [PMID: 22233585]

[7] Bartoloni A, Zammarchi L. Clinical aspects of uncomplicated and severe malaria. Mediterr J Hematol Infect Dis 2012; 4(1)e2012026. [http://dx.doi.org/10.4084/mjhid.2012.026] [PMID: 22708041]

[8] Nadjm B, Behrens RH. Malaria: An update for physicians. Infect Dis Clin North Am 2012; 26(2): 243-59. [http://dx.doi.org/10.1016/j.idc.2012.03.010] [PMID: 22632637]

[9] Ferri FF. Protozoal infections Ferri'sColor Atlas and Text of Clinical Medicine. Elsevier Health Sciences 2009; p. 1159. [http://dx.doi.org/10.1016/B978-1-4160-4919-7.50334-0]

[10] Taylor WRJ, Hanson J, Turner GDH, White NJ, Dondorp AM. Respiratory manifestations of malaria. Chest 2012; 142(2): 492-505. [http://dx.doi.org/10.1378/chest.11-2655] [PMID: 22871759]

[11] Korenromp EL, Williams BG, de Vlas SJ, *et al.* Malaria attributable to the HIV-1 epidemic, sub-Saharan Africa. Emerg Infect Dis 2005; 11(9): 1410-9. [http://dx.doi.org/10.3201/eid1109.050337] [PMID: 16229771]

[12] Hartman TK, Rogerson SJ, Fischer PR. The impact of maternal malaria on newborns. Ann Trop Paediatr 2010; 30(4): 271-82. [http://dx.doi.org/10.1179/146532810X12858955921032] [PMID: 21118620]

[13] Matteelli A. CastelliF. Life cycle of malaria parasites. Institute of Infectious and Tropical Diseases.University of Brescia, Italy 2005.

[14] Garnham PCC. Malaria parasites and other Haemosporidia. Oxford: Blackwell Scientific publication 1966.

[15] Coatney GR, Cooper WC, Young MD. Studies in human malaria. XXX. A summary of 204 sporozoite-induced infections with the Chesson strain of Plasmodium vivax. J Natl Malar Soc 1950; 9(4): 381-96.
[PMID: 14804098]

[16] Garham PCC. Malaria parasites of man: Life-cycles and morphology (excluding ultrastructure).Malaria - Principles and practice of malariology. Churchill Livingstone 1988; Vol. I: pp. 65-96.

[17] Carter R, Gwadz RW. Infectiousness and gamete immunization in malaria.Kreser JP, Eds Malaria. New York Academic Press 1980; 3: p. 263-97.
[http://dx.doi.org/10.1016/B978-0-12-426103-7.50013-6]

[18] World Health Organisation. Guidelines for the treatment of malaria. 3rd ed., 2005.

[19] David B, Jacoby RMY. Encyclopedia of Family Health. Third 2005.

[20] Quinine. http://www.discoveriesinmedicine.com/Ni-Ra/Quinine.html.

[21] Cinchona bark. http://historyofmalaria.com/2010/02/cinchona-bark/.

[22] Achan J, Talisuna AO, Erhart A, *et al.* Quinine, an old anti-malarial drug in a modern world: Role in the treatment of malaria. Malar J 2011; 10: 144.
[http://dx.doi.org/10.1186/1475-2875-10-144] [PMID: 21609473]

[23] Dobson SMaM. The history of antimalarial drugs.Antimalarial Chemotherapy: Mechanisms of Action, Resistance, and New Directions in Drug Discovery. Totowa PIR, Ed. New Jersey: Humana Press 2001; pp. 15-25.

[24] Aden Abdi Y. L Lars G, Ericsson O, Hellgren U. Handbook of Drugs for Tropical Parasitic Infections. 1995.

[25] Salako LA, Sowunmi A. Disposition of quinine in plasma, red blood cells and saliva after oral and intravenous administration to healthy adult Africans. Eur J Clin Pharmacol 1992; 42(2): 171-4.
[http://dx.doi.org/10.1007/BF00278479] [PMID: 1618248]

[26] White NJ. Antimalarial pharmacokinetics and treatment regimens. Br J Clin Pharmacol 1992; 34(1): 1-10.
[http://dx.doi.org/10.1111/j.1365-2125.1992.tb04100.x] [PMID: 1633062]

[27] Karlsson KK, Hellgren U, Alván G, Rombo L. Audiometry as a possible indicator of quinine plasma concentration during treatment of malaria. Trans R Soc Trop Med Hyg 1990; 84(6): 765-7.
[http://dx.doi.org/10.1016/0035-9203(90)90069-Q] [PMID: 2096500]

[28] White NJ. The treatment of malaria. N Engl J Med 1996; 335(11): 800-6.
[http://dx.doi.org/10.1056/NEJM199609123351107] [PMID: 8703186]

[29] Okitolonda W, Delacollette C, Malengreau M, Henquin JC. High incidence of hypoglycaemia in African patients treated with intravenous quinine for severe malaria. Br Med J (Clin Res Ed) 1987; 295(6600): 716-8.
[http://dx.doi.org/10.1136/bmj.295.6600.716] [PMID: 3117315]

[30] Looareesuwan S, Phillips RE, White NJ, *et al.* Quinine and severe falciparum malaria in late pregnancy. Lancet 1985; 2(8445): 4-8.
[http://dx.doi.org/10.1016/S0140-6736(85)90056-X] [PMID: 2861481]

[31] Antimalarial Martindale. The Extra Pharmacopoeia. London: Pharmaceuitical Press 1993; p. 30.

[32] Uganda Malaria Surveillance Project. UMSP sentinel site malaria surveillance report. 2010.

[33] Wasunna B, Zurovac D, Goodman CA, Snow RW. Why don't health workers prescribe ACT? A

qualitative study of factors affecting the prescription of artemether-lumefantrine. Malar J 2008; 7: 29. [http://dx.doi.org/10.1186/1475-2875-7-29] [PMID: 18252000]

[34] Sabchareon A, Chongsuphajaisiddhi T, Sinhasivanon V, Chanthavanich P, Attanath P. *In vivo* and *in vitro* responses to quinine and quinidine of *Plasmodium falciparum.* Bull World Health Organ 1988; 66(3): 347-52.
[PMID: 3048758]

[35] de Vries PJBN, Bich NN, Van Thien H, *et al.* Combinations of artemisinin and quinine for uncomplicated falciparum malaria: Efficacy and pharmacodynamics. Antimicrob Agents Chemother 2000; 44(5): 1302-8.
[http://dx.doi.org/10.1128/AAC.44.5.1302-1308.2000] [PMID: 10770766]

[36] Alecrim MG, Lacerda MV, Mourão MP, *et al.* Successful treatment of Plasmodium falciparum malaria with a six-dose regimen of artemether-lumefantrine versus quinine-doxycycline in the Western Amazon region of Brazil. Am J Trop Med Hyg 2006; 74(1): 20-5.
[http://dx.doi.org/10.4269/ajtmh.2006.74.20] [PMID: 16407341]

[37] WHO. Malaria treatment guidelines. 2010.

[38] Lell B, Kremsner PG. Clindamycin as an antimalarial drug: Review of clinical trials. Antimicrob Agents Chemother 2002; 46(8): 2315-20.
[http://dx.doi.org/10.1128/AAC.46.8.2315-2320.2002] [PMID: 12121898]

[39] Philipson A, Sabath LD, Charles D. Erythromycin and clindamycin absorption and elimination in pregnant women. Clin Pharmacol Ther 1976; 19(1): 68-77.
[http://dx.doi.org/10.1002/cpt197619168] [PMID: 1245094]

[40] Sparkes C, Roland V. Sparkes C, Roland V. Antimalaria medication. Article, www.belmonthistory.org 2010; pp. 2203 -2213.

[41] https://patient.info/medicine/chloroquine.

[42] https://pubchem.ncbi.nlm.nih.gov/compound/amodiaquine.

[43] https://www.webmd.com/drugs/2/drug-5911/pyrimethamine-oral/details.

[44] https://patient.info/medicine/proguanil-for-malaria-prevention.

[45] https://medlineplus.gov/druginfo/meds/a603030.html.

[46] https://www.rxlist.com/mepron-drug.htm#description.

[47] https://chealth.canoe.com/drug/getdrug/malarone.

[48] Markus MB. Biological concepts in recurrent *Plasmodium vivax* malaria. Parasitology 2018; 145(13): 1765-71.
[http://dx.doi.org/10.1017/S003118201800032X] [PMID: 29564998]

[49] www.eurekalert.org2008.

[50] http://apps.who.int/medicinedocs/en/d/Jh2922e/2.5.6.html.

[51] van Vugt M, Brockman A, Gemperli B, *et al.* Randomized comparison of artemether-benflumetol and artesunate-mefloquine in treatment of multidrug-resistant falciparum malaria. Antimicrob Agents Chemother 1998; 42(1): 135-9.
[http://dx.doi.org/10.1128/AAC.42.1.135] [PMID: 9449273]

[52] https://www.healthline.com/health/doxycycline-oral-tablet.

[53] LellB, Kremsner PG. Clindamycin as an Antimalarial Drug Review of Clinical Trials 2002.

[54] https://www.drugs.com/condition/malaria.html.

[55] Jonville MC, Kodja H, Humeau L, *et al.* Screening of medicinal plants from Reunion Island for antimalarial and cytotoxic activity. J Ethnopharmacol 2008; 120(3): 382-6.

[http://dx.doi.org/10.1016/j.jep.2008.09.005] [PMID: 18848979]

[56] do Céu de Madureira M, Paula Martins A, Gomes M, Paiva J, Proença da Cunha A, do Rosário V. Antimalarial activity of medicinal plants used in traditional medicine in S. Tomé and Príncipe islands. J Ethnopharmacol 2002; 81(1): 23-9. [http://dx.doi.org/10.1016/S0378-8741(02)00005-3] [PMID: 12020924]

[57] Karamati SA, Hassanzadazar H, Bahmani M, Rafieian-Kopaei M. Herbal and chemical drugs effective on malaria. Asian Pac J Trop Dis 2014; 4 (Suppl. 2): S599-601. [http://dx.doi.org/10.1016/S2222-1808(14)60686-1]

[58] Heidarian E, Rafieian-Kopaei M, Ashrafi K. The effect of hydroalcoholic extract of *Allium latifolium* on the liver phosphatidate phosphatase and serum lipid profile in hyperlipidemic rats. Majallah-i Danishgah-i Ulum-i Pizishki-i Babul 2013; 15(4): 37-46.

[59] Batista R, Silva AdeJ Jr, de Oliveira AB. Plant-derived antimalarial agents: New leads and efficient phytomedicines. Part II. Non-alkaloidal natural products. Molecules 2009; 14(8): 3037-72. [http://dx.doi.org/10.3390/molecules14083037] [PMID: 19701144]

[60] Hilou A, Nacoulma OG, Guiguemde TR. *In vivo* antimalarial activities of extracts from *Amaranthus spinosus* L. and *Boerhaavia erecta* L. in mice. J Ethnopharmacol 2006; 103(2): 236-40. [http://dx.doi.org/10.1016/j.jep.2005.08.006] [PMID: 16171960]

[61] Boyom FF, Kemgne EM, Tepongning R, *et al.* Antiplasmodial activity of extracts from seven medicinal plants used in malaria treatment in Cameroon. J Ethnopharmacol 2009; 123(3): 483-8. [http://dx.doi.org/10.1016/j.jep.2009.03.008] [PMID: 19442463]

[62] Esmaeili S, Naghibi F, Mosaddegh M, Sahranavard S, Ghafari S, Abdullah NR. Screening of antiplasmodial properties among some traditionally used Iranian plants. J Ethnopharmacol 2009; 121(3): 400-4. [http://dx.doi.org/10.1016/j.jep.2008.10.041] [PMID: 19059470]

[63] Okokon JE, Antia BS, Igboasoiyi AC, Essien EE, Mbagwu HO. Evaluation of antiplasmodial activity of ethanolic seed extract of *Picralima nitida.* J Ethnopharmacol 2007; 111(3): 464-7. [http://dx.doi.org/10.1016/j.jep.2006.12.016] [PMID: 17234375]

[64] Abdel-Sattar E, Harraz FM, Al Ansari SM, *et al.* Antiplasmodial and antitrypanosomal activity of plants from the Kingdom of Saudi Arabia. J Nat Med 2009; 63(2): 232-9. [http://dx.doi.org/10.1007/s11418-008-0305-5] [PMID: 19067114]

[65] Tona L, Cimanga RK, Mesia K, *et al. In vitro* antiplasmodial activity of extracts and fractions from seven medicinal plants used in the Democratic Republic of Congo. J Ethnopharmacol 2004; 93(1): 27-32. [http://dx.doi.org/10.1016/j.jep.2004.02.022] [PMID: 15182900]

[66] Bah S, Jäger AK, Adsersen A, Diallo D, Paulsen BS. Antiplasmodial and GABA(A)-benzodiazepine receptor binding activities of five plants used in traditional medicine in Mali, West Africa. J Ethnopharmacol 2007; 110(3): 451-7. [http://dx.doi.org/10.1016/j.jep.2006.10.019] [PMID: 17126508]

[67] Okokon JE, Nwafor PA. Antiplasmodial activity of root extract and fractions of *Croton zambesicus.* J Ethnopharmacol 2009; 121(1): 74-8. [http://dx.doi.org/10.1016/j.jep.2008.09.034] [PMID: 18996464]

[68] Ndjakou Lenta B, Vonthron-Sénécheau C, Fongang Soh R, *et al. In vitro* antiprotozoal activities and cytotoxicity of some selected Cameroonian medicinal plants. J Ethnopharmacol 2007; 111(1): 8-12. [http://dx.doi.org/10.1016/j.jep.2006.10.036] [PMID: 17141994]

[69] Waako PJ, Gumede B, Smith P, Folb PI. The *in vitro* and *in vivo* antimalarial activity of *Cardiospermum halicacabum* L. and *Momordica foetida* Schumch. Et Thonn. J Ethnopharmacol 2005; 99(1): 137-43. [http://dx.doi.org/10.1016/j.jep.2005.02.017] [PMID: 15848033]

[70] Khaomek P, Ichino C, Ishiyama A, *et al. In vitro* antimalarial activity of prenylated flavonoids from Erythrina fusca. J Nat Med 2008; 62(2): 217-20.
[http://dx.doi.org/10.1007/s11418-007-0214-z] [PMID: 18404327]

[71] Okokon JE, Udokpoh AE, Antia BS. Antimalaria activity of ethanolic extract of *Tetrapleura tetraptera* fruit. J Ethnopharmacol 2007; 111(3): 537-40.
[http://dx.doi.org/10.1016/j.jep.2006.12.030] [PMID: 17236733]

[72] Iwalewa EO, Omisore NO, Adewunmi CO, *et al.* Anti-protozoan activities of *Harungana madagascariensis* stem bark extract on trichomonads and malaria. J Ethnopharmacol 2008; 117(3): 507-11.
[http://dx.doi.org/10.1016/j.jep.2008.02.019] [PMID: 18372133]

[73] Philippe G, Angenot L, De Mol P, *et al. In vitro* screening of some *Strychnos* species for antiplasmodial activity. J Ethnopharmacol 2005; 97(3): 535-9.
[http://dx.doi.org/10.1016/j.jep.2004.12.011] [PMID: 15740892]

[74] Okokon JE, Ita BN, Udokpoh AE. Antiplasmodial activity of *Cylicodiscus gabunensis.* J Ethnopharmacol 2006; 107(2): 175-8.
[http://dx.doi.org/10.1016/j.jep.2006.03.002] [PMID: 16635557]

[75] Abosl AO, Mbukwa E, Majinda RR, *et al. Vangueria infausta* root bark: *In vivo* and *in vitro* antiplasmodial activity. Br J Biomed Sci 2006; 63(3): 129-33.
[http://dx.doi.org/10.1080/09674845.2006.11732732] [PMID: 17058713]

[76] Tolu OO, Odunayo RA, Ibukun EA, Peter OF. Medicinal plants useful for malaria therapy in Okeigbo, Ondo State, Southwest Nigeria. Afr J Trad CAM 2007; 4(2): 191-8.

[77] Lategan CA, Campbell WE, Seaman T, Smith PJ. The bioactivity of novel furanoterpenoids isolated from *Siphonochilus aethiopicus.* J Ethnopharmacol 2009; 121(1): 92-7.
[http://dx.doi.org/10.1016/j.jep.2008.10.007] [PMID: 18996179]

SUBJECT INDEX

A

K. Tamreihao, Saikat Mukherjee and Debananda S. Ningthoujam (Eds.)
All rights reserved-© 2019 Bentham Science Publishers

B

C

D

E

F

G

K

S

T

www.ingramcontent.com/pod-product-compliance
Lightning Source LLC
LaVergne TN
LVHW070948210926
848482LV00002B/141